Current Developments in
Anthropological Genetics

Volume 3

BLACK CARIBS

A Case Study in Biocultural Adaptation

Current Developments in Anthropological Genetics

A Continuation Order Plan is available for this series. A continuation order will bring
delivery of each new volume immediately upon publication. Volumes are billed only upon
actual shipment. For further information please contact the publisher.

Current Developments in Anthropological Genetics

Volume 3

BLACK CARIBS

A Case Study in Biocultural Adaptation

EDITED BY

MICHAEL H. CRAWFORD

University of Kansas
Lawrence, Kansas

PLENUM PRESS · NEW YORK AND LONDON

The Library of Congress cataloged the first title in this series as follows:

Main entry under title:

Current developments in anthropological genetics.

Includes index.
   CONTENTS: v. 1. Theory and methods.
   1. Human population genetics—Addresses, essays, lectures. 2. Human evolution—
Addresses, essays, lectures. 3. Human genetics—Addresses, essays, lectures. I. Mielke,
James H. II. Crawford, Michael H., 1939–

GN289.C87   573.2   79-24900

ISBN-13: 978-1-4612-9652-2   e-ISBN-13: 978-1-4613-2649-6
DOI: 10.1007/978-1-4613-2649-6

©1984 Plenum Press, New York
Softcover reprint of the hardcover 1st edition 1984
A Division of Plenum Publishing Corporation
233 Spring Street, New York, N.Y. 10013

Contributors

V. Bach-Enciso, Laboratory of Biological Anthropology, University of Kansas, Lawrence, Kansas 66045

R. M. Baume, School of Dental Medicine, The University of Connecticut Health Center, Farmington, Connecticut 06032

Rebecca Brown, American National Red Cross, Bethesda, Maryland 20814

Pamela J. Byard, Department of Anthropology, University of Kansas, Lawrence, Kansas 66045; present address: Department of Anthropology, Case Western Reserve University, Cleveland, Ohio 44106

Sheila Cosminsky, Department of Anthropology, Rutgers University, Camden, New Jersey 08102

Michael H. Crawford, Laboratory of Biological Anthropology, University of Kansas, Lawrence, Kansas 66045

Ramon Custodio, Laboratorio Custodio, S. de R. L. Pathologia Clinica y Anatomia Pathologica, 1229 Tegucigalpa, D. C., Honduras

William V. Davidson, Department of Geography and Anthropology, Louisiana State University, Baton Rouge, Louisiana 70803

Eric J. Devor, Department of Psychiatry, Washington University School of Medicine, Washington University, St. Louis, Missouri 63178

Dale D. Dykes, Minneapolis War Memorial Blood Bank, Minneapolis, Minnesota 55404

Brian Sank Firschein, Human Genetics and Biological Variations Laboratory, N. S. Kline Psychiatric Research Institute, Orangeburg, New York 10962

I. Lester Firschein, Department of Anthropology, Hunter College–City University of New York, New York, New York 10021

Henry Gershowitz, Department of Human Genetics, University of Michigan, Ann Arbor, Michigan 48104

Nancie L. Gonzalez, Department of Anthropology, University of Maryland, College Park, Maryland 20742

C. J. M. R. Gullick, Department of Anthropology, Durham University, Durham DHI 3HN, England

R. G. Huntsman, Canadian Red Cross, Blood Transfusion Services, St. John's, Newfoundland, Canada A1B 4A4

Janis Hutchinson, Laboratory of Biological Anthropology, University of Kansas, Lawrence, Kansas 66045

Carol Jenkins, Institute of Medical Research, P.O. Box 378, Madang, Papua New Guinea

Virginia Kerns, Department of Sociology, Virginia Polytechnic Institute and State University, Blacksburg, Virginia 24061

A. C. Kopeč, Serological Population Genetics Laboratory, London, England

Francis C. Lees, Department of Anthropology, State University of New York at Albany, Albany, New York 12222

Paul M. Lin, Institute of Social and Behavioral Pathology, and Psychiatric Research Unit, Department of Psychiatry, Pritzker School of Medicine, The University of Chicago, Chicago, Illinois 60637

J. M. Lord, British Museum (Natural History), Sub-Department of Anthropology, London SW7, England

J. H. Mielke, Laboratory of Biological Anthropology, University of Kansas, Lawrence, Kansas 66045

R. M. Newton, Canadian Red Cross, Blood Transfusion Services, St. John's, Newfoundland, Canada A1B 4A4

D. H. O'Rourke, Department of Anthropology, University of Utah, Salt Lake City, Utah 84112

H. F. Polesky, Minneapolis War Memorial Blood Bank, Minneapolis, Minnesota 55404

John H. Relethford, Department of Anthropology, State University of New York at Albany, Albany, New York 12222; present address: Department of Anthropology, State University of New York at Oneonta, Oneonta, New York 13820

Derek F. Roberts, Department of Human Genetics, University of Newcastle upon Tyne, England NE2 4AA

Diane Sank, Department of Anthropology, The City College, City University of New York, New York, New York 10031, and Human Genetics and Biological Variations Laboratory, N. S. Kline Psychiatric Research Institute, Orangeburg, New York 10962

Moses S. Schanfield, American National Red Cross, Bethesda, Maryland 20814; present address: Genetic Testing Institute, Atlanta, Georgia 30308

K. Skradsky, Minneapolis War Memorial Blood Bank, Minneapolis, Minnesota 55404

D. Tills, British Museum (Natural History), Sub-Department of Anthropology, London SW7, England

A. Warlow, British Museum (Natural History), Sub-Department of Anthropology, London SW7, England

Hazel Weymes, Department of Anthropology, University College London, London WC1E 6BT, England

Emory Whipple, Department of Anthropology, Indiana University–Purdue University at Fort Wayne, Fort Wayne, Indiana 46805

Preface

While the previous two volumes in this series were based upon methodology, theory, and the relationship between ecology and population structure, this book can be viewed as an in-depth case study. The population genetics of a multitude of diverse groups geographically distributed throughout the world was examined in the first two volumes. In contrast, this volume focuses upon a single ethnic group, the Black Caribs (Garifuna) of Central America and St. Vincent Island, and explores the interrelationships among the ethnohistory, sociocultural characteristics, demography, morphology, and genetic structure of the group. This volume offers a broad and intensive treatment of the Black Caribs and their interactions with surrounding populations.

My interest in the genetics of the Black Caribs was sparked by an accidental meeting in Amsterdam, Holland, in March 1975. A conversation with Nancie Gonzalez at the Applied Anthropology Meetings revealed the "truth-is-stranger-than-fiction" history of the Black Carib peoples of the Caribbean. This was a population with a small-sized founding group and a unique biological success story. Nancie Gonzalez was particularly interested in estimating the Carib Indian admixture in the contemporary Garifuna population. Given my previous experience in estimating Spanish and African admixture in the Tlaxcaltecan population (whose gene pool consisted predominantly of Indian alleles), a group that appeared to be primarily African with some Indian admixture was of great interest. Aside from the ethnohistorical interest, I believe that such a population may add considerably to our understanding of the inheritance of complex morphological traits.

The first fieldwork on the Black Caribs was performed during the summer of 1975 in Livingston, Guatemala. The primary focus of those investigations was to estimate the Carib Indian contribution to the formation of the Black Carib gene pool. P. M. Lin and I joined Nancie Gonzalez in the field for a short time during the summer to collect blood specimens, dermatoglyphics, some dental casts, and anthropometric data. Nancie Gonzalez collected genealogical and sociocultural data from Livingston from 1956 to 1976. Her knowledge of the

Carib peoples of Livingston provided valuable background for the interpretation of the genetic and biological data.

Following the 1975 fieldwork, a more intensive field research program was envisaged for the summer of 1976 in Belize. Researchers and research support from five different institutions formed the core of a 6-week multidisciplinary effort. Nancie Gonzalez, assisted by Loretta St. Louis, was responsible for the sociocultural anthropology and fertility aspects of the project. Francis Lees and a graduate student, Pamela Byard, both from State University of New York in Albany, collected skin color reflectometry data. One of the innovative features of their study was the collection of reflectance data by means of both the British E.E.L. and the U.S. Photovolt reflectometers. This approach permitted the development of conversion formulas for the comparative utilization of data from both machines by using different wavelength filters. Eugenie Scott collected anthropometric measurements of children and adults, particularly for purposes of comparing those with normal and abnormal hemoglobins. Paul Lin, from Wichita State University, measured a sample of children and made dermatoglyphic prints on a series of Belize City Creoles. These data formed the backbone of a comparison with the Caribs of Livingston, Guatemala. Three researchers came from the University of Kansas: M. H. Crawford, E. Murray, and D. H. O'Rourke. Murray was responsible for screening for abnormal hemoglobins with a modified microchromatographic technique. The purpose of the identification of HbAS heterozygous women was to retest Firschein's (1961) conclusion that under malarial conditions sickle cell trait women are more fertile than their HbAA counterparts. O'Rourke made dental impressions from a select sample of people from the community who had a fairly complete dental set. M. H. Crawford tested for anomalous color vision and collected some of the blood specimens. In all of our studies during the last decade we have always tried to return to the community as much as possible in return for its cooperation. In Belize, the physician on the research team, David Hiebert, provided free medical care and radiological consultations. He worked in close cooperation with the local physicians, Dr. J. Miranda at Stann Creek and Dr. von Hienkel at Punta Gorda.

Field investigations were begun on St. Vincent Island during the summer of 1979, when Paul Lin, Janis Hutchinson, and I spent 1 month investigating three villages on the windward side of the island. Blood pressure, anthropometric measurements, genealogies, and blood specimens were collected from 450 persons representing three villages – Owia, Sandy Bay, and Fancy. St. Vincent Island plays a pivotal role in the understanding of the population structure of the Black Caribs, since they originated from this island from a small founding group.

Frank Livingstone informed me of another research group (consisting of University College, London and Memorial University of Newfoundland) working with Black Carib populations in Honduras. After contacting this group, and following a visit to Lawrence by Richard Huntsman, they agreed to provide several chapters so that a more complete overview of Black Carib research would be available under a single set of covers. Thus, Chapters 14, 15, and 17, on the blood genetics of Honduras and Belize Black Caribs, were subsequently added to this volume. Since the British/Canadian and U.S. Groups worked independently, there is some overlap as to the data collected. However, this redundancy should be viewed as a unique strength of the volume because it provides an opportunity to evaluate the results of a series of sampling procedures. A nagging question in population biology concerns the representative nature of samples taken from large human populations and the possibility of bias.

Many colleagues and associates aided in the organization and realization of this Black Carib research program. Drs. Nancie L. Gonzalez and Paul M. Lin were instrumental in the development of the research program and participated in several of the field investigations. Similarly, I would like to acknowledge the aid of Drs. Francis Lees, Pamela J. Byard, David Hiebert, and Dennis H. O'Rourke for their participation in the fieldwork in Belize. Without the assistance and support of the public health officers and nurses in Belize, Guatemala, and St. Vincent, this study would not have been possible. In particular, I acknowledge the cooperation, help, and good will of Drs. Kibukomusoke, Naidas, Castillo von Heinkel, and Father Anthony Briskey.

I would like to thank Marcia Early for her considerable typing, editing, and administrative skills. Laura Poracsky provided the illustrations for many of the chapters. I thank Pamela Byard for her critical evaluation of a number of manuscripts and her useful recommendations for their improvement.

This research was supported in part by the following grants: PHS Research Career Development Award K04 DE028-05; National Institute of Dental Research #DE04115-02; Biomedical Sciences Research Grants #4349-5706, 4309-5706, and 4932-x706-4; and Faculty Senate Research Grant #3507-x038.

Michael H. Crawford

Contents

Chapter 7.   Ethnicity and Mating Patterns in Punta Gorda, Belize
              Sheila Cosminsky and Emory Whipple

PART II: MORPHOLOGICAL SECTION

Chapter 8.   Nutrition and Growth in Early Childhood among the
                Garifuna and Creole of Belize
              Carol Jenkins

Chapter 9.   Skin Color of the Garifuna of Belize
              Pamela J. Byard, Francis C. Lees, and John H. Relethford

PART III: GENETIC SECTION

Chapter 16. Blood Group, Serum Protein, and Red Cell Enzyme
             Polymorphisms, and Admixture among the Black Caribs
             and Creoles of Central America and the Caribbean
             *Michael H. Crawford, Dale D. Dykes, K. Skradsky, and
             H. F. Polesky*

Chapter 17. Abnormal Hemoglobins among the Black Caribs
             Ramon Custodio and R. G. Huntsman

Chapter 18. Immunoglobulin Allotypes in the Black Caribs and Creoles of Belize and St. Vincent

Moses S. Schanfield, Rebecca Brown, and Michael H. Crawford

Chapter 19. Genetic Population Structure of the Black Caribs and Creoles

Eric J. Devor, Michael H. Crawford, and V. Bach-Enciso

Chapter 20. Anthropogenetics in a Hybrid Population: The Black Carib Studies

Derek F. Roberts

1

Problems and Hypotheses
An Introduction

MICHAEL H. CRAWFORD

1. Introduction

The University of Kansas research program described in this volume is a continuation of a theoretical interest that I initiated in 1969 with the study of genetic, demographic, and morphological microdifferentiation of transplanted Tlaxcaltecan populations of Mexico. The primary objective of the Tlaxcaltecan project, performed between 1969 and 1975, was to measure evolutionary changes in human populations transplanted from their valley of origin (approximately 400 years ago) into markedly diverse environments. The complicating variable in that study was the gene flow from the Spanish colonial administration and from the surrounding indigenous peoples into the transplanted communities (Crawford, 1976). Only limited and conservative conclusions could be drawn concerning evolutionary rates and genetic microdifferentiation.

As a result of the findings in the Tlaxcaltecan project, geographically isolated populations that migrated into the New World at least 4000 years ago were selected for the next series of investigations. A study was initiated in 1978 to compare Alaskan and Siberian Eskimos for purposes of measuring microdifferentiation provided by a greater time dimension. The preliminary results suggest a clear-cut differentiation of Alaskan and Siberian groups along the first scaled eigenvector, following the Harpending and Jenkins (1973) method of R-matrix analysis (Crawford et al., 1981; Crawford and Enciso-Bach, 1982). The population structure of the Eskimos genetically documents the movements of Siberian groups into the New World and reflects an apparent

MICHAEL H. CRAWFORD • Laboratory of Biological Anthropology, University of Kansas, Lawrence, Kansas 66045.

concordance among ethnohistory, geography, linguistics, and genetic patterns of the Arctic peoples.

This relationship, among time of divergence, history, and degree of micro-differentiation, is of concern in this volume. While the Eskimo study provides a time dimension of transplantation of several thousand years, the Mexican Indian groups diverged only 300—400 years ago, and the Black Caribs underwent fission 180 years ago.

This chapter provides background information on the Black Caribs in regard to their unique ethnohistory (particularly facts of genetic interest) and their distinctive biological, demographic, and social characteristics. In addition, the central evolutionary hypotheses examined by this volume are summarized. Finally, the reasons for the internal organization of this volume into three sections are discussed.

2. Ethnohistory

The Black Caribs (Garifuna) form a biological and cultural amalgam of Arawak and Carib Indians with West African slaves. The African component was added to the original Amerindian population of St. Vincent from 1517 to 1646 in the form of runaway slaves from European-held islands, through Carib raids on various settlements, and possibly the wreckage of a slave ship. Although the traditional accounts describe the wreckage of Spanish galleons enroute to Barbados from the coast of Nigeria, Gullick (1979) argues that if the slave ship had come directly from Africa, the culture of the survivors would have been African oriented. Yet, the slaves acquired the language (Island Carib) and assumed a major portion of the culture of the Amerindians on St. Vincent.

After an initial period of slavery under the Carib Indians, the African—Carib hybrids eventually founded their own villages in the interior of the Island of St. Vincent. They came under British jurisdiction by a treaty of 1668 and proceeded to war with the British forces of occupation. In 1676 approximately 3000 Black Caribs resided on the island and they forced the surviving Red Caribs (Amerindians) into relinquishing land to them. The Black Caribs increased numerically until 1683, when a British expeditionary force killed a large number of Caribs. After a series of wars with the British, instigated by the French, the Black Caribs were first relegated to a small portion of the island and, after a disastrous defeat in 1795, were deported.

On February 25th, 1797, the *H.M.S. Experiment* arrived at Balliceaux accompanied by naval transport brought to carry the Caribs to Roatan (Gullick, this volume, Chapter 3). One hundred or fewer of the Black Caribs managed to evade the British, and their descendants constitute the contemporary population. Gullick (this volume, Chapter 3) estimates on the basis of Colonial Office Files

(#260/13–15, WO 1/85, and 690) that only 2500 Caribs were deported to Roatan (Chapter 4, this volume, the number is re-estimated at 2045). Other estimates vary between 4000 and 5080 (Davidson, this volume, Chapter 2; Taylor, 1951). Don Jose Rossi y Rubra, the leader of the Spanish force sent to Roatan to recapture the island from the Black Carib "invasion," estimated the presence of 2000 Black Caribs on Roatan in May 1797. The Caribs unceremoniously surrendered the island to the Spanish and rapidly emigrated to the Central American mainland.

Fewer than 2500 Black Caribs migrated to the mainland in 1797 or 1798 and established the initial settlement in Trujillo, Honduras. The coast of Honduras already contained some Creole settlements founded by slaves brought to work in the mines and, later, fruit plantations. Thus, there was genetic admixture, particularly between the Creoles of Haiti and the Black Caribs during the initial colonialization of the Mosquito coast of Central America. It is highly likely that the Creole–Carib unions contributed to the rapid growth of the Black Caribs from 2000 to 75,000–80,000 in 180 years. The Black Caribs are now found from Stann Creek, Belize, to LaFe, Nicaragua, in a total of 54 towns and fishing villages.

Those Black Caribs who avoided the British deportation of 1797 gave issue to the estimated 1100–2000 Garifuna on St. Vincent Island. The 1960 census, thought to be an underestimate by Gullick (this volume, Chapter 3), enumerated 1265 Caribs on the island, of whom 518 were at New Sandy Bay, 368 at Rose Bank, 70 at Owia, 59 at Fancy, and the remainder in a nunber of smaller towns. However, Gullick (this volume, Chapter 3) estimated 880 Black Caribs in New Sandy Bay, 340 in Owia, and 180 in Fancy.

There is disagreement among the earliest ethnographers as to the degree of reproductive isolation and gene flow into the Black Carib communities. Conzemius (1928) notes, "they seldom intermarry with other races." Taylor (1951) describes the Garifuna as a "society apart, whose members rarely intermarry or have any social dealings with the other, non-Carib communities with which they come in contact." Gonzalez (1969) concurs that some "mixed marriages" do take place, but primarily with Creoles. Both she and Firschein (1961) maintain that the Caribs express a preference for an ethnic endogamy. Kerns did not find such a preference among the Black Caribs of Belize. Firschein (1961) further maintains that Black Caribs constitute a genetic isolate, a point disputed by Kerns (this volume, Chapter 6). Combining early genealogies with censuses and records, Kerns argues that interethnic crosses were always occurring and cites the 1861 census for British Honduras, which enumerates 23% of the Black Caribs as being of mixed ancestry. Likewise, Ghidinelli (1976) documents considerable admixture among the Caribs of Livingston, Guatemala. These numerous interethnic crosses may be less prevalent in the small, isolated villages of St. Vincent Island, for which no estimates are available.

3. Unique Characteristics of the Black Caribs

The black Caribs are a distinct population created by a series of unique historical events. A population geneticist could not have "designed" an evolutionarily better adapted colonizing population than is found among the Black Caribs. A number of features are useful for the successful radiation of such a group. These include considerable genetic variability, some mechanism to sustain this variability, and adaptions to the diseases prevalent in the area; colonization groups should also have a culture that ameliorates some environmental pressures. All of these population features or characteristics are present among the Black Caribs.

The Black Carib gene pool consists of a complex amalgam of a number of different racial, ethnic, and populational components. The original Amerindian population of St. Vincent Island was a combination of Arawak and Carib Indians. The added African component, based upon a heterogeneous sampling of the west coast of Africa, undoubtedly included many tribes, geographical regions, and languages. The Black Caribs from St. Vincent also incorporated additional African and Creole groups during their expansion, first from Roatan, then through Honduras, British Honduras, Guatemala, and Nicaragua. European components were added along the way, primarily through hybridization with Haitians or various Creole groups. Finally, some Central American Indians, possibly Maya or even Ladino, in British Honduras and Mosquito Indians in Honduras contributed genetically to this highly heterozygous gene pool. The richness of the genetic variation maintained in the Black Carib gene pool is important evolutionarily because, in the process of fissioning or subdivision of groups under colonization, there is a reduction of genetic variability. This reduction would be maladaptive among small groups that are expanding into a diverse range of environments.

The social organization of the Black Caribs provides a rapid "reshuffling" of genes throughout the population. The Black Carib family is consanguineal (coresidential kinship that includes no regularly present male in the role of husband—father) and matrifocal. Solien de Gonzalez (1965) defines a matrifocal family as "a type of family or household grouping in which the woman is dominant and plays the leading role psychologically." This type of family structure is common among the Garifuna, who practice "serial polygyny," in which men periodically reside in a consanguineal household and then move into another household. Gonzales estimates that 55% of the households in Livingston, Guatemala practice serial polygyny, while the remainder exist in relatively permanent extended families. One result of this form of social organization is that the male genetic material is rapidly recombined within the population to produce new genotypes. Thus, many new genetic combinations are possible as the males mate with a large number of females and often produce half-sibs. In addition, immunological maternal blood group incompatibility should occur less frequently in such populations, given the mating structure.

Because of the African ancestry of the Black Caribs, they possess a number of genetic adaptations to malaria. Thus, abnormal hemoglobins in the form of heterozygotes HbAS and HbAC provide resistance to *Plasmodium falciparum.* The Duffy African genotype *(FyFy)* and glucose-6-phosphate dehydrogenase deficiency (G6PD deficiency) also increase resistance against malaria. The Amerindians, lacking the hemoglobinopathies, often live inland in highland regions to avoid parasitization by the *Plasmodium* organism. Malaria extracts high mortality from those Indians who reside in areas infested with *Anopheles* mosquitos or visit lowland and coastal towns for trade.

Besides being a biological amalgam of African/Amerindian, the Black Caribs also exhibit a hybrid culture in the extractive efficiency, nutrition, and belief systems. Solien (1959) notes the similarities of Black Carib and West Indian Negro cultures. Taylor (1951) described Black Carib culture as "a Negro cake composed of Amerindian ingredients." The Black Carib economy consists primarily of fishing and horticulture. Among the agriculture products grown by the women is cassava, a root, which contains high levels of thiocyanates. Jackson (1981) summarized the evidence in support of cassava being used in Liberia to ameliorate the effects of sickling on individuals with sickle cell anemia. Thus, the cassava consumption/sickle cell anemia amelioration may provide an example of biocultural interaction and adaptation to the mortality costs associated with the hemoglobinopathy balanced polymorphism.

4. Central Research Problems

This volume examines a number of biocultural research problems associated with Black Carib and Creole populations of Central America and St. Vincent Island. These central foci include the following:

1. The relationships among ethnohistory, particularly unique historical events, genetics, and evolution of human populations. This volume documents the importance of unique historical events, migration, and marriage patterns on the genetics of the Black Caribs. Without knowledge of the origins and history of these people, the observed genetic variation makes little evolutionary sense. However, the concurrent application of these diverse methodologies to sociocultural, genetic, and ethnohistorical questions results in unique answers.

2. A measure of West African and Amerindian hybridization in the creation of Black Carib and Creole gene pools. This research focus is closely related to the first one, since the parental gene frequencies must be identified on the basis of historical records of archeological evidence. Thus, based on archeological excavations, we infer that at the time of contact the original

Amerindians of St. Vincent Island were a cultural and biological amalgam of Carib and Arawak groups. The presence of albumin Mexico in Belizean Black Caribs reveals that the Amerindian component was not limited to the founding South American groups, but that some gene flow from contemporary New World populations occurred after the Black Carib transplantation to Central America. These data support Kern's contention (see Chapter 6) that the Black Carib gene pool was not reproductively isolated, as has been claimed by earlier researchers, and that there is a high incidence of interethnic marriages. It is in this fashion that biological and cultural information have a synergistic effect; each discipline contributes to the resolution of controversial issues in the other field.

3. To measure genetic microdifferentiation of Black Carib communities, given short periods of geographical separation — less than 180 years. These approaches to the study of microdifferentiation are complicated by differential levels of hybridization and gene flow and the small sizes of the founding groups. As a result, caution must be exercised in the interpretation of traditional estimates of microdifferentiation in subdivided populations, such at R_{ST} or F_{ST}, genetic distances, or even R-matrix analyses. The results of these evolutionary methods of analysis must be interpreted in conjunction with historical, socio-cultural, demographic, and geographical information.

4. With few exceptions, most of the population structure estimates that have been published are based upon gene frequency data. The morphologically based ascertainment of population structure almost invariably utilizes the Malécot model, and, to my knowledge, the Harpending and Jenkins (1975) R-matrix technique has not been applied. Thus, two of the chapters in this volume, namely Chapter 10 (dental structure) and Chapter 13 (dermatoglyphics) examine the population structure of the Black Caribs through R-matrix analysis. In addition, Chapter 18 contains the application of immunoglobulin data for the estimation of population structure.

5. One of the central hypotheses that we had planned to test concerns a comparison of achieved reproduction of females who have an HbAS versus HbAA genotype. Thus, the null hypothesis can be stated in the form: $H_{AS} = H_{AA}$, i.e., there are no differences in fertility between women 45 years of age or greater with HbAS genotype and those with HbAA genotype. This is a reconsideration of Firschein's (1961) conclusion that differential fertility, rather than differential mortality, maintains the hemoglobin polymorphism among Black Caribs.

Unfortunately, insufficient reliable demographic data were collected by our field team. Thus, the retesting of this hypothesis was left to Custodio and Huntsman, and their results conflict with Firschein's. However, these results must be considered preliminary given the small sample sizes.

5. Contents of This Volume

This volume is subdivided into three parts, each contributing to the understanding of Black Carib evolutionary biology. The first division, entitled "Sociocultural and Demographic Section," includes a series of chapters that provide background information and grist for the interpretation of biological data. The chapter by William Davidson, a geographer, arms the reader with information on the distribution of the Black Caribs and some historical reconstruction of their colonization of the coast of Central America. Charles Gullick presents an overview on the ethnohistory of the Black Caribs on St. Vincent Island, with special reference to the sizes and locations of settlements formed by those who evaded the British "roundup" in 1797. The third chapter in Part I, by Nancie Gonzalez, provides insight into the household and family structure among the Black Caribs of Livingston. Dr. Gonzales is uniquely qualified to include a time dimension and the social changes experienced by the Livingston community, since she initiated the study of this group over 25 years ago. In a similar vein, I. Lester Firschein (Chapter 5) performed his fieldwork in British Honduras in 1955–1956 and offers a unique biological and demographic perspective on the Black Caribs of 1956. Virginia Kerns (Chapter 6) and Sheila Cosminsky and Emory Whipple (Chapter 7) examine the mating patterns of Black Caribs and demonstrate the absence of significant reproductive isolation. Both studies document, using different techniques, the relatively high incidence of interethnic matings and provide a sociocultural measure of gene flow.

The second part of this book, entitled "Morphological Section," consists of six chapters, all focused upon a series of quantitative traits. The first contribution to this section (Chapter 8), by Carol Jenkins, analyzes nutritional differences between the Black Caribs and Creoles of Belize and documents their effects on growth and development. This chapter provides some insight into the environmental–genotypic interactions that produce the adult phenotypes that are measured and discussed in subsequent chapters. Chapter 9, on the skin color of the Black Caribs of Belize, by Pamela Byard, Francis Lees, and John Relethford, provides another measure of admixture – but one based upon a morphological trait. They demonstrate a high concordance between skin color and blood group measures of genetic admixture in human populations.

Chapters 10 and 13 in Part II apply dental and dermatoglyphic traits to the measure of population structure. The Harpending and Jenkins (1973) R-matrix method of analysis used in these chapters indicates similar genetic affinities as seen for estimates based upon blood group markers. In addition, factor analysis of dermatoglyphic traits reveals the existence of "universal factor structures," which had been noted previously for other human groups. These underlying factor structures, associated with the vascular and innervation patterns, have been verified for African, European, Amerindian, Siberian, and Oceanic populations – with no exceptions.

The last two chapters of this section, Chapters 11 and 12, deal with the Black Carib physique and the relationship between body build and risk of hypertension. Paul Lin, in Chapter 11, anthropometrically compares two populations of Black Caribs with varying degrees of Amerindian ancestry. He examines the morphological consequences of admixture by comparing St. Vincent Island Caribs, whose gene pool consists of almost equal contributions of Amerindian and African genes, with Livingston Caribs, who are predominantly West African but contain 20% Amerindian genes. Chapter 12 examines the relationship between various anthropometric variables and the level of blood pressure. In addition, this chapter also tests the hypothesis that a relationship exists between the "degree of Africanness" and risk of hypertension.

The third portion of this volume, entitled "Genetic Section," contains six chapters on blood marker genetics and on population genetic analysis. Chapters 15 and 17 are the fruits of a collaboration among a Honduranian physician, Dr. Ramon Custodio, Dr. Richard Huntsman (Memorial University of Newfoundland), and an English blood research group, which includes D. Tills, H. Weymes, A. Warlow, A. C. Kopeč, and J. M. Lord. Chapter 15 summarizes the blood group genetic variation observed among Honduranian Black Carib populations. Custodio and Huntsman, in Chapter 17, attempt to retest Firchein's (1961) conclusion that the increased fertility, and not decreased mortality, of Black Carib females with hemoglobin AS genotype is what maintains hemoglobin polymorphism in a malarial environment. Chapter 14 is the product of Hazel Weymes' (University College, London) dissertation research performed in several communities of Belize.

Chapters 16, 18, and 19 resulted from fieldwork by University of Kansas research groups from 1975 through 1979. Chapter 16, by M. H. Crawford, Dale Dykes, and Herbert Polesky, examines the genetic variation for blood groups, red blood cell proteins, and serum proteins in 10 populations residing in seven communities. In addition, this chapter estimates the relative proportions of West African, Amerindian, and European genes in the Black Carib and Creole gene pools. The incidence of immunoglobulin allotypes in Black Carib and Creole populations is summarized in Chapter 18. This chapter, authored by M. S. Schanfield, R. Brown, and M. H. Crawford, also estimates admixture and population structure on the basis of these Gm and Km frequencies. Chapter 19, by E. J. Devor, M. H. Crawford, and V. Bach-Enciso, combines the historical and demographic characteristics of the Black Carib communities with the observed genetic variation.

The final chapter is an overview of this compendium and its theoretical implications. Professor Derek F. Roberts' research spans three generations and provides him with a time perspective on the field of anthropological genetics.

References

Conzemius, E., 1928, Ethnographical notes on the Black Carib (Garif), *Am. Anthropol.* **30** (2):183–205.

Crawford, M. H. (ed.), 1976, *The Tlaxcaltecans: Prehistory, Demography, Morphology and Genetics*, University of Kansas Publications in Anthropology.

Crawford, M. H., and Enciso, V. B. 1982, Population structure of the circumpolar people of Siberia, Alaska, Canada, and Greenland, in: *Current Developments in Anthropological Genetics: Ecology and Population Structure*, Vol. 2 (M. H. Crawford and J. H. Mielke, eds.), pp. 51–91, Plenum Publishing, New York.

Crawford, M. H., Mielke, J. H., Devor, E., Dykes, D.D. and Polesky, H. F., 1981, Population structure of Alaskan and Siberian indigenous communities, *Amer. J. Phys. Anthrop.* **55**:167–185.

Firschein, I. L., 1961, Population dynamics of the sickle-cell trait in the Black Caribs of British Honduras, Central America, *Am. J. Hum. Genet.* **13**:233–254.

Ghidinelli, A., 1976, La Familia entre los Caribes Negros, Ladinos y Kekchies de Livingston, *Guatemala Indigena* **11**(3–4):1–315.

Gonzales, N. L., 1969, *Black Carib Household Structure*, University of Washington Press, Seattle.

Gullick, C. J. M. R., 1979, The Black Caribs in St. Vincent: The Carib War and aftermath. *42 Centres International des Americanistes* **6**:451–465.

Harpending, H. C., and Jenkins, T., 1973, Genetic distance among southern African populations, in *Methods and Theories of Anthropological Genetics* (M. H. Crawford and P. L. Workman, eds.), pp. 177–199, University of New Mexico Press, Albuquerque.

Jackson, L., 1981, The relationship of certain genetic traits to malaria in Liberian children and mothers, *Am. J. Phys. Anthropol.* **54**:236.

Solien, N. L., 1959, West Indian characteristics of the Black Carib, *Southwest. J. Anthropol.* **15**:300–307.

Solien de Gonzalez, N. L., 1965, The consanguineal household and matrifocality, *Am. Anthropol.* **67**:1541–1549.

Stewart, J., and Faron, L., 1959, *Native Peoples of South America*, McGraw-Hill, New York.

Taylor, D., 1951, *The Black Caribs of British Honduras*, Viking Fund Publications in Anthropology, no. 17, Wenner-Gren Foundation, New York.

PART I

SOCIOCULTURAL AND DEMOGRAPHIC SECTIONS

2

The Garifuna in Central America

Ethnohistorical and Geographical Foundations

WILLIAM V. DAVIDSON

1. Introduction

So-called "Carib" populations have inhabited three major areas of the New World tropics (Map 1). *South American Caribs*, the most prominent aboriginal family north of the Amazon, consist of several widely distributed, but linguistically related, tribes, such as the Galibi of the Guyana coast and the Yukpa of the Colombian–Venezuelan borderlands. Today they number approximately 25,000 (Basso, 1977). Caribs who migrated from the mainland onto the Lesser Antilles a few centuries before the arrival of the Europeans, in spite of acquiring the language of the Arawak Indians of the islands (Taylor, 1951; Durbin, 1977), eventually became known as the *Island Caribs* (Rouse, 1948). After two centuries of European depredations, they were confined to only two islands, Dominica and St. Vincent, where even now small remnant populations live: about 2000 on the Reserve in Dominica (Layng, 1976) and nearly 2000 in 11 villages on St. Vincent (Gullick, 1975). A third Carib population descended from the St. Vincentian group currently lives in Central America. These are known in the English language literature as Black Caribs, but perhaps more properly should be labeled *Garifuna*, the name by which they know themselves. Other names often attached to the group are *morenos*, Trujillianos, Vincentinos, and Karif. It is the

WILLIAM V. DAVIDSON • Department of Geography and Anthropology, Louisiana State University, Baton Rouge, Louisiana 70803.

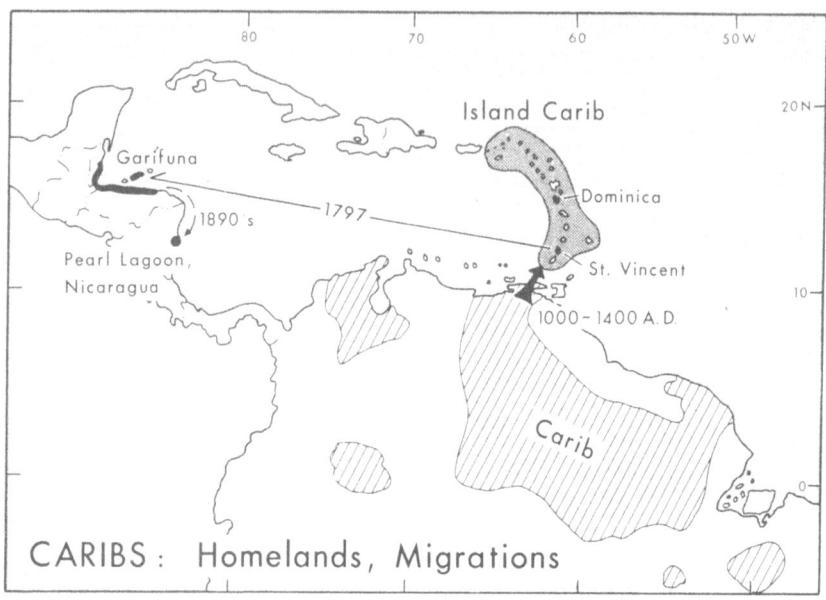

MAP 1. Carib homelands and migrations. Generalized from Chamberlain (1913), Steward and Mason (1950), Loukotka (1967), and Basso (1977, 1978).

intent of this introductory chapter to relate briefly the ethnohistorical and geographical background of the Garifuna since their arrival in Central America from St. Vincent.

2. St. Vincent Origins

The generally accepted version of Garifuna ethnogenesis is that during the 17th century black Africans from slave ships wrecked on St. Vincent were joined later by runaway slaves from nearby upwind plantations (such as those on Barbados) and gradually mixed with the native islanders, the so-called "Red Caribs" (W. Young, 1795; Taylor, 1951; Gonzalez, 1969; Gullick, 1977). Although details of the fusion and early activities are slight, the enlarging hybrid group, physically Negroid but with an Amerindian culture, dominated the Indians of the island by 1700 (Labat, 1970). At least by 1763, they were labeled "Black Caribs" by the Englishmen on the island (W. Young, 1795) and were a large and cohesive enough body to challenge the English masters for control of St. Vincent. Finally, after a lengthy period of conflicts, the 2-year Carib—English War (1795—1796) ended Carib resistance, and in the spring of 1797 virtually the entire Black Carib community of St. Vincent was exiled to the western Caribbean. Subsequently, they spread around the Bay of Honduras, where they live today in 52 coastal villages and number 60,000—70,000.

3. Dispersal in Central America

The dispersal seems to have occurred in five temporal–territorial units:

1. St. Vincent to Roatan Island, Honduras, 1797.
2. The Trujillo core, 1797–1810.
3. Honduran Mosquitia, 1803–1814.
4. Belize, 1802–1832.
5. Western Honduras and Guatemala, 1821–1836.

By 1836, one-third of the modern villages had been established, and the extent of settlement around the Bay of Honduras had been reached. After that date, with the exception of the two villages at Pearl Lagoon, Nicaragua, founded in the late 19th century (Davidson, 1980), new sites and relocations have taken place within the 1836 limits.

3.1. St. Vincent to Roatan Island, Honduras, 1797

The first Garifuna settlement in Central America was on Roatan, largest of the Bay Islands, just off the north coast of Honduras. At Port Royal, the large natural harbor on the south side of the island, the British Navy stranded a few thousand Black Caribs in April 1797 (Barrett, 1797). "A few thousand" may be as close to a certain figure as will ever be available to answer the critical question of how many Caribs were transported from St. Vincent. The primary sources, both Spanish and English, are confusing and inconsistent, and may never divulge an acceptable figure. The lowest figures, reported in Spanish sources, are derived from the area of disembarkation. An English sailor captured by a Spanish fleet while en route to Roatan said "1600 Black Caribs" were being transported (Saenz, 1797); the leader of the Spanish reconnaissance to the island learned from Carib chiefs there that "2000, more or less," were left by the British (Rossi y Rubi, 1797). Transcriptions of the 1801 census taken by Governor Ramon Anguiano in Trujillo are even more confusing: his record (Anguiano, 1801) lists "4000 caribe negros," while the 1804 rendition of the same census shows "5500." Del Castillo (1813) thought 4000 were exiled to Roatan. De Tornos (1816) learned that 2000 were deposited on the island.

English estimates for the population of exiled Caribs cluster near 5000. Southey (1827) gave a precise count of 4633 Carib prisoners on St. Vincent during October 1796. Bryan Edwards (1819), premier historian for the British islands for the period, reported that 5000 lived at the end of the war. Shepard (1831) recorded that 5080 were transported to Roatan. Unfortunately, the best records of the deportation, the letter and ship's log of Captain Barrett (1796–1797, 1797), commander of the naval expedition, contain no population figures.

Once on Roatan, the Garifuna seem to have split into at least two camps, one of which formed a village on the north coast of the island at a spot now called Punta Gorda. Although the bulk of the exiles passed to the Honduran mainland within a couple of years, Punta Gorda apparently remained settled until the present.

3.2. The Trujillo Core, 1797-1810

Bewildered by the sudden presence of shiploads of recently warring people deposited on their colonial doorstep, the Spanish government in Guatemala City dispatched a small force to reconnoiter the situation on Roatan. Jose Rossi y Rubi, commander of the expedition, quickly arranged a peaceful transfer of most of the Garifuna to the adjacent coast near Trujillo (Rossi y Rubi, 1797). Trujillo was the obvious choice for relocation because it was the only center of Spanish settlement on the Bay of Honduras.

The Garifuna migrants immediately dominated and transformed the hinterland of Trujillo Bay. The 4000 or 5000 Caribs listed in the census of Anguiano must have overwhelmed the previous residents of the port: 480 Spaniards, 300 English-speaking Negroes, probably captured during Spanish raids on the English colonies at Black River and on Roatan in 1782 (Davidson, 1974), and 200 French-speaking blacks recently arrived from Haiti via Cuba (Houdaille, 1954). The degree to which the new arrivals mixed with the inhabitants of Trujillo is unknown in detail, but the deportees from St. Vincent were acquainted with the French language and must have felt some common bond with the Haitian blacks. Garifuna were also soon comprising the bulk of the military at Trujillo (Roberts, 1827) and taking surnames from their Spanish hosts (Beaucage, s.f.).

The most restless Caribs began outward movements as soon as they reached the mainland: some few went to the east into Mosquitia, others established [by 1810 (Vallejo, 1893)] some of the five villages near Trujillo (Rio Negro, Cristales, Santa Fe, San Antonio, Guadalupe). But the overwhelming majority of the population remained intact (Roberts, 1827; Rochester, 1828) until the 1830s, when the Republican Wars in Central America scattered the Garifuna losers (Galindo, 1833; T. Young, 1842). Afterward, Trujillo housed only about 1000 (Montgomery, 1839). Because of its early role as their first center in Central America, Trujillo is still considered the "national capital" and mother settlement of the modern Garifuna.

3.3. Honduran Mosquitia, 1803-1814

Detailed reconstructions of the third movement of Garifuna, from Trujillo east into Mosquitia, are hindered by contradictions in the oral and written records. Beaucage (1970), using the oral tradition of the Garifuna, suggested that the eastward migration was motivated by a desire to return along the coast to St. Vincent. Reporters from earlier times (T. Young, 1842) wrote that the Garifuna moved to end "the unceasing demands upon their labour" at Trujillo.

It is also possible that the tremendous population pressure on the lands near Trujillo simply made a dispersal imperative.

Whatever the reasons for moving, the historical record indicates that the mouth of the Black River (Rio Negro, Tinto) was the effective eastern limit of settlement. A few Garifuna had journeyed the shore as far as the Patuca River (Patook) by late 1804 (Henderson, 1809; Bancroft, 1887), but 4000–5000 Caribs were still in Trujillo at the time (Anguiano, 1804), and evidently remained there until at least 1811, when 6000 were counted (del Castillo, 1813). There is a questionable report of a Garifuna agricultural colony at the mouth of the Chapagua River in 1803 (Anon, 1803), and a fairly reliable account of the establishment of a village at Sangrelaya (Zachary Lyon, Sacrelien, Sacraliah) by 1814 (Anon, 1938). One could speculate that the founding of Sangrelaya, traditionally inhabited by the family with the best claim to leadership since the days on St. Vincent (the Sambulas), might have provided sufficient impetus to assure permanent settlement outside the realm of Trujillo control.

The eastern frontier of Garifuna settlement, across the Black River, was irregularly the scene of Garifuna intrusions into lands occupied by the Miskito Indians. Following the 1804–1807 trek to the Patuca, other attempts at settlement near Cape Gracias a Dios in 1821 (AGCA 1821) and on Carataska Lagoon in the mid-1850s (Bell, 1899) failed, and retreats westward back across the Black River were reportedly caused by storms (T. Young, 1842) and the oppression of a Miskito chief (Roberts, 1827). The area of Garifuna control remained west of the Black River and was obviously recognized as theirs by 1820: the Poyais Colonization Scheme of Gregor McGregor (Hasbrouck, 1927) included maps (Vandermaelen, 1827) that labeled the region "Caribania," and the Spaniards named a Carib leader as the political power for the area (Beaucage, 1970) in a probable attempt to reduce Miskito influence.

Although Caribs were present in Mosquitia for three decades in small numbers, no large influx took place until the defeat of Garifuna forces by the Central American Republican armies in 1832. Then, as one contemporary reported, the Garifuna fled eastward to escape "their subsequent discomfiture" (Galindo, 1833).

3.4. Belize, 1802-1832

The fourth realm of expansion was British Yucatan, or modern Belize. Settlement there should be considered in light of whether the migrants intended temporary or permanent settlement. From the earliest days on Roatan and at Trujillo, Carib sailors, with (Henderson, 1809) and without (Burdon, 1933) British companions, were cruising Belizean waters in their homemade dugout watercraft. Although some came to Belize to fish as independents and others sailed there as trader/smugglers, they also accompanied their recent enemies, the British, as loggers (Henderson 1809). There is no evidence that for three decades Garifuna intended permanent settlement in Belize.

Dangriga, formerly Stann Creek Town, has always been the center of Garifuna settlement in the colony. It is the site of the first permanent village and is today the largest Carib settlement, with over 7500 inhabitants, mostly Carib-speakers. Dunn (1828) recognized it as a Carib village as early as 1827, but we know that by August 1823 at least 25 Garifuna laborers were there to clear land for British settlers recently from the Poyais Colony at Black River (Hasbrouck, 1927). Because the settlers completely abandoned the site within 8 months, it is feasible to expect the workers to remain as permanent residents and to reap the harvest of their farmlands. Whatever the exact origins of the settlement, there is widespread agreement that the early rapid growth of the village resulted from the in-migration of Honduran Garifuna fleeing Republican reprisals following the losing Loyalist insurrection of 1832 in the vicinities of Omoa and Trujillo (Squier, 1855). Within 5 years, the settlement at Stann Creek and to the south at Punta Gorda had several hundred residents who had refused amnesty and evidently planned to remain in British territory away from the capricious military behaviour of the Central Americans. By 1840, Stann Creek had over 1000 inhabitants (Allen, 1841; Blunt, 1864); Punta Gorda was home for half as many (Stephens, 1841).

3.5. Western Honduras and Guatemala, 1821–1836

Garifuna occupation of the final stretch of coast, in western Honduras and Guatemala, is difficult to unravel historically because non-Carib, free Negroes lived in the area previous to Garifuna entry. There are observations of Negro settlers, reportedly Haitian but perhaps with Garifuna, at the mouth of the Rio Dulce for 1802 (Termer, 1936), for 1804 (Coelho, 1955), and for about 1806 (Gonzalez, 1969). At fort Omoa, Negroes were reported there as soldiers in 1801 (Abarca, 1898) and as general settlers by 1808 (Juarros, 1823). However, no evidence is present that these were Garifuna, and other references to Negro population in the area do not occur until the 1820s. In fact, the coast between Trujillo and Omoa is consistently known as being virtually deserted (Urrutia, 1818).

Any large number of Garifuna in the region might be traced to the contingents brought from Trujillo to Omoa to fight for the Spanish Crown during the wars of independence and the later civil war of 1832. After losing battles to the Central Americans, Garifuna fled to the safety of British lands in Belize (Galindo, 1833; Squier, 1855), and probably returned to western Honduras when amnesty was granted in 1836 (Salazar, 1932). In the same year lands along the Motagua River were offered for logging (Ibid., p. 415), and this new opportunity for wages may have lured more Garifuna.

The major Carib settlement of the region, at Livingston, Guatemala, was probably permanently established about 1830. Situated atop a prominent bluff on the western bank at the mouth of the Rio Dulce, the site was well known to

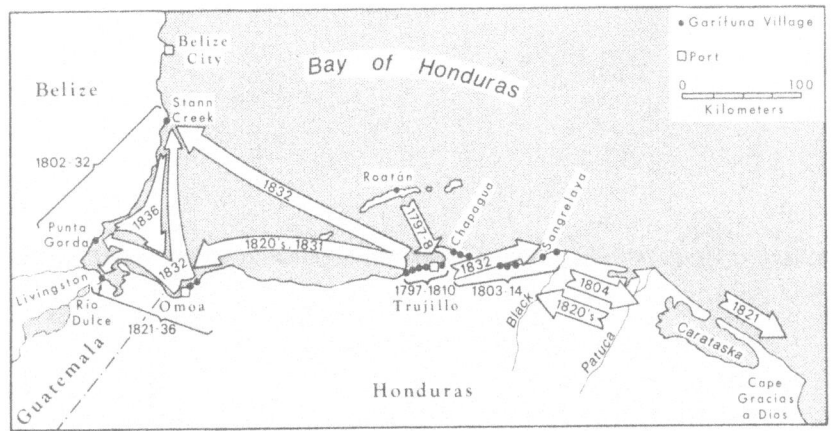

MAP 2. Dispersal of the Garifuna in Central America, 1797–1836.

travelers of the 1820s, who invariably ran their ships aground on the shallow, shifting sand bar just offshore. None of the travelers delayed at the bluff [for examples see Henderson (1809), Dunn (1829), Thompson (1829), Wilson (1829)] specifically mention the presence of Garifuna before 1832, when, as Castañeda (1909) learned, 150 Caribs from Honduras settled there. Obviously, the village encountered difficulties during the period of early growth: only 100 souls lived there in 1836 (Salazar, 1932), and the 40–50 huts there in 1838 (Montgomery, 1839) were probably burned in the fire of 1840 (Page, 1840).

After four decades of relatively intense movements, the Garifuna had established about 20 villages around the Bay of Honduras from Stann Creek, British Honduras, to the Black River in Honduran Mosquitia (Map 2). The dispersal opened new lands and fishing grounds, and thereby reduced the tremendous pressure on the resources of Trujillo. Life in the new locations must have eased for the Garifuna, and their movements, although never ceasing, seem to have relaxed. Now, more than a generation away from their homeland on St. Vincent, the Garifuna began organizing for permanence in Central America. How they arranged themselves in their new habitat is the theme of the following section.

4. Patterns of Settlement

The modern spatial organization of the Garifuna can be illustrated as a scaled hierarchy of five regions. In order of decreasing size they are (1) culture realm, (2) trade area, (3) village subsistence region, (4) settlement proper, and (5) family compound. The following areal sketches will indicate the variety of ways the Garifuna orient themselves to the physical world around the Bay of Honduras.

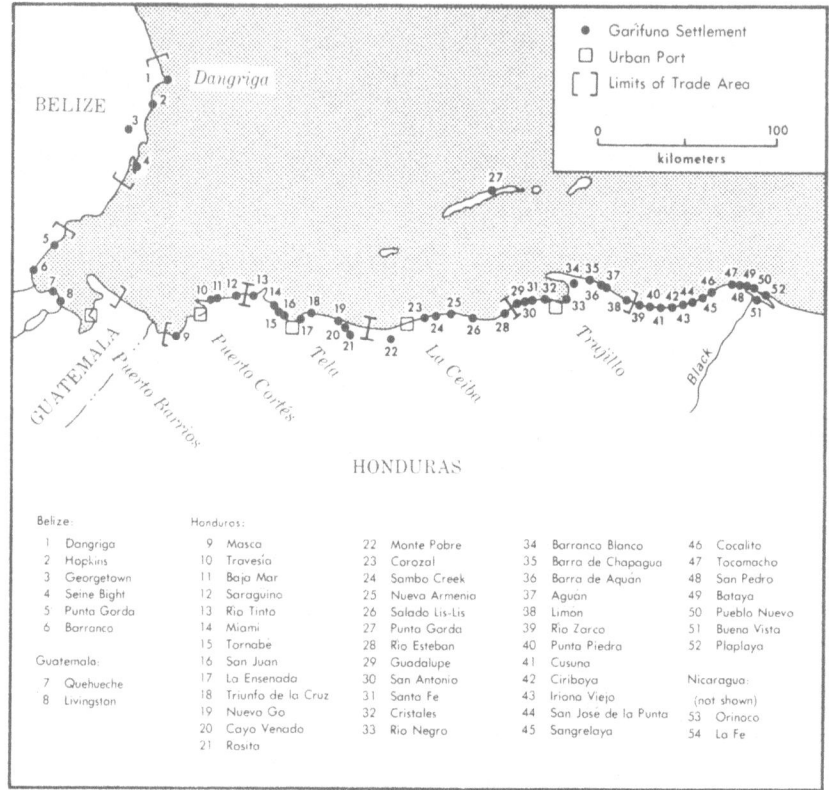

MAP 3. Garifuna in Central America, settlements and trade areas, 1978.

4.1. Garifuna Culture Realm

Garifuna villages and their nearshore lands dominate the rural landscape of the Caribbean littoral for 400 miles — central Belize to eastern Honduras. Distances between the settlements are slight (averages: 15 miles in Belize, less than 5 miles in Honduras), but urban ports interrupt Carib lands in five instances (Map 3). No village is farther than 10 miles inland; all but three touch coastal waters. Thus, the long chain of beach villages gives the Garifuna realm a narrow, discontinuous configuration. Because of the consistent selection of coastal sites for settlement, the dominant aspects of physical geography for each village are relatively similar.

In the western Caribbean, trade winds blow onshore from the east and northeast. So consistent are these winds that in lieu of directions, Hondurans refer to east as "up" [wind], west as "down." In Belize, "up" is north, "down" is south. The winds, which blow ashore over warm currents of the Bay, moderate temperatures of the coastal lands. Because of the slight variation in temperature throughout the year, seasonality is expressed most clearly in the distribution of rainfall: June to December is the rainy period, December to June is dry. Of course, local habitats vary in topography, soils, sources of fresh water, etc., but nowhere in the realm are differences so great that subsistence production is significantly affected (see Section 4.3 on village subsistence region).

Although it is improbable that any single Garifuna knows all settlements in his or her culture realm, contacts are considerable throughout the area, and Garifuna knowledge of the extent of settlement is widespread. Within the tropical, wet–dry, windy fringe of the Bay of Honduras, some 65,000* Garifuna know (see Table 1) they can travel and visit, without invitation, and be assured that the warmth of family awaits their arrival. In many instances actual relatives will greet travelers in far-flung settlements. For example, the Sambula family, before mentioned as one of leadership on St. Vincent, has a representative in at least 34 Garifuna villages. Other prominent surnames that are typically Garifuna include Alvarez, Arana, Arzu, Bernardez, Casildo, Castillo, Centeno, Crisanto, Flores, Gonzalez, Lopez, Martinez, Melendez, Morales, Palacio, Velasquez, and Zenon.

4.2. Trade Areas

Within the larger culture realm seven trade areas can be delimited[†] (Map 3). Each commerical network is composed of a large, non-Garifuna port (Dangriga is an exception) and a hinterland that includes several Garifuna villages. To be within a trade area contact between a village and the urban center must occur at least weekly. Only in eastern Honduras are settlements so isolated that frequent trade contacts do not occur on a scheduled basis, but even there traders pass occasionally.

Beachwalks are the normal mode of transportation between village and port, but frequently, particularly when heavy produce is involved, the trips are in small watercraft or truck-buses. The exchange of produce normally consists of coconuts, palm oil, fish, coconut bread, and cassava from the villages, and fuel, ice, citrus, dry goods, and hardware from the ports. Also, a fleet of Garifuna-

---

* I once calculated the Garifuna population in Central America to be about 77,000 (Davidson, 1976). That figure was based on census material from Belize and Guatemala, and on aerial photography flown in 1973 and ground-checked in 1974. Several Garifuna researchers questioned the total population, primarily because dwellings that appeared on the photographs were thought to be unoccupied. The revised lower figure used here, 65,000, was derived after taking the criticisms into account.

† Since the trade area framework was first presented (Davidson, 1976), Lundberg (1978) has correctly pointed out that the Punta Gorda–Barranco network should not be considered a unit apart from Livingston. Here I have included these three settlements with Puerto Barrios. Still, one must realize that while contacts between southern Belize and Livingston are frequent, and those between Livingston and Barrios are daily, Belizean contacts with Barrios are minimal.

Table 1. Garifuna in Central America: Settlements and Populations[a]

Country	Garifuna population	Garifuna as percent of country population
Belize	11,000	7.85
In six settlements	8,700	
Elsewhere	2,300	
Guatemala	5,000	0.083
In two settlements	3,100	
Elsewhere	1,900	
Honduras	48,000	1.71
In 44 settlements	42,750	
Elsewhere	5,250	
Nicaragua	1,000	0.05
In two settlements	750	
Elsewhere	250	
Total population	65,000	

[a] Approximate values for 1978.

produced trading vessels ply the coast to carry Ladino foodstuffs to the port markets.

The relationship of trade center and Carib village is of importance beyond the economic exchange that takes place. Trade areas are economic "mesohabitats," but they also provide the framework for the incorporation of the Garifuna into Central American life. It is from the urban ports that non-Garifuna ways are introduced into the villages. It is from the ports that Garifuna men are drawn onto the merchant ships that carry them to the U.S. and elsewhere over the globe.

4.3. Village Subsistence Region

A third spatial system envelops the village and provides a resource base from which the local inhabitants receive their daily sustenance. The cultivated lands that lie behind the settlement are included, as are the offshore waters and nearby coastal lagoons that serve as fishing grounds. The Garifuna have so consistently chosen similar physical environments for their villages that an idealized habitat can be reconstructed. Judging from the compilation of features found in all settlements (Table 2), the ideal site is one located less than 100 yards from the sea on beachland very near the mouth of a small stream or river. Preferably, the settlement is backed by a narrow, freshwater lagoon, across which cultivable hill lands are easily reached by dugout.

Cultivated lands are often several miles from the village, usually on national

Table 2. Prominent Physical Features for 54
Garifuna Settlements, 1978

Feature	Occurrences
Beach	47
Stream or river mouth	33
Hill land	25
Lagoon	16
Protected bay	9

territory. In their use of shifting field, slash-and-burn farming techniques, some Garifuna travel several miles to plots, while others farm relatively near home. The amount and location of cleared land (but not necessarily farmed) have varied greatly historically. For example, small "plantations" of the residents of Barranco, Belize, during the period of commercial banana operations before World War II, were extensive, covering a few thousand acres and ranging 12 miles from the village. Today, that area has shrunk to about 140 acres within 1.5 miles of town (Map 4). Nicaraguan Caribs have also reduced their plantings recently

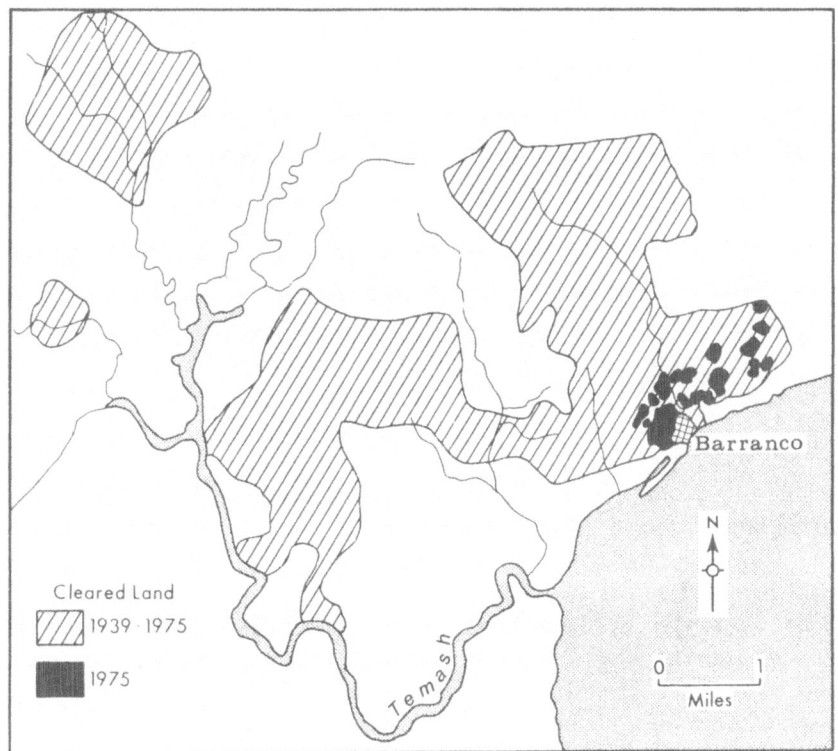

MAP 4. Land clearing for agriculture, Barranco, Belize, 1939–1975 (Lundberg, 1978).

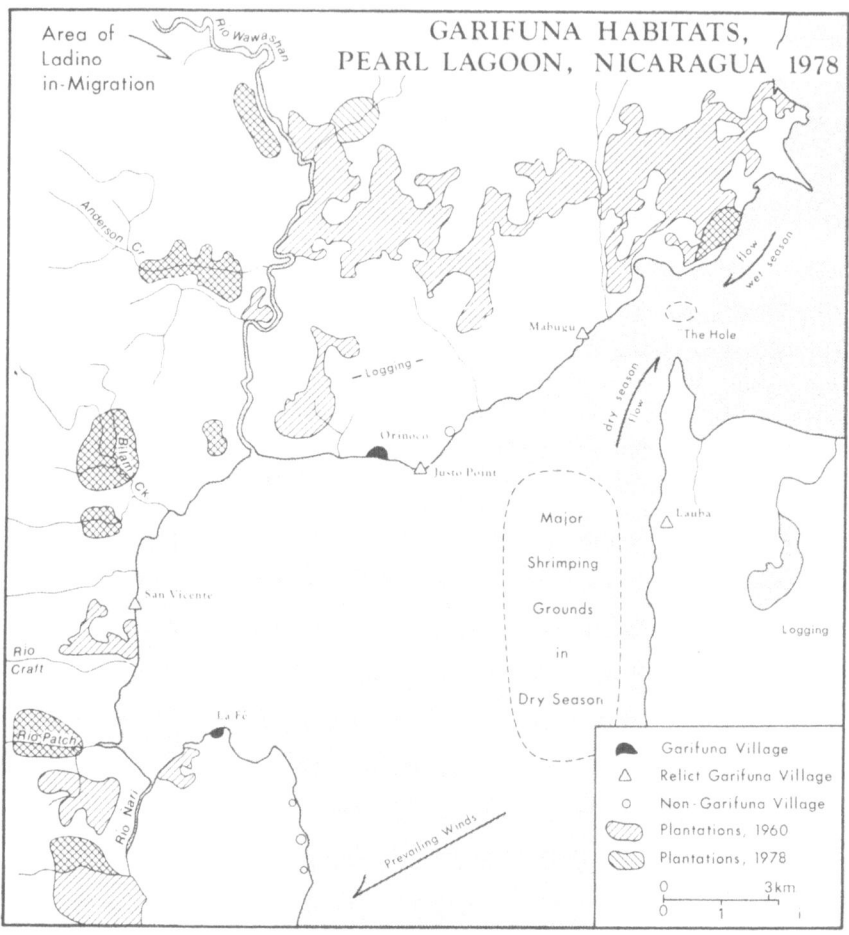

MAP 5. Garifune habitats, Pearl Lagoon, Nicaragua, 1978.

and are in eminent danger of losing more lands unwillingly to Ladino farmers moving onto their lands (Map 5).

This native turf is the region of primary subjective significance. The area might be envisioned as two hemispheric bulbs — one to the seaward and one inland — separated by the elongated shoreline, beachland, coconut fringe, and linear village. The seaward is the male sphere; there he fishes in a light, open, fluid environment. There his watercraft can ease the burden of backborne loads. Inland is the domain of the female. There she cannot escape the more difficult and dark, heavily vegetated and firm zone where she practices her agriculture and gathers firewood (Fig. 1).

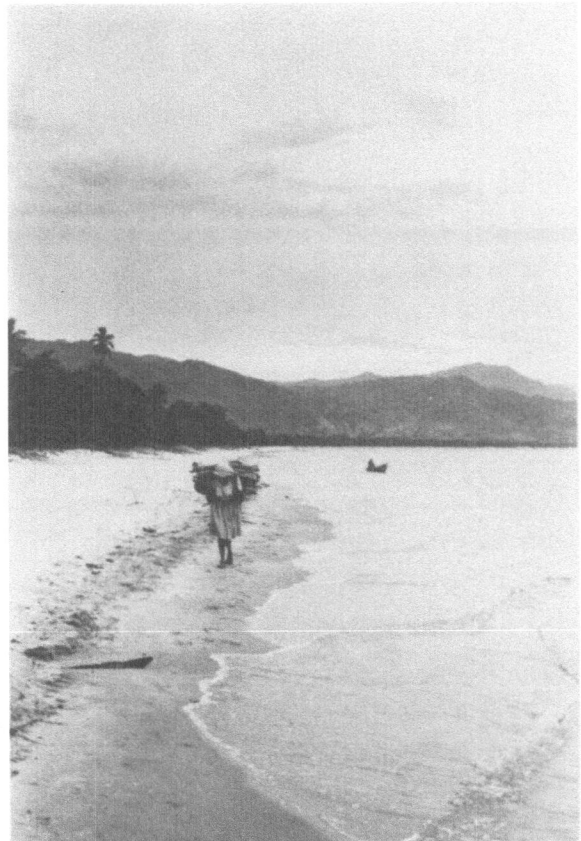

FIGURE 1. Bringing firewood to the settlement: elderly female walks the beach, her grandson follows offshore in a dugout.

4.4. Settlement Proper

Fifty-four settlements are inhabited predominently by Garifuna-speaking people. The range of congregations is large, from urban centers possessing an array of services (Dangriga) to small collections of fishing huts dug into the beach sand (Rio Zarco, Miami) (see Figs. 2 and 3). Because they are delimited by the distribution of dwellings, settlements are the most easily recognized and bounded space in the hierarchy of Garifuna settlement patterns. Here are concentrated the material expressions of Garifuna culture.

Generally, houses and outbuildings are closely clustered; such agglomeration probably reflects the highly social nature of the residents. Smaller villages are linear, with the ridge poles of the houses parallel to the sea. As settlements enlarge, a few rows of houses develop inland, and further growth normally brings

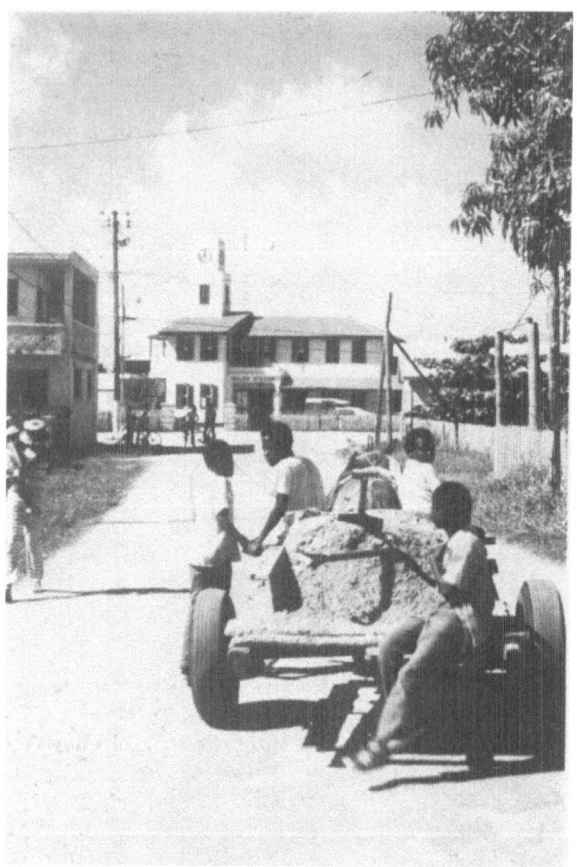

FIGURE 2. Selling beach sand throughout urban Dangriga, Belize.

nucleation near the middle of the linear village (Fig. 4). Settements large enough to support public buildings exhibit centrality in the location of schools, churches, and stores (Map 6).

Settlement landscapes are dominated by Garifuna dwellings, which traditionally are constructed in two distinctive forms. Both have cahoon palm thatching for the roof, but one has walls of wattle-and-daub, the other has horizontal strips of royal palm bark (*yagua*). Partitioned into two rooms (for eating and for sleeping), these houses are unusual in folk design for Central America because their roofs have a high pitch and are rectangular in form.

Other prominent features of the landscape include the artifacts of a subsistence orientation based on fishing and the cultivation of cassava. Also, settlements display a variety of intense human activities that occur regularly. Settlements abound with social places where residents *from anywhere within the village* are welcome to sit and chat: men build and repair dugouts under the

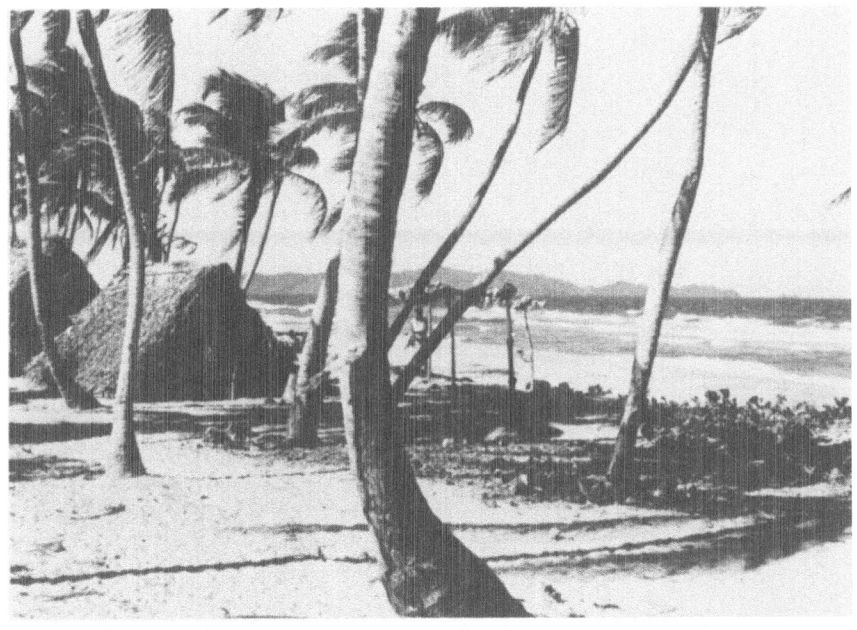

FIGURE 3. Fishing huts atop the beach at Miami, Honduras.

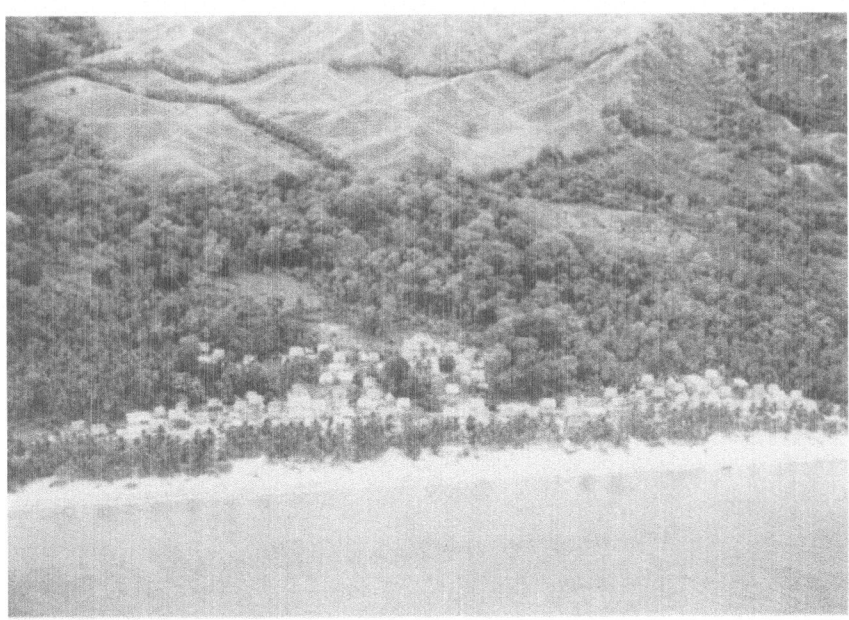

FIGURE 4. A nucleating village, Guadalupe, Honduras.

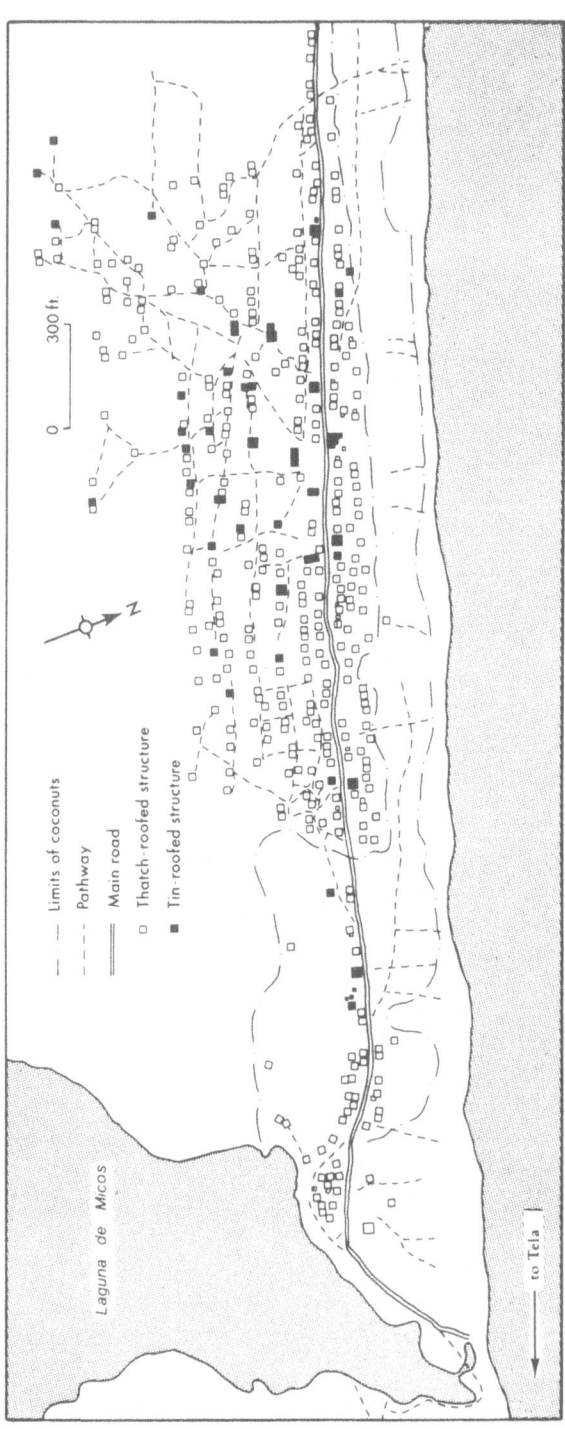

MAP 6. Tornabe, Honduras, settlement features, 1973. From aerial photograph

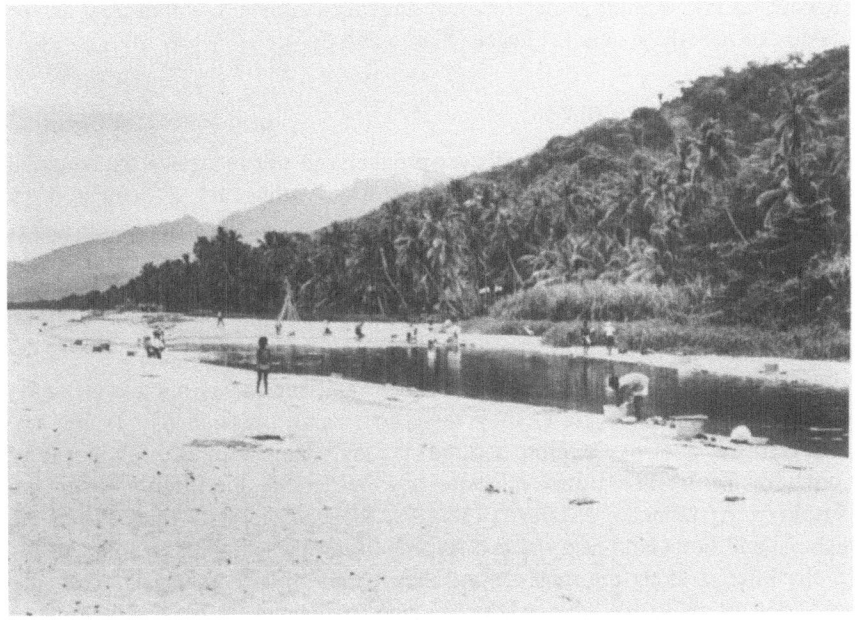

FIGURE 5. Wash day on the beach at San Antonio, Honduras.

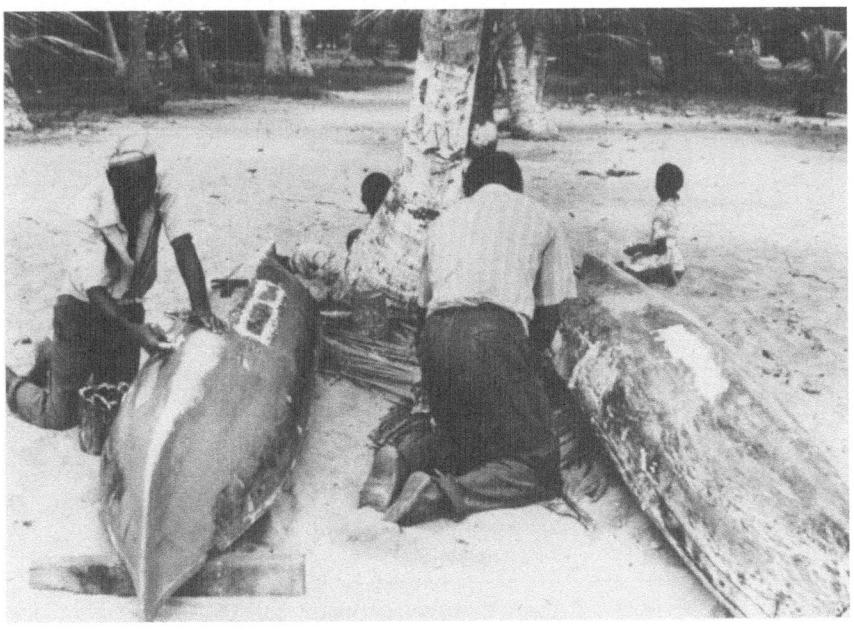

FIGURE 6. Boat repair under the coconut palms.

coconut palms, women gather to wash and dry clothing, children play on the margins of the village near the beach (Figs. 5 and 6).

4.5. Family Compound

Most visitors to Garifuna villages probably do not recognize that internal subdivisions, here called family compounds, exist within each settlement. Very little can be seen in the landscape to distinguish one sector from another. Yet inhabitants categorize sections of their villages primarily on the basis of family residence. In size, compounds range from a small cluster of dwellings and out-buildings belonging to the local members of an extended family to *barrios*, or neighborhoods, of over 100 homesteads.

Because settlement usually occurs first along the waterfront and is family-related, as compounds grow, they seem to enlarge perpendicular to the sea. Access to the water is therefore assured via family land. Also, later entrances by nonfamily (or non-Garifuna) relegates new settlers to the interior or on the periphery. At Orinoco, Nicaragua (Map 7), the two oldest families settled the highest (and best) land near the sea. As generations passed, younger folks settled to the interior along the ridge behind their parents. Newcomers were left only lands downslope to the west, where flooding is frequent. Tornabe, Honduras, a

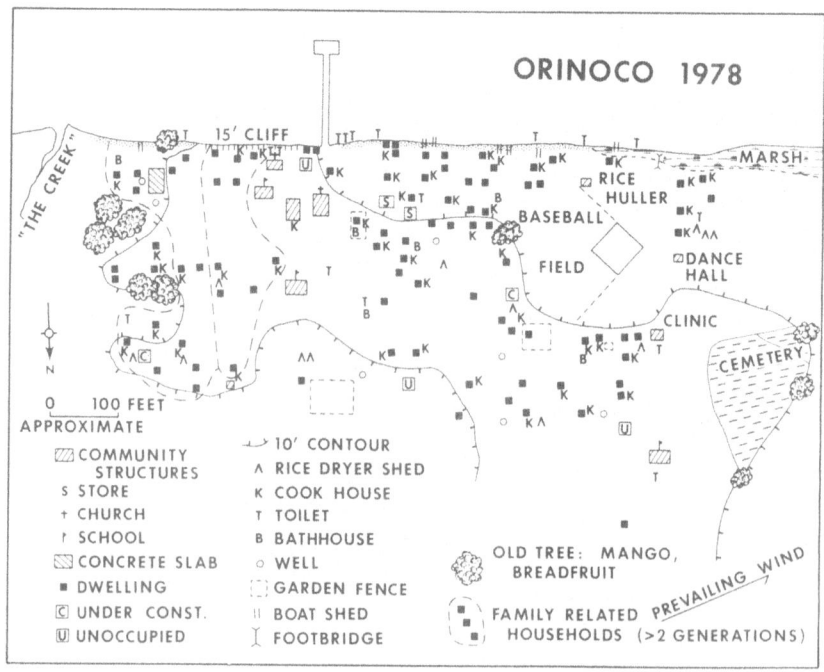

MAP 7. Orinoco, Nicaragua, settlement features.

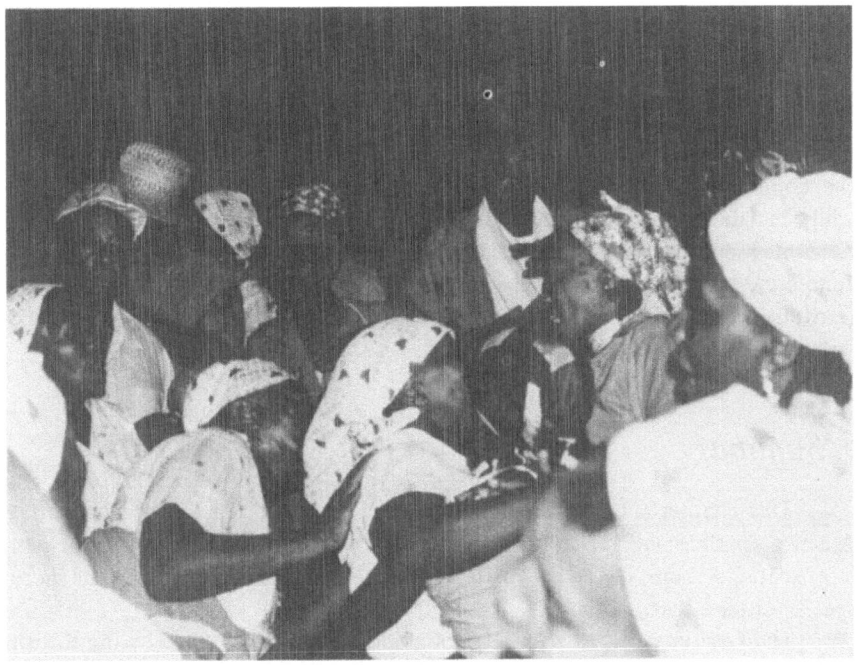

FIGURE 7. New Year's dance at Cristales, Honduras.

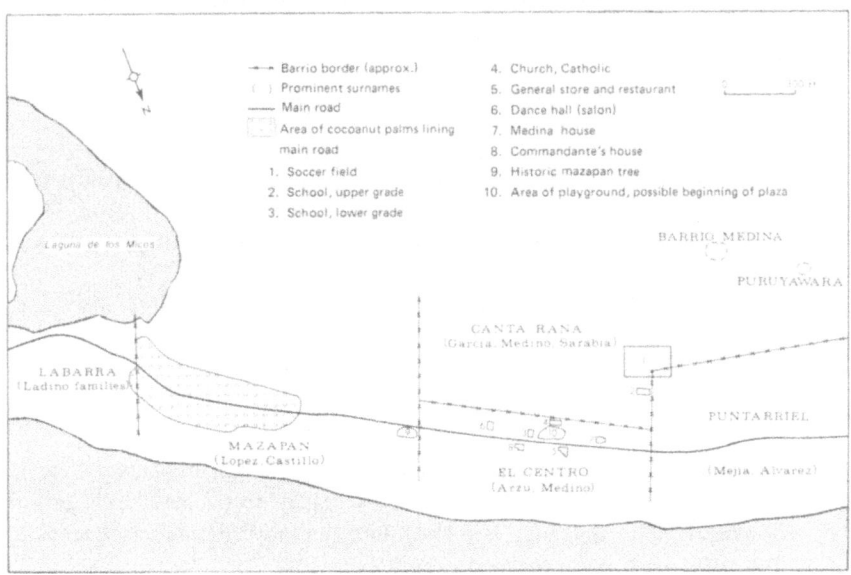

MAP 8. Tornabe, Honduras, *barrio* subdivisions, approximate for 1976. After King (1976).

village of about 1800 inhabitants, has five locally recognized internal sections, including one recently occupied by Ladino migrants [see Map 8 and King (1976)].

Clearly, it is through the agency of family-related activities of the compound that Garifuna maintain their cultural continuity. Within the borders of the compounds children receive their socialization and attachment to family, adult females gather for processing cassava and food preparation, and *barrio* residents sponsor dance groups (Fig. 7) and host ritual observances. The compound-based reverence for ancestors is the primary matrix that allows Garifuna ways to persist in a modernizing world along the shores of the east coast of Central America.

5. Summary

This chapter sets the Garifuna-speaking population of Caribbean Central America in time and place. Descriptions of the major historical episodes and large spatial domains of the group are here presented as background for the more specific studies that follow.

The Garifuna arrived at the Bay of Honduras in 1797, exiled by the British from their homeland on St. Vincent Island in the far southeast Caribbean. During the next four decades they dispersed along the littoral of Belize, Guatemala, and Honduras, moved by their own initiative, as laborers for British loggers, and as victims of local wars. The movement of individuals continues, particularly among males, and amounts to a type of coastal nomadism.

The present areal organization of the Garifuna can be illustrated as a hierarchy consisting of five scales.

1. The Garifuna Culture Region is a narrow, discontinuous band of 52 villages and near-shore lands that rims the Bay of Honduras from Stann Creek, Belize, to Plaplaya, Honduras, Also, a two-village enclave is isolated at Pearl Lagoon, Nicaragua.
2. Most Garifuna participate in one of seven Commercial Trade Areas. Each network is composed of a large, usually non-Garifuna port that is connected to several nearby villages by at least weekly contacts.
3. The Village Subsistence Region includes a Garifuna settlement and its surroundings, from which the local inhabitants receive daily foodstuffs. This homeland is the region of primary subjective significance.
4. Linear Coastal Villages are the most easily recognized units in the pattern of settlement. Here are found the most intense expressions of Garifuna culture in the landscape.
5. Within villages a final spatial component can be seen in the Family Compounds. They are homesteads of the local members of an extended

family and vary in size from a few dwellings and associated outbuildings to large *barrios*.

References

Abarca, R., 1898, Plan de ahorras en el gobierno militar de Guatemala (1801), in *Costa Rica y Costa de Mosquitos* (M. M. Peralta, ed.), pp. 295–326, Imprenta general de Lahure, Paris.

AGCA (Archivo General de Centro America), 1821, Caribes con otros en Cabo de Gracias a Dios, Sig. B5.4, Leg. 8859, exp. 1373, Guatemala City.

Allen, B., 1841, Sketch of the east coast of Central America, *J. R. Geog. Soc.* 2:76–89.

Anguiano, R., 1801, Poblición de las provincias de Honduras matricula del año 1801, Ms., Guatemala Indiferente 1525, Num. 11, Archivo General de Indias, Sevilla.

Anguiano, R., 1804, Población de las provincias de Honduras matricula del año de 1801 de Comayagua, 1 de mayo de 1804, Ms., Guatemala 5ª III, 501, Num. 9, Archivo General de Indias, Sevilla.

Anon, 1803, Progresos de la agricultura en Trugillo, *Gazeta de Guatemala* (Guatemala City), 1803 (December 19):469–470.

Anon, 1938, Limites entre Honduras y Nicaragua . . . 1938, s.i., New York.

Bancroft, H. H., 1887, *History of Central America*, Vol. 3, A. L. Bancroft, San Francisco.

Barrett, J., 1796–1797, Journals of the Proceedings of His Majesty's Ships: *Experiment*, 24 Aug 1796–4 Aug 1797, Ms., Public Record Office, Adm. 51, 1226, London.

Barrett, J., 1797, Letter of Captain John Barrett, July 7, 1797. Halifax Harbour, Nova Scotia, Ms., Public Record Office, London, Adm. 1, 1515, Cap B131.

Basso, E. B., 1977, *Carib-speaking Indians: Culture, Society, and Language*, University of Arizona Press, Tucson.

Beaucage, P. (s.f.), *Historia del pueblo Garifuna y su llegada a Hondruas en 1796*, Editorial Paulino Valladares, s.l. (1964).

Beaucage, P., 1970, *Economic Anthropology of the Black Carib of Honduras*, Ph.D. dissertation, University of London.

Bell, C. N., 1899, *Tangweera*, Edward Arnold, London.

Blunt, E., 1864, *The American Coastal Pilot*, Edmund and George Blunt, New York.

Burdon, J. A., 1933, *Archives of British Honduras*, Vol. 3, Sifton Praed, London.

Castañeda, F., 1909, *Guia del viajero en la República de Guatemala*, Artes Graficas "Electra," Guatemala.

Chamberlain, A. F., 1913, Linguistic stocks of South American Indians, with distribution map, *Am. Anthropol.* (n.s.) 15:236–247.

Coelho, R., 1955, The Black Carib of Honduras, Ph.D. dissertation, Northwestern University, Evanston, Illinois.

Davidson, W. V., 1974, *Historical Geography of the Bay Islands, Honduras*, Southern University Press, Birmingham, Alabama.

Davidson, W. V., 1976, Black Carib (Garifuna) habitats in Central America, in *Frontier Adaptation in Lower Central America* (M. Helms and F. Loveland, eds.), pp. 85–94, Institute for the Study of Human Issues, Philadelphia.

Davidson, W. V., 1980, The Garifuna of Pearl Lagoon: Ethnohistory of an Afro-American enclave in Nicaragua, *Ethnohistory*, 27(1):31–47.

Del Castillo, F., 1813, Dictamen de Florencio del Castillo 31 de agosto de 1813, Cadiz, Ms., Archivo General de Guatemala, A.1.22.4, Leg. 2648, Exp. 22122, Guatemala City.

De Tornos, J., 1816, Informe de la provincia de Honduras despues de hecha su visita de ordenanza, Comayagua, 20 de febrero de 1816, Ms., Guatemala 501, Archivo General de Indias, Sevilla.

Dunn, H., 1828, Guatimala, or the United Provinces of Central America, in 1827–1828, Ms. copy, Tulane Library, New Orleans.

Dunn, H., 1829, Guatimala, or the United Provinces of Central America, in 1827–1828, G. and C. Carvill, New York.

Durbin, M., 1977, A survey of the Carib language family, in Carib-Speaking Indians (E. B. Basso, ed.), pp. 23–38, University of Arizona Press, Tucson.

Edwards, B., 1819, The History, Civil and Commercial, of the West Indies, Vol. 4, T. Miller, London.

Galindo, J., 1833, Notice of the Caribs in Central America, J. R. Geog. Soc. 3:290–291.

Gonzalez, N. S., 1969, Black Carib Household Structure, University of Washington Press, Seattle.

Gullick, C. J. M. R., 1975, The Caribs at St. Vincent, a historical background and research bibliography, National Studies (Belize) 3(May):22–27.

Gullick, C. J. M. R., 1977, Black Carib origins and early soceity, in Proceedings of the International Congress of Study of Pre-Columbian Culture of Lesser Antilles, pp. 1–10, Caracas, Venezuela.

Hasbrouck, A., 1927, Gregor McGregor and the colonization of Poyais, Hispanic Am. Hist. Rev. 7:438–459.

Henderson, G., 1809, An Account of the British Settlement of Honduras, C. and R. Baldwin, London.

Houdaille, J., 1954, Negroes Franceses en América Central a fines del siglo XVIII, Antropol. Histo. Guatem. 6:65–67.

Juarros, D., 1823, A Statistical and Commercial History of the Kingdom of Guatemala, J. Hearne, London.

King, P., 1976, A descriptive and comparative study of the barrios of Tornabé, Honduras, in Field Studies in Central America I: Tela and Vicinity, Honduras (W. V. Davidson, compiler), pp. 71–79, Department of Geography and Anthropology, Louisiana State University, Baton Rouge, Louisiana.

Labat, P., 1970, The Memoirs of Père Labat, 1693–1705, Frank Cass, London.

Layng, A., 1976, The Carib population of Dominica, Ph.D. dissertation, Case Western Reserve University.

Loukotka, C., 1967, Ethno-linguistic distribution of South American Indians, Ann. Am. Assoc. Geog. 57(2):map supplement.

Lundberg, P. A., 1978, Barranco: A sketch of a Belizean Garifuna (Black Carib) habitat, M. S. thesis, University of California, Riverside.

Montgomery, G. W., 1839, Narrative of a Journey to Guatemala, in Central America in 1838, Wiley and Putnam, New York.

Page, E. L., 1840, Notes on a Journey from Belize to Guatemala in 1834, London.

Roberts, O., 1827, Narrative of Voyages and Excursions on the East Coast and the Interior of Central America, Constable, Edinburgh.

Rochester, W., 1828, Letter to Henry Clay, from Truxillo, 15 May 1828, U.S. National Archives, MC-219, roll 2 (Vol. 1), Washington, D.C.

Rossi y Rubi, J., 1797, Diario de 23 mayo, Gazeta de Guatemala (Guatemala City), 21(26 junio):164–168.

Rouse, I., 1948, The Caribs, in The Circum-Caribbean Tribes, Vol. 4, Handbook of South American Indians (J. H. Steward, ed.), Bureau of American Ethnology, Bulletin 143, pp. 547–565, Washington, D.C.

Saenz, P., 1797, Informe de Pedro Saenz, Gazeta de Guatemala (Guatemala City), 16(22 mayo):127–129.

Salazar, C., 1932, *Guatemala–Honduras Boundary Arbitration: The Case of Guatemala*, n.p., Washington, D.C.

Shepard, C., 1831, *An Historical Account of the Island of Saint Vincent*, W. Nicol, London.

Southey, T., 1827, *Chronological History of the West Indies*, Vol. 3, Rees, Orme, Brown, and Green, London.

Squier, E. G., 1855, *Notes on Central America*, Harper, New York.

Stephens, J. L., 1841, *Incidents of Travel in Central America, Chiapas, and Yucatan*, Vol. 1, Harper and Row, New York.

Steward, J. H. and J. A. Mason, 1950, Tribal and linguistic distributions of South America, in *Handbook of South American Indians*, Vol. 6 (map in back pocket), Bureau of American Ethnology, Bulletin 143, Washington, D.C.

Taylor, D., 1951, *The Black Carib of Honduras*, Viking Fund Publications in Anthropology, no. 17, Wenner-Gren Foundation, New York.

Termer, F., 1936, *Zur geographie der republik Guatemala*, De Gruyter, Hamburg.

Thompson, G., 1829, *Narrative of an Official Visit to Guatemala from Mexico*, John Murray, London.

Urrutia, C., 1818, Letter of Octubre 3 from President and Captain-General-de Guatemala, in *Guatemala–Honduras Boundary Arbitration (1932)* (C. Salazar, ed.), pp. 180–181, Washington, D.C.

Vallejo, A., 1893, *Primer Anuario Estádistico correspondiente el año de 1889*, Tipográfia National, Tegucigalpa, Honduras.

Vandermaelen, P., 1827, *Atlas Universal* (sheet 72), H. Ode, Bruxelles.

Wilson, J., 1829, *Brief Memoir of the Life of James Wilson . . . During a Residence in Guatemala*, A. Panton, London.

Young, T., 1842, *Narrative of a Residence on the Mosquito Shore*, Smith, Elder, and Co., London.

Young, W., 1795, *An account of the Black Caribs in the Island of St. Vincent's*, J. Sewell, London.

3

The Changing Vincentian Carib Population

C. J. M. R. GULLICK

1. Introduction

Estimates of the number of Black Caribs living in St. Vincent demonstrate some of the problems resulting from varying systems of ethnic classification used by Caribs and non-Carib observers. Thus population figures based on Vincentian Carib views differ from those of outside observers. In addition, population figures according to any one group for any one point in time tend to be vastly different from those of the same group at another time. Problems in assessing Carib population size are compounded by other factors. Before 1797 few figures can be assigned any degree of accuracy, because of their having been put forward with a view to propaganda. In the 19th century this complication disappeared, but despite the availability of official censuses, nominally based on actual head counts, Carib numbers are uncertain due to a paucity of information about the classification system used. However, because of a lack of other evidence, these official counts generally have to be considered at face value. In the 20th century numerous official figures are available, but they frequently disagree with one another and with other evidence. This chapter will consider the differing estimates of the founding populations appearing in these three periods and from them try to produce a demographic characterization of the Black and Yellow Carib residents of St. Vincent. The emphasis will be placed on periods having least secondary analysis, while those frequently analyzed elsewhere will be discussed in less detail.

C. J. M. R. GULLICK • Department of Anthropology, Durham University, Durham DHI 3HN, England.

2. Prior to 1797

The period before 1797 saw the origins of the Black Caribs and the battles against the European colonists by them and the Yellow Caribs. Information on the history and population numbers before the British annexation of St. Vincent in 1763 is sparse. As I have demonstrated elsewhere (Gullick, 1978*b*), the black component of the Black Caribs could have come at any time during the period 1517–1646, but was probably a gradual phenomenon that has continued to the present day. The African component seems initially to have been made up of runaway slaves from European-held islands and captives taken on raids in those islands. There may also have been a major influx of blacks from a wrecked slaver in the area. The evidence for this wreck is, however, inconclusive. In later periods, intermarriage took place with the freed Afro-American population of St. Vincent.

2.1. Population Estimates

Once the British annexed the island, numerous estimates of the Carib population size began to appear. These tend to be of two distinct orders of magnitude. Estimates of between 2000 and 3000 were used in arguments claiming that the Carib half of the island was underutilized and should be taken over. To bolster this case Yellow Carib numbers were put in the low hundreds, and it was then maintained that they alone had any rights to land in St. Vincent. Other figures in the 5000–6000 range did not differentiate between Black and Yellow Caribs and were normally included in claims for war damage or in pleas for the removal of the Caribs from St. Vincent. Both sets of numbers were of propaganda value and therefore suspect. Various estimates based upon ecological factors, such as the carrying capacity of the island, would favor the lower range of figures. The number of Caribs deported after the Carib Wars support the lower group of estimates, though many Caribs died in these wars, so that there may have been more than 5000 originally [see Gullick (1976*a*, 1978*a*) for details]. The Carib Wars have been discussed in great detail (e.g., Kirby and Martin, 1972; Gullick, 1969, 1974, and 1976*b*). The second Carib War (1795–1805) resulted in the deportation to Central America of 2500 Caribs, both Black and Yellow (Colonial Office 260/13–15, War Office 1/85, and 690). Other estimates of the number captured reached as high as 5080, but such high estimates are included in claims for damages caused by the Caribs and may well be overinflated (see Chapter 4, this volume). This high figure certainly does not fit in with ecological and archeological evidence (Gullick, 1978a; Bullen and Bullen, 1972).

3. Post-1797

This deportation occurred in 1797 but did not include all the Caribs, and the war limped on until 1805. A second minor expulsion occurred in 1801, when about 60 Caribs, mainly women and children, were either sent to Trinidad or pressed onto a ship. The location of the Carib combatants at this phase is uncertain, but they were probably at a village near Morne Ronde, and another group made up of Black Caribs and Maroons were at a place called Lapiton, somewhere in the mountains above Gordons. There were also communities of noncombatant Yellow Caribs in the North Windward (Colonial Office 160/17–19). In 1804 an act was passed stating that the Caribs had forfeited their claims to the lands left them in the treaty of 1773. According to the Colonial Office files (260/17) and to the Map of Carib Grant Lands,* when the Caribs of Morne Ronde surrendered in 1805, they were only granted about 230 acres of land in that region. Their numbers were listed as 16 men, nine women, and 20 children. There may have been another community of Caribs in the upper Massariaca Valley (now known as Greiggs), but it has been difficult to date the foundation of this community (Gullick, 1976b). Figure 1 provides a geographical location of settlements on the island.

From 1804, when the Black Caribs lost most of their lands in St. Vincent, much of the propaganda value in their population figures and descriptions of their culture disappeared, and thus the little evidence of their condition in the 19th century tends to be more reliable. The first census that could have included them was held in March 1812 (St. Vincent, 1812). No specific heading for Caribs was given, but they may have made up the majority of the 60 freemen of color in St. David's, which included Morne Ronde, and some of the 72 in Charlotte Parish, which included both the North Windward and Greiggs. The Yellow Caribs were less likely to have been included under this heading than the Black Caribs, but there was no other apparent rubric that might have included them. If this census was at all accurate and if the Black Caribs were included, there were probably fewer than 132 of them on the island. Their numbers were further reduced by the eruption of the Soufriere volcano in June 1812, in which 56 individuals are said to have died. How many Caribs were included in this number is uncertain. However, the Morne Ronde Caribs are reported to have fled before the lava flow hit the area and thus probably survived. Some of the surviving Caribs are known to have left the island for Trinidad.

The location of the Caribs in the North Windward during the first third of the 19th century is uncertain. However, Bayley, after a trip to the Carib "king" sometime between 1826 and 1829, said that "the Caribs reside together in a fine quarter of the island called the Carib Country (the North Windward)" (Bayley, 1833, p. 285). He described this land as "the only really level ground in St. Vincent" (p. 285). This suggests that he did not reach Owia and that the Carib settlement was south of New Sandy Bay. He described the settlement as "little" and thought that the total Carib population was "hardly" 1000 and that "there numbers decrease yearly" (Bayley, 1833). I suspect that this figure was a

* Co 260/17 and from a "Map of the Grant Lands" in the Lands and Survey Department, St. Vincent.

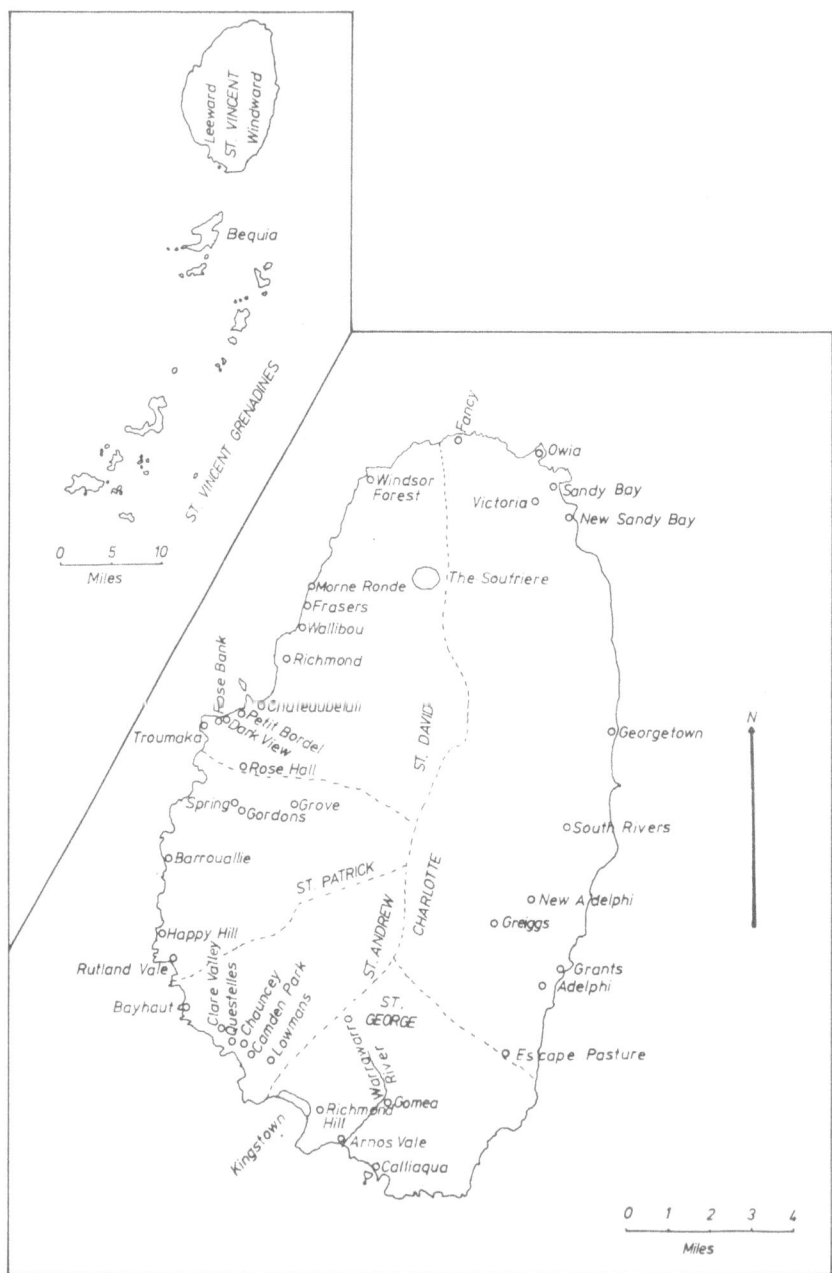

FIGURE 1. Location of St. Vincent Island in the Lesser Antilles. This map also locates the major communities of the island that are discussed in the text.

slight exaggeration, especially when viewed in the context of the 1812 and 1844 censuses.

3.1. 1844 Census

The 1844 census (St. Vincent, 1844) listed "178 Charibs residing to Windard . . . 95 Charibs residing to Leeward . . . making the total number of these people 273." The Black Caribs of the Leeward were counted as "Black," while the Yellow Caribs of the Windward were "Coloured." The census report noted "this was all that remained of these Aborigines. They have the occupancy of 230 acres, granted for their subsistence." Of the Windward Caribs 106 were given as living in Sandy Bay, and the rest may have been residing in Greiggs (population at that time was 54) or possibly Owia (population 81), as they were found there at later dates. Most of the Leeward Caribs must have lived at Morne Ronde, which had a population of 84.

This census was after emancipation, when contact between the Caribs and the black population of the island increased, and intermating may have resumed. The Black Caribs were sufficiently integrated into the island to have been involved in a smallpox epidemic in 1849, although few seem to have died from it. The 1851 census (St. Vincent, 1851) mentioned "167 Charibs residing to Windward." Davy (1854), who visited Sandy Bay at about that time, thought that there were still about 106 at Sandy Bay. No figures of the Carib population in St. David's were given by either source. Thus they may have been more affected by the epidemic than were the Windward Caribs. In fact, the census suggests that the disease had a negligible effect on the whole island's population. As a result the Governor decided that the census was inaccurate. There was also an epidemic of yellow fever in 1852, but this seems to have been most virulent among the whites, and the Caribs may have escaped its ravages. They were, however, caught by the 1854 cholera outbreak and were indeed blamed for having introduced it from other islands (Horsford, 1856). As many as 2200 died of cholera in St. Vincent, but despite this the Carib population remained numerically static in official figures, the 1861 census (St. Vincent, 1861) listing 169 in Charlotte Parish, 22 in St. David's, and one in both Kingstown and St. George's.

3.2. Carib-Creole Contact

It is probable that by this time there was considerable communication between the Carib and black populations of St. Vincent. Thus if one can judge by surnames, one (or perhaps two) of the leaders of the 1862 riot was Carib and one of the witnesses was probably the same. The main locale of the fighting was on the Windward, south of Georgetown [see Gullick (1974) for details]. That integration and intermarriage were taking place is demonstrated by a report of the Attorney General for 20 March 1882 (Attorney General, St. Vincent, 1882).

In it he decided that

> the rule that a Carib woman marrying a stranger should leave the
> settlement [of Morne Ronde] and live with her husband seems just and
> necessary and is moreover agreeable to the common law of England . . . .
> In the present case Henrietta Thompson is of mixed birth – her father
> Joseph Olivierre, being a native of Gomea, her mother a Carib. It is not
> stated when or where she was born; but I am of the opinion that she
> cannot be regarded as a Black Carib under the King's Grant. She should
> therefore have no right to be located on the settlement and it is clear
> that her husband cannot have such a right

This is especially interesting, as it is highly probable that her father, Joseph
Olivierre, was at least part Yellow Carib. The Attorney General continued,
"under the law of the settlement, also Mrs. Thompson would forfeit her right of
residence (if any) by her marriage with Joseph Thompson." Another manuscript
of 1887 (St. Vincent 87/267) mentions another expulsion of a non-Carib from
the settlement.

Likewise, in the North Windward, contact between Caribs and Creoles
seems to have taken place. When Chester visited the island just after the riots, he
reported that the Caribs lived "to the extreme North of the island . . . . (They)
are but few in number, and have almost entirely forsaken their ancient habits.
They live like the negroes in houses and a Carib belle may even be seen in a
crinoline. Few of the original colour now exist; the greater number being called
'Black Caribs.' These last are of mixed race . . . who in physical characteristics
are rather African than American" (Chester, 1869). Chester's omission of Sandy
Bay, Greiggs, Morne Ronde, and perhaps Bequia is peculiar, especially when his
description is ,compared with Musgrave's (1891), who said "the true Caribs, who,
in contradiction to the Black Caribs, are locally called the Yellow Caribs [rent]
land at a place called Sandy Bay on the Windward coast under the nominal
control of a headman . . . . The Black Caribs reside on the Leeward side of the
island at Morne Ronde . . . . There is also another settlement of Black Caribs at a
place called Greiggs."

Contemporary accounts do not mention the Carib community on Bequia,
the island to the south of St. Vincent, despite petitions in 1888 from the fishermen of Bequia that included the statement that "they represented a race of men
who had been in the habit of fishing (in a disputed area) from time immemorial"
(262 a/88). It has not been possible to trace the history of this community
before this date, but I have been able to collect some oral histories on the
subject. Some claim that the Caribs escaped there from the boats deporting them
to Central America and from the internment camp on the two neighboring
islands. Others think that they were descendants of the original Island Carib
inhabitants of the island. Yet others claim that they were French and not Carib,
but do mention being held prisoner by the British on Baliceaux.

In 1877 the first anthropologist to visit the Caribs, Ober, visited Sandy

Bay, which he considered "the most secluded (village) in the island." The Caribs were squatters there under a chief who was "a pure Carib." He also mentions a Black Carib who "had married a Yellow Carib, a woman of uncontaminated Indian blood." He considered "scarcely 200 or only six families to be pure Caribs" (Ober, 1880).

3.3. Population Effects of Cataclysms

None of the published travelers' tales mention the formation by then of yet another Carib community. This was due to some Morne Ronde Caribs moving to Frasers after 1875. Nor do they record that after the storms of 1876 the Caribs of the North Leeward moved temporarily to Chateaubelair. A similar exodus from the North Windward may have occurred after the 1886 hurricane devastated the area. A more disastrous event was a land slip at Sandy Bay in 1896, which killed 11. This was, however, minor compared to the damage done by the 1898 hurricane and the 1902 volcanic eruption. The death toll of the hurricane was 300, and many Caribs must have been included, as the north of the island was worst hit. Afterwards some of the Morne Ronde Caribs moved to Frasers and the government set about rehousing the Morne Ronde and Frasers Caribs. After some disputes they were eventually in 1899 given house lots at Rose Bank. Few, however, had moved there before the eruption of 1902. During this eruption the Morne Ronde Caribs were the most sensible of those living in the area, and most of them fled before the eruption, so were not included among the dead. The North Windward Caribs fared less well.* This eruption caused most of the major changes in the Caribs' location and undoubtedly affected their numbers. It also marks a divide in the types of population statistics available. Up to the time of the eruption, statistics, as already stated, were mainly dependent on censuses and travelers' estimates, the latter normally being somewhat larger than the former. After the eruption there were, in addition to these, various lists of inhabitants of houses and land, which, with a knowledge of modern Carib kinship networks, can be used to estimate more closely the size of the Carib population. Such calculations of modern Vincentian Carib numbers produce somewhat larger figures than those given in the censuses. I, having compiled my own census of the Carib community of Petit Bordel, decided that official censuses tend to include many people normally considered Carib as mixed. I thus tend to prefer these less official figures and suspect, but cannot be certain, that this is true of most previous censuses. Thus I would tend to believe travelers' estimates of the Carib population in the 19th century, but only if they were about one-third above census count.

This brings us to one of the major problems of at least 20th century Carib statistics: the protean nature of the classification "Carib." I have explored this in detail elsewhere (Gullick, 1976c), but must point out here that claims to be

* PP 1899 LXI, PP 1902 LXVI, PP 1904 LX, PP 1911 LII and Anderson and Flett (1903).

Carib depend on circumstance, and interrogation by officialdom as in a census certainly does not provide an occasion for claiming Caribness. In the end I decided to count as Carib anybody who was accepted as such in any major Carib community, as much of this rested on kinship and, in particular, surnames. I consider that my use of such names to determine ethnicity in various lists of Vincentians is as accurate, if not more so, than the censuses. However, I do not feel that such figures can be used to work backward to before the eruption, because of uncertainties as to how many Caribs were among the 2000 dead in the eruption and because historically the definition of Carib could have been different. In any event, the survivors from Fancy, Owia, Sandy Bay, Morne Ronde, Frasers, and Rose Bank fled to the south of the island, and the government had to deal with them along with other refugees. They were, however, the most vociferous. There were various attempts to persuade the inhabitants of Owia and Fancy who had "a certain amount of Carib in them" (though the ones from Fancy had slightly less) to emigrate to Jamaica, Tobago, St. Lucia, Dominica, or British Honduras, but to no avail. They were eventually settled in the south of the island at Camden Park (mainly from Sandy Bay and Wallibou), Clare Valley (a sizable proportion from Frasers), Rutland Vale (mainly from Richmond), Rose Bank (from Morne Ronde), and Barrouallie (temporarily from Morne Ronde). Sundry other refugees were settled at Troumaka, Richmond Hill, Park Hill, Arnos Vale, New Adelphi, and Mount Wynne. The refugees were, however, listed under their home villages. Thus it can be calculated that the following numbers of adult Caribs escaped from the following villages: Morne Ronde and Frasers, 44–48; Rose Bank, 44–54; Wallibou, three; Richmond, 7–13; Fancy, four; Owia, 34; Sandy Bay, 36–39. Thus between 172 and 195 adult Caribs had survived the eruption. In addition, the Greiggs Caribs were south of the danger zone. Given the number of tracts produced in the split-up of the Carib settlement at Greiggs, it is probable that 33 households of Caribs lived there in addition to the refugees.*

3.4. Population Movements

Morne Ronde was never resettled following the eruption; all its surviving Caribs moved south, mainly to Rose Bank. However, they eventually cultivated the land at Morne Ronde by commuting there by boat or occasionally on foot. None of the other villages were abandoned for long.

In the wake of the eruption, another anthropologist, Sapper, visited. He observed the Camden Park Caribs and stated that only four or five were pure-bred (Sapper, 1903). The remainder, he thought, were mixed with either blacks and/or Asiatics. He added that they were unhappy in their new homes. These probably made up the bulk of the Caribs who had returned to their old lands at

---

* See preceding footnote and also PP 1906 LXXV, and "List of Refugees" uncatalogued manuscript in the St. Vincent Government Archives.

Owia and Sandy Bay by 1905 (Sapper, 1903; Parliamentary Papers 1906 LXXV).

There was perhaps another population movement at this period. In June 1903, the Carib reserve in Dominica was created and Rouse (1949) claims that some of the Vincentian Caribs joined the Dominican Caribs there. If this happened, not many stayed; the Domincan census of 1921 (Dominica, 1921) shows that only nine persons of Vincentian birth were found in the whole of the island.

The next major movement of the Caribs in St. Vincent was the gradual return to the North Windward of the scattered refugee communities of the south of the island. This return is reflected in the St. Vincent Land and House Tax Rolls. These list only the better off Caribs and are not entirely satisfactory in locating the Caribs of the tax-free North Leeward grant. As there may be multiple holdings by some Caribs, the following figures are for the number of taxable lands and houses held by Caribs and not for the number of Caribs taxed. The rolls were sampled at 10-year intervals, commencing in 1910 (St. Vincent, 1910, 1920, 1930). At that date there were 109 taxable lands and houses in Charlotte Parish, of which 35 were in the Owia district, 19 at Sandy Bay, 10 at Greiggs, and six at Victoria. In St. David's, which, as pointed out, was under-represented in this sample, there were 73, of which 45 were at Rose Bank and 21 at Rose Hall. In the chief location of Carib refugees, St. Andrew's Parish, there were 102, of which 44 were at Camden Park, 28 at Questelles, seven at Clare Valley, and five at Lowmans. In the other major refugee area, St. George's Parish, there were 49, of which eight were at Richmond Hill and seven at Meeks. In St. Patrick's Parish there were 33, of which 12 were at Grove, 11 at Happy Hill, and six at Spring. Surprisingly, there were only eight in the Grenadines, six of which were on Bequia.

The situation, as given for 1910, was soon changed as the result of the Caribs of the Clare Valley–Questelles area expressing their desire to return to the Carib Country. Thus in 1911 a small estate at Sandy Bay was purchased by the government and divided into 50 rural and 60 urban lots, and Caribs in the St. Andrew's area were allowed to exchange their lands there for these new lands. Others purchased these new sites (PP 1912–1913 LVIII).

In 1912 Fewks, another anthropologist, briefly visited the Caribs in the south of the island and reported that "the mixed-blood survivors of the St. Vincent Caribs who once lived at Morne Ronde, near the Soufriere, but who are now settled at Camden ... still retain some of their old customs."* While some of the Morne Ronde Caribs were at Camden Park, most were in fact at Rose Bank, which Fewks did not visit.

* While the quote is from the 34th Annual Report of the Bureau of American Ethnology 1912–1913, most of the information about Fewks' visit to St. Vincent is to be obtained from his diaries in the National Anthropological Archives, the Smithsonian Institution.

There was little permanent depletion of the Caribs in World War I, as only three or four of them died in combat, although many of them saw service in France or in Palestine. The position of the Caribs in 1920 is shown by the taxable land and houses possessed by them (St. Vincent, 1920). In Charlotte there were 105 holdings, 56 of which were at Sandy Bay with its new township, nine at Greiggs, seven at Owia, and five each at Victoria and Grants. In St. David's there were 53, 33 of which were at Rose Bank and 15 at Rose Hall. The depletion of numbers in St. David's probably indicates the returning use of their tax-free grant lands near Morne Ronde. The refugee area was similarly depleted. There were 53 in St. Andrew's, with 21 at Camden Park, 12 at Questelles, and five at Clare Valley; and in St. George's there were 36, 11 of which were at Richmond Hill. In St. Patrick's there were only 14, with seven at Grove. The Grenadines had increased to their more likely level of 29, 25 of which were on Bequia. Similar movements continued during the next decade, and in 1930 (St. Vincent, 1930) there were 130 in Charlotte Parish; 55 were at Sandy Bay, 21 at Greiggs, 10 at Owia, six at Victoria, and five at Grants. In St. David's, with its accustomed underrepresentation, there were 47, 27 of which were at Rose Bank and 13 at Rose Hall. The south was yet more depleted, with 41 in St. Andrew's; 17 were at Camden Park, nine at Questelles, and five at Lowmans; there were 36 in St. Goerge's, with 12 at Richmond Hill and 12 in St. Patrick's. The Grenadines had 32, 26 of which were on Bequia.

3.5. Census of 1931

The census of 1931 (St. Vincent, 1931) was the first for over 40 years in which the rate of the population was included. The only headings used were "Negro," "Coloured," "White" or "European," and "Others." The last presumably included a few Syrians (only seven in 1945), East Indians, and Caribs. Persons born of East Indian parents and persons born in India were also enumerated. The island had 623 males and 616 females described as "Others," 301 males and 327 females born in St. Vincent of East Indian parents, and 12 males and 13 females born in India, which would mean that the Carib and perhaps Syrian population would have been 586 in all, made up of 310 men and 276 women. If, however, the same calculations are done by districts, the Indians more than account for the "Others," and if these areas are assumed to have contained no Caribs, then there were 637 (339 males and 297 females) Caribs and Syrians on the island. These were mainly in Areas E (Escape Pastures and above Greiggs to Windsor Forest), with 309 males and 285 females (total 594); B (Byahaut Ridge to Warrawarro River with the exception of Kingstown), with 22 males and 12 females (total 34); and A (Kingstown), with eight males only. Other Caribs probably came under the headings "Negro" and "Coloured" if this census resembled later ones. Thus the total number of Caribs at this date is questionable [see Gullick (1974) and Kuczynski (1953) for more details].

At about the same time as this census, some new house lots for Caribs were prepared at Dark View. This hamlet seems to have been counted as part of Rose Bank for official purposes, and thus this move is not revealed in the most recent and accessible house and land tax roll (St. Vincent, 1937). Furthermore, this one is not strictly comparable with previous lists, as water rates are also included. It, however, did show the distribution of Caribs in the island more accurately than did the immediately preceding census. Thus in 1937 there were 170 Carib holdings in Charlotte Parish, 51 of which were at Sandy Bay, 36 at Owia, 26 at Greiggs, 16 at Victoria, seven at South Rivers, six at Grants, and five at New Adelphi. There were 66 in St. David's, with 53 at Rose Bank and 10 at Rose Hall, but, as ever, these figures underrepresent their presence in that area. In the south of St. Vincent there were 42 at St. Andrew's, with 16 at Camden Park, nine at Questelles, and six at Lowmans; 60 in St. George's, with 15 at Richmond Hill, six at Stubbs, and five at Gomea; and 14 in St. Patrick's with five at Spring. The Grenadines had 34, 30 of which were in Bequia.

4. Current Population Estimates

There were few Carib population movements during World War II despite the purchase by the government of 24.5 acres at Delves Level to act as an overspill for the neighboring village of Sandy Bay, which had become over-crowded. There was no census in 1941 as would have been expected. The most important Carib migrations of this period were those of individuals to the oil works of Aruba and Trinidad. The Caribs tended to prefer the latter. Many of the better off modern Caribs earned much of their money there during this boom period. The postwar years produced a wave of self-generated resettlement schemes for the Caribs. Gullick (1975) has analyzed their effect on Carib ethnicity elsewhere, and thus all that need be pointed out here is that such moves seem to have strengthened family ties, which in turn reinforced "Caribness." It resulted in many persons who previously had claimed to be Afro-Americans claiming to be Caribs, and thus resulted in a great increase in the Carib population. The resettlement schemes [described in detail in Gullick (1974, 1975)] involved the removal of Sandy Bay to New Sandy Bay with the eventual inflow of persons from Owia to a later extension to this new village. Similarly, the Rose Bank Caribs were moved to a new village at Petit Bordel, which was just north of their old village, making it slightly easier for them to commute to their lands at Morne Ronde. Greiggs only received some assistance with repairing homes. The situation before these moves is shown by the 1945 census (St. Vincent, 1945). According to this there were 242 Caribs on the island, the major concentrations being in the regions of Chateaubelair (including Rose Bank) with 117, Sandy Bay (including Owia) with 77, Layou with 16, Barrouallie with nine, and Calliaqua with five. There were lesser numbers in other areas. It is noteworthy that the region including Greiggs did not number among the more Carib areas. This makes me highly suspicious of this census and its definition of Carib. Likewise, the number of Caribs in the Grenadines was low. The situation of the Caribs in the midst of these moves is indicated by the 1960 census (St. Vincent, 1960) despite its undercounting of Caribs. It was after the initial Sandy Bay moves and before the one to Petit Bordel. According to this census there were 1265 Caribs on the island, 518 of whom were at New Sandy Bay, 368 at Rose Bank (including Dark View), 70 at Owia (including Old Sandy Bay), 59 at Fancy, 42 at Greiggs, 30 at both Wallibou and Windsor Forest, 10 at Camden Park, nine in the Petit Bordel–Sharps area, and four on Bequia. I did my fieldwork after the relocation was completed, and although a census was taken in 1970, I prefer my own estimates of Carib populations at that time. In these I used the aforementioned criteria of being accepted as a Carib in Sandy Bay, Petit Bordel, Rose Bank, Greiggs, or Owia. My figures are thus far greater than those of official statistics. I estimate that there are 5000 such Caribs on St. Vincent, and that the major concentrations are at New Sandy Bay (880), Owia (340), Rose Bank (260), Petit Bordel (260), Greiggs (210), Fancy (180), Dark View (80), and Windsor Forest (25). The slightly less accurate estimates of other major Carib groupings include South Side, Bequia (460), Camden Park (180), Chateaubelair (140), Clare Valley (80), Questelles (60), Lowmans, Leeward (60), Chauncey (40), and, least certain of all, Gomea (40). These figures are based on fieldwork observations and on projections based on the known age structure of the Caribs combined with the analysis of electoral lists in St. Vincent (St. Vincent, 1970–1973). These figures show how many Caribs seem to have remained at their refuges in the south of St. Vincent and not returned to the north with the other Caribs. They also show a minor growth point at Gomea, which I have been unable to explain, though I realize that Caribs have been there since the middle of the 19th century.

5. Conclusion

The size of these population estimates in comparison with earlier official statistics makes me suspicious of the official statistics. Thus I must admit that I feel that Luke's (1950) estimates of the 900 Caribs in the North Leeward and 1000 in the North Windward to be nearer the truth than the 1945 census. I fear he did not attempt to estimate the Greiggs, South Leeward, and Bequia Carib populations. However, as already pointed out, the Carib grouping is dependent on contemporary classifications, and I suspect that even if there were no descendants of the Caribs on the island, groups would claim to be so, as has happened in both St. Lucia and Trinidad. I thus look forward to the results of genetic analyses by physical anthropologists of the various Carib and possibly Carib populations. This has been started by the Department of Anthropology at

Durham University, where Vincentian palm and finger prints are being analyzed to compare and contrast with its extensive collection of Central American Carib prints. The next stages are obviously to study both the major Carib communities in St. Vincent and the areas where they settled as refugees and compare and contrast these with other Carib populations and other Afro-American ones both in St. Vincent and elsewhere. The population of Bequia poses another topic for study. These analyses should be made more meaningful by the research work being done on Central American Carib genetics, and I look forward to seeing if current research confirms my views as to the relative sizes of populations and the extent of interethnic mariages among the Caribs in St. Vincent.

ACKNOWLEDGMENTS

This paper is based on fieldwork in St. Vincent in 1970, 1971, 1974, and 1976. Some of the ethnohistorical research was done with the aid of a Smithsonian STV Fellowship, for which I extend many thanks. References to Crown Copyright records appear by permission of the controller of Her Majesty's Stationary Office and to those in the Vincentian Government Archives by permission of the Secretary to the Cabinet.

References

Anderson, T., and Flett, J. S., 1903, Report on the eruptions of the Soufriere, in St. Vincent in 1902, *Philos. Trans. R. Soc.* **200**(1).

Annual Report of the Bureau of American Ethnology, 1912–1913, No. 34, pp. 10–11.

Attourney General, St. Vincent, 1882, Mrs. Thompson's case, unnumbered ms. in the St. Vincent Government Archives.

Bayley, F. W. N., 1830, *Four years' Residence in the West Indies from 1826*, 2nd ed., William Kidd, London.

Bullen, R. P., and Bullen, A., 1972, *Archaeological Investigations on St. Vincent and the Grenadines, West Indies*, The William L. Bryant Foundation, American Studies Report no. 8.

Chester, G. J., 1869, *Transatlantic Sketches in the West Indies, South America, Canada and the United States*, Smith, Elder and Co., London.

Colonial Office files 260/13–19 as per catalogue number, the Public Record Office, London.

Davy, J., 1854, *The West Indies before and since Emancipation.* F. G. Cash, London.

Dominica, 1921, Census.

Fewks, J., 1913, Diary, Ms. 4408, The National Anthropological Archives, The Smithsonian Institution, Washington, D.C.

Gullick, C. J. M. R., 1969, The changing society of the Black Caribs, B. Litt. thesis, Oxford University.

Gullick, C. J. M. R., 1974, Tradition and change amongst the Caribs of St. Vincent, Ph.D. thesis, Oxford University.

Gullick, C. J. M. R., 1975, Political policies and interethnic relations in St. Vincent and Malta, paper at the Society for Applied Anthropology, 34th annual meeting.

Gullick, C. J. M. R., 1976a, Exiled from St. Vincent: The development of Black Carib culture in Central America up to 1945. Progress Press, London.

Gullick, C. J. M. R., 1976*b*, The Black Caribs in St. Vincent: The Carib War and aftermath, in: *The Actes du Congres international des Americanistes* 6:451–465.

Gullick, C. J. M. R., 1976*c*, Carib ethnicity in a semi-plural society, *New Community* 5(3): 250–258.

Gullick, C. J. M. R., 1978*a*, The ecological background to the Carib Wars, *J. Belizean Affairs* 6:51–61.

Gullick, C. J. M. R., 1978*b*, Black Carib origins and early society, in: *The Proceedings of the 1977 International Congress for the Study of the Pre-Columbian Cultures of the Lesser Antilles*, pp. 283–290, Université de Montréal, Montreal.

H 87/267 St. Vincent Government Archives, as per catalogue.

Horsford, J., 1856, *A Voice from the West Indies*, A. Heylin, London.

Kirby, I. E., and Martin, C. I., 1972, The rise and fall of the Black Caribs of St. Vincent The Development Corporation, St. Vincent.

Kuczynski, R. P. (ed. Long, B.), 1953, *Demographic Survey of the British Colonial Empire*, Vol. 3, Royal Institute of International Affairs. Oxford University Press, London

List of Refugees, 1902, St. Vincent Government Archives.

Luke, H., 1950, *Caribbean Circuit*.

Musgrave, T. B. C., 1891, *Historical and Descriptive Sketch of the Colonies of St. Vincent in The West Indies*, The Jamaica Exhibition, Jamaica.

Ober, F., 1880, *Camps in the Caribbees*. Lee and Shephard, Boston.

Petition of Bequia Fishermen, 1888, St. Vincent Government Archives catalogue No. 262 a/88.

Parliamentary Papers, 1899–1913, reference numbers as in Parliamentary Catalogues.

Rouse, I., 1949, The Caribs, in *The Circum-Carribean Tribes*, Vol. 4, *Handbook of South American Indians* (J. H. Steward, ed.), Bureau of American Ethnology, Bulletin, 143, pp. 547–565, Smithsonian Institution, Washington, D.C.

Sapper, K., 1903, St. Vincent, Die Karaiben, *Globus* 84:379–383.

Shephard, C., 1831, An historical account of the island of St. Vincent, Ridgway and Sous, London.

St. Vincent, 1812, Census.

St. Vincent, 1844, Census.

St. Vincent, 1851, Census.

St. Vincent, 1861, Census.

St. Vincent, 1871, Census.

St. Vincent, 1910, Land and House Tax Roll.

St. Vincent, 1920, Land and House Tax Roll.

St. Vincent, 1930, Land and House Tax Roll.

St. Vincent, 1931, Census.

St. Vincent, 1937, Land, House and Water Rates Roll.

St. Vincent, 1945, Census.

St. Vincent, 1960, Census.

St. Vincent, 1970–1973, List of Electors.

WO 1/85 and 690 War Office Files as per catalogue number, the Public Record Office, London.

4

Garifuna (Black Carib) Social Organization

NANCIE L. GONZALEZ

1. Introduction

Migration is today a topic of major social anthropological interest, probably largely stimulated by the massive movement of peoples from the lesser to the more highly developed nations of the world. Interestingly, although the world has experienced such major population shifts before, they have usually been in the other direction, and anthropologists have long been among the chroniclers of colonial impact upon indigenous sociocultural systems everywhere. Still, relatively few studies have focused upon the effect of migration per se in shaping a system over time — perhaps because we have tended to choose geographical or political entities as our units of analysis. We can then document the impact of migration upon a *village*, for example, or even upon the nation-state as sender or receiver of migrants.

This perspective, valuable though it is for many purposes, misses the fact that some societies may actually be *products* of an ongoing migratory process that is best understood in historical and global terms. Sometimes, as with the Chinese, there may remain a major cultural and geographical center with which the migrants continue to identify for ethnic purposes. In others, ethnicity may be created or enhanced by the diaspora. The African peopling of the Caribbean and other parts of the New World spawned a range of new societal types, with cultural components derived from the various African heritages, mixed with elements from Europe and indigenous America. Herskovits pioneered in the study of these "reinterpretations," as he called them (1938).

NANCIE L. GONZALEZ • Department of Anthropology, University of Maryland, College Park, Maryland 20742.

However, it is increasingly clear that migrations in some important senses do not have definite beginnings or endings, and that the *expectation* of living in more than one location during one's lifetime may be an imporant part of one's cultural heritage in many societies. If so, the process is bound to have both social and biological implications for the individual, as well as for society. We will leave it to others to document the psychological and medical effects upon *people* – in this book we address ourselves to the sociocultural biological systems.

In the pages that follow, I shall try to demonstrate that Garifuna culture and society cannot be understood apart from the process of migration. Like many small Caribbean nations, the Garifuna have long been dependent upon cash brought or sent back by members of the society who have migrated elsewhere in search of work. The Garifuna, however, have been affected by migration for a much longer period of time than most, and were launched upon this way of life by an entirely different set of historical circumstances. For most of the smaller islands, emancipation created a situation in which there was simply not enough land for the freed slaves to carve out holdings upon which they could support themselves and their families. Therefore, the men began to move to other areas of the Caribbean as well as to North America and Europe in search of work. Within the area itself they found it on large plantations and on the docks, or, later, on the Panama Canal and in the oil refineries of Aruba and Curacao. Britain, Canada, and the U.S. have provided both seasonal and permanent employment opportunities, especially since 1940.

2. St. Vincent Background

The Garifuna, on the other hand, were never enslaved. Their forebears on St. Vincent engaged in horticulture, fishing, and small-time trading with nearby islands. Their Amerindian ancestors were noted navigators, quite familiar with both the heavens and the waters of the southern Caribbean, and also adept in the manufacture and use of canoes. As we shall see, this familiarity with and dependence upon the sea has been a continual theme from the earliest days up to the present in their cultural history.

Early descriptions of St. Vincent suggest that the Garifuna lived in scattered households throughout the interior of that island. Polygyny was clearly acceptable, but certainly not universal. Kinship terminology used until recently suggests that matrilateral cross-cousin marriage may have been a common feature, but we actually have very little evidence of the early details of their social organization. The language, today called Island Carib, is basically Arawakan, with large numbers of loan words from French, English, and Spanish. The fact that there are still traces of different linguistic forms to be used by men and women has been interpreted to mean that the Carib invaders took Arawakan women as wives in the earliest days, long before there was any African influx. It is noteworthy that the language shows no evidence of significant African influence. This is consistent with the view that their African ancestors joined the Indians sporadically and in small numbers over a fairly long period of time. At any given moment, the Indians must have dominated numerically, though succeeding generations became more and more African phenotypically as new blacks married in. As I suggested earlier (Gonzalez, 1959b), it is likely that the so-called Black Caribs have not always been as uniformly "black" as they appear today. We are able to document a certain amount of admixture with blacks from Haiti, other parts of the West Indies, and the U.S. over the past century.

New information acquired during a search of the British and Central American (Guatemalan) archival materials in 1982–1983 has finally solved some of the problems and mysteries associated with the final days in, and departure from, St. Vincent. After their final defeat in July, 1796, most of the Garifuna surrendered in small groups and were detained on the island of Baliseau until March, 1797, when they were transported to the island of Roatan off the coast of Honduras. A total of about 4200 surrendered, but between October and March they were devastated by an epidemic – perhaps typhus – and only 2026 actually arrived. Some were still ill, so it is likely that even more succumbed before they were transferred to Trujillo by mutual agreement with the Spanish authorities (May).

At that time, a company of about 300 so-called "French" blacks lived in Trujillo, and served the Spanish as mercenary soldiers. These were ex-slaves who were fugitives not only from Haiti, but from other French islands in the Caribbean. Although intermarriage between this group and the Garifuna has not been documented, it seems almost certain that it occurred, as it probably did to some extent with the Miskito Indians (also a hybrid Indian/African group living on the Mosquito Shore).

As Kerns suggests (this volume, Chapter 6) there has probably been more admixture with various other groups than the Garifuna have traditionally admitted. Although most of the surnames today are Spanish, presumably adopted during the earliest years in Honduras, many can be traced to specific non-Garifuna individuals, usually European or American white males who lived in Central America during the late nineteenth or early twentieth century.

A list of slaves from the nearby fort at Omoa in 1776 includes names which seem suspiciously similar to some found today in Livingston, and still other names are identical to those of certain Creole families in Belize. At the time of arrival in Roatan all their names were French, and in many cases no surnames were given at all. This may account for the fact that today many of their surnames are those ordinarily used as Christian names by modern Spanish- and English-speaking peoples.

3. Garifuna Social Organization, Central America

Since 1797, when the Garifuna were brought to Central America, the settlement pattern has been exclusively coastal (Davidson, 1974). Typically, houses are clustered along the shore, with the slash-and-burn gardens conveniently located in the bush from 1 to 5 miles inland. Women have long been primarily responsible for these gardens, with seasonal help from the men, who spent more of their time fishing and traveling to seek part-time wage-paying jobs. The more the men stayed away, the more the women left behind took over domestic decision-making, maintenance of the religious culture, and general responsibility for the care and socialization of the children. Elsewhere, one can find fuller ethnographic details on the kinship system (Gonzalez, 1960), the nonunilineal descent group (Gonzalez, 1959a), customs relating to childbearing and child-raising (Cosminsky, 1976; Kerns, 1977; Gonzalez, 1979b; Munroe, 1964; Sanford, 1971), family and household organization (Gonzalez, 1969, 1970), and changes occurring in all of these as a result of increasing urbanization (Gonzalez, 1965, 1979a). In addition, Kerns (1983) has recently completed a study of the role of older women, which has advanced both our knowledge of the Garifuna and our understanding of the social meaning of aging. Here, therefore, I will simply describe the various concrete social structures as they existed in 1979, showing how they serve the needs of this migratory people, as well as how they articulate with each other and with those of the larger societies with which the Garifuna are inextricably enmeshed.

Among the Garifuna, as is also true in most other parts of the Caribbean, it is necessary to distinguish conceptually between the family and the household. The former includes all persons related by blood or marriage ties as traced through both parents and as far back as memory serves. The skew toward matrifocality is reinforced by the fact that children have more contact with their maternal relatives, and with women more than with men. Thus, the family-related memories of the women tend to be more vivid, and the genealogical relationships on that side more exactly recalled. Although family ties are generally considered important, and kin are expected to be of assistance to each other, in fact, bitter feuds often lead to broken ties and the loss of genealogical knowledge. As I have shown elsewhere (Gonzalez, 1959a), certain religious rituals may function to reinforce some ties at the expense of others, depending upon how individuals choose to align themselves at different times of their lives.

The household, on the other hand, although it contains a core of kin, also frequently contains persons who are unrelated, or whose relationship is only very distantly remembered. Surveys done in 1956 and again in 1975 showed that approximately 45% of the households in the town of Livingston, Guatemala, contained no marital pair. Rather, they included a core of consanguineally related women and children, assisted by brothers, uncles, and adult sons of those women. Although many of the husbands/fathers of these women and children were temporarily absent in search of work, others had apparently abandoned the households, and the women were dependent upon their own labor and contributions from family members either in Livingston or elsewhere.

3.1. Households in Livingston, 1956

So that the reader may better understand the extreme flexibility of Central American Garifuna domestic groups and how they allow for change over time, I will describe the household in which I lived as it was in 1956, and as I found it when I returned in 1975. The central woman, Victoria, was legally married to Joseph, who had been born in Dangriga (then Stann Creek), Belize. Although he had long before moved "permanently" to Livingston, he actually resided in another neighborhood (barrio; see Section 3.4), where he ran a small tavern. The house itself was owned by Victoria, and was built upon land she had inherited, along with several siblings, from her mother. In 1956 each of the siblings inhabited a house in what I have referred to as "the compound," and lived there with some of his or her children and grandchildren. Only one of these siblings had a coresident spouse, although the eldest male had a wife who lived elsewhere in town.

In Victoria's household there also lived her four adult children, including a pair of 18-year-old male twins (Patrick and Ernest), a 30-year-old legally married but childless eldest daughter (Ruth), and a 26-year-old daughter (Sally), who at that time had already borne three sons, each by a different father, none of whom had ever actually resided with her. Ruth's husband lived and worked in another town, and when he visited Livingston he spent his time partly in this household and partly in that of another woman with whom he had several children, whom Ruth referred to as his "outside" children.

Ernest was involved in a liaison with a young woman from another neighborbood who bore him a child during my stay, but who continued to live with her own mother. Patrick, although he had had a number of temporary sexual experiences, had not yet contracted anything the townspeople might have seen as a "real" marital relationship.

Upon my return in 1975, Ruth had died, and her husband was no longer thought of as in any way related to this household, perhaps because his wife had never borne any children. The second daughter, Sally, had moved out of her mother's house into that of one of Victoria's siblings who had also died in the interim. Her new residence was only about 500 feet from that of her mother, and there was constant coming and going between the two units. Sally now had what appeared to be a stable relationship with the man who had fathered the last four of her now eight living children. Although they coresided, there was no legal marriage tie.

With Victoria, now an enfeebled woman in her late 70s, there was Tamara, the daughter of Ernest, who by this time had emigrated to New York, where he was living with a woman other than Tamara's mother. Tamara, only 16, had already borne two children, both of whom lived with her although their father still resided with his own mother in another neighborhood. Although he occasionally slept with Tamara in Victoria's house, and quite frequently ate dinner there, he kept most of his belongings and ate most of his meals at his mother's house.

There also resided in Victoria's house in 1975 Tamara's uncle, Patrick, now in his late 30s. He had never actually set up housekeeping with any woman, and he recognized only one son, a teenager who lived in Los Angeles with his mother. In 1975 Patrick was involved with a much younger woman, who, although having borne him two children, still lived with her own mother in another barrio. Patrick was now the primary supporter of Victoria's household. He had a thriving tailor shop, where he made shirts and trousers for men and slacks for women. In addition, he worked at various odd jobs about town whenever he could. His eldest sister, Ruth, had been the major "administrator" within the household, but he had become the apparent "head" after her death in 1956. However, it was clear that Victoria herself was the ultimate authority regardless of whether Ruth or Patrick was the dominant figure.

Victoria's household could not have functioned in 1975 without the assistance of several of her grandchildren, sons and daughters of Sally and Ernest. In addition to Tamara, who cooked, the smaller children took turns helping to clean the house, take food to Victoria, and run errands. They also usually slept there at night. Although largely confined to her chair, Victoria sat most of each day in the primary living room of her house, from which vantage point she could observe and comment upon daily domestic and community events. She helped "mind" the younger children, who generally responded dutifully to her commands.

During the course of my second stay in 1975, Tamara, together with her two children, moved out to take up residence with the mother of her children's father.* The small bedroom occupied by Tamara was now turned over to a female cousin of Victoria's deceased husband, visiting from Belize. In addition, a youth also related to Victoria through her husband slept in her kitchen upon occasion, making a bed on top of a pile of cement blocks that were stored there by Ernest, who hoped one day to return from New York and build his own house in the family compound. By 1975, Victoria's two elder brothers, as well as the sister formerly mentioned, were deceased. The house of one of them had been removed from its site by his widow, who set it up again on her own family land in another neighborhood. The widow of the second brother emigrated to New York City with her children, where she later remarried and still resides. It

---

* Patrick had also moved out to make room for me, the ethnographer. He was able to rent a house down the street for considerably less than what I was paying the family for my quarters. He was also able to run back and forth several times daily and still manage the household affairs very nicely.

was Ernest's intention to build on the site vacated by the removal of his uncle's house. The other house had been rented to a nonrelative, the cash money going to help support Victoria and the household in general.

In January 1978, when my research assistant visited Livingston again, Victoria had passed away, and the main house was now occupied by Sally, her six youngest children (including one who had been born since 1975), and the man who by this time seemed to have become her permanent partner. In addition, Tamara and her two children had also moved back in, her union having apparently been terminated, at least for the time being. Patrick had moved back into the small adjoining house, which had previously been occupied by this ethnographer. He remained the senior authority, although Sally and her partner were also important administrators.

3.2. Consanguineal Households

Thus, it becomes clear that households and families among the Garifuna are both fluid and extended. Relatives freely come and go, and space within the various households is repeatedly rearranged and refurbished in order to accommodate needs as these shift through time. There seems always the possibility of squeezing in one or two more, and children especially are freely moved about, sleeping in first one house and then another. Adults seem most closely tied to their natal units, and although some couples achieve fairly long-lasting unions, even these may drift apart in later life, each person returning to his or her own kin.

The strongest and most enduring social unit, then, is the sibling group with a mother in common. Children may go back and forth between the maternal relatives of their mother and those of their father, but most, in the long run, seem to be more closely attached to their mother's relatives, with some exceptions, of course. Exceptions tend to occur in those cases where the mother's relatives have an extraordinarily large group to care for, or where the mother has gone off to New York City or elsewhere and not returned for a long period of time. The latter was the case for Tamara and her half-siblings, also children of Ernest. Their mothers and their maternal grandmothers were all in New York. I have dubbed households like this "consanguineal." They consist of a core of consanguineally related adults plus children and are accompanied by a mating system often referred to as "serial polygyny." Little emphasis is placed on formal or legal marriage ties, and even when marriages do take place, husbands and wives often reside separately, as the above example makes clear. Furthermore, when viewed over time, a given household changes not only in response to births and deaths, but also in relation to the migratory behavior of the core group, their mates, and their kin.

In 1956 I postulated that this type of household and mating system could be interpreted as a response to certain economic and demograhic conditions. In

Table 1. Sex Ratios by Decade of Life among Caribs in Livingston, Guatemala, 1956

	Males			Females			Excess of females over males	Sex ratio
Age	Present	Absent	Total	Present	Absent	Total		
0–1	39	2	41	55	0	55	14	0.7454
2–10	174	8	182	171	10	181	−1	1.0055
11–20	109	30	139	188	21	209	70	0.6651
21–30	72	36	108	115	23	138	30	0.7826
31–40	72	21	93	113	21	134	41	0.6940
41–50	59	18	77	102	9	111	34	0.6937
51–60	49	24	73	77	5	82	9	0.8902
61–70	27	3	30	55	0	55	25	0.5455
>70	19	0	19	35	0	35	16	0.5426
Total	620	142	762	911	89	1000	238	–

particular, I focused on the fact that the Garifuna were by that time dependent on cash wages as a supplement to gardening, fishing, and petty trade. Since wage-paying jobs for men were very scarce in the village and the immediate vicinity, they increasingly went farther afield to find work. As can be seen in Table 1, the migration of males created a distinct imbalance in the sex ratio. I reasoned then that women, left behind when the men traveled, were by default left in charge of the domestic domain. The consanguineal household seemed to provide a kind of stability that allowed the society to survive longer than it otherwise might have in the face of increasing modernization brought about by the introduction of new goods and values from the outside. The Garifuna culture, including the language, religious ceremonies, the value system, and the like, was successfully promulgated by this institution. Children living in consanguineal households did come into contact with men, but these were more often their older brothers, uncles, and temporary partners of their mothers than their own fathers. Thus, the loss of any single "father figure" did not seem to be so serious as it would in a system where the nuclear family household was the ideal. In addition, the fact that all these different men had some responsibility for providing economic resources to the household decreased the chance that the unit would be seriously impaired if any one of them lost his job or failed to return.

3.3. Household Changes in 1975

In 1975 when I returned to Livingston after a 13-year absence, I was eager to learn whether the frequency of consanguineal households had remained the same. I reasoned that if this type of domestic unit and its associative mating patterns was adaptive, it should either remain the same or increase. Table 2 compares the frequency of different types of households in 1956 and in 1975.

Table 2. Frequency of Various Household Forms in Livingston, Guatemala, 1956 and 1975

| | 1956 | | 1975 | |
	Number	Percentage of total	Number	Percentage of total
Consanguineal households				
One woman plus children	84	23.20	23	18
Two or more women and children	40	11.05	17	13
One or more women and children and consanguineally related male	40	11.05	16	13
Subtotal	164	45.03	56	44
Single-person households	0		6	5
Affinal households				
One couple and children	104	28.73	36	29
One couple, no children	49	13.54	12	10
One couple plus children of the woman only	27	7.46	8	6
One couple plus children belonging to neither	18	4.97	8	6
Subtotal	198	54.70	64	51
Total	362	100.00	126	100

It seems clear that no major change has occurred, and I would thus conclude that it is an adaptive pattern.

However, my 1975 survey did present some surprises. The data on migration showed that now many women as well as men leave the village to work, and that New York is an ever more popular destination (see Table 3). Furthermore, reproductive histories suggest that although serial polygyny has long been an acceptable pattern, its frequency may also be increasing. Thus, it appears that the younger women may be undergoing more changes in marital patterns than did their mothers and grandmothers at their age (see Table 4).*

---

* Preliminary evidence suggests that in New York City more of these early liaisons are sanctioned by law. If this is the case, and if the marriages fail, a high divorce rate might be predicted. Since divorce and all of its concomitant problems is likely to be more psychologically traumatic for both partners than mere separation of "partners," this probably has some implications for Garifuna mental health. I am not aware that this subject has been studied systematically yet.

Table 3. Sex and Location of Relatives Reported as Living Outside Livingston at Time of Survey of 126 Households, 1975

	Guatemala City	Other Guatemala	New York	Other North America	Belize	Total
Females	6	17	31	1[a]	11	66
Males	13	46	25	1[b]	15	100
Total	19	63	56	2	26	166

[a] Canada.
[b] Los Angeles.

Table 4. Percentage of Women Having Had Two or More Mates, by Age Cohort, in Livingston, 1975

Age cohort	Teens	20s	30s	40s	50s	60s	70s
Percentage	50	49	62.5	48	50	25	39
Number	4	18	16	25	16	20	18

3.4. The Neighborhood

After the family and household, the next most important social unit is the neighborhood. As alluded to several times, a large village or town is further divided into sections comprising loosely organized groups of households. In some cases these various parts of the village are formally recognized, as in Livingston, where there are some 15 different named *barrios*, or neighborhoods. In the case of smaller villages, the entire population may behave as a single neighborhood. Although there are no formal "self-help" neighborhood associations, often sports and religious clubs bear the names of the *barrios*. Generally speaking, groups of households in neighborhoods tend to be mutually supportive in times of crises, and the designation "neighbor" suggests fairly strong affective bonds. Neighbors are second only to kin, and in cases where one is feuding with some kin, neighbors may even receive hospitality first. The strength of these bonds carries over during the migratory process, so that in New York City, for example, two people from the same neighborhood may be seen as "almost kin" *vis-à-vis* other Garifuna.

In both Central America and in New York there are various voluntary associations to which both men and women may belong. Some carry the names of neighborhoods, villages, or towns in Central America, even when their membership is more broadly based. Sometimes a "storefront" locale is rented and operated by a few entrepreneurs, as a private club. Interestingly, although these *are* businesses in many ways, they actually *do* serve to attract people from the same part of the "homeland" and provide a measure of psychological well-being for Garifuna in an otherwise strange and hostile world. Private homes may also serve on weekends as centers where friends may gather to eat, drink, dance, and converse. The hostess charges for food and liquor, but payment is unobtrusive and the atmosphere of the gathering is more social than commercial. Other associations derive from and promote religious activity, and these include both those sodalities associated with the Catholic Church and other groupings having to do with the traditional Garifuna religious and philosopical beliefs, including a strong element of respect for (if not worship of) the ancestors. In Livingston, the church sodalities are themselves partly organized along neighborhood lines, and they tend to include a strong component of mutual aid among the members, as well as support of the church. In New York City membership in these religious sodalities seems to have declined, probably because they are largely organized by the churches themselves, with which the Garifuna do not yet feel closely aligned.* It is primarily women, children, and the oldest men who participate in these activities, both in Central America and in New York. The men's involvement is minimal, however, even among the elderly.

Sports, especially soccer and basketball, are of great interest in both Central America and in New York, and many clubs are formed to promote these activities. Not only do the clubs sponsor teams, buying their jerseys and some other equipment, but they arrange games with other teams both at home and elsewhere, and sponsor trips for players and spectators. In New York groups of friends meet on Sundays in public parks to play against other teams, both Garifuna and non-Garifuna. Women also attend and set up tables nearby where they sell homecooked Caribbean foods, not necessarily of Garifuna tradition. Sometimes dances and other social events will also be arranged, largely to earn money for equipment and team transportation costs.

Finally, there are what can best be described as ethnic-related associations. In Central America there has been celebrated for a very long time, on November 19, the supposed arrival of the first Garifuna in Belize. This has come to be known as Settlement Day and it has now been made an official Belizean holiday. Garifuna from all over Central America, as well as those who now live in U.S. and elsewhere, try to return home to celebrate, and if they are unable to do that they have some kind of commemoration wherever they may be. The day has come to be a major holiday in both New York and in Los Angeles, for example. Although they are called a "committee," the group of people who arrange the

---

* I have a suspicion that in New York there is greater interest in Protestantism than there is in Central America, where probably 90% or more of the Garifuna are Roman Catholics. This subject has not been well explored, but given the nature of the larger world in which they now find themselves, such a shift would not be surprising. If it does turn out to be true, we might wonder what the effect will be upon the ancestral rites still so important in Central America. The tolerant attitudes of the Catholic Church toward such ancillary practices may well have been a factor in its retaining so many Garifuna "souls." On the other hand, the New York environment does not seem the most ideal in which to maintain the ceremonies either. More attention needs to be paid to this matter.

festivities in effect form a kind of voluntary association. The preparations go on for most of the year, and involve planning of dances, preparation of costumes, election of a queen, and in some cases the sponsoring of excursions, including arrangements for feeding and housing visitors.

In Dangriga, Belize, the largest Garifuna settlement in that country, there is also an association of older women who are the self-appointed protectors of the old ways. They object to some of the newer choreographic experimentation of the young people who dominate the Settlement Day committee, and meet regularly throughout the year to practice dancing as they believe their ancestors did. They also take part in the official Settlement Day activities.

Another type of association is that represented by the Carib Development Society, which informants say has been in existence in Dangriga for as long as anyone can remember. It is basically a mutual aid society, the members of which pay 25 cents per week for burial insurance. In addition, in recent years members of this group have lobbied in Belize to achieve better conditions for their ethnic group within the government. They have also promoted remedial education for those Garifuna who are unable to read and write, and have helped others of their ethnic group to acquire land.

In New York City there have appeared over the last few years several groups whose expressed purpose is to help the home communities in Central America. Although in some cases it was difficult to ascertain what, if any, benefits had accrued to those left at home, it was said that the Dangriga Development Association, for example, had sent money to help the survivors of hurricanes, and to sponsor students, in addition to sponsoring excursions for New Yorkers to return home for Settlement Day. Money is raised in New York not only through requests for direct donations, but by holding dances to which the entire Garifuna community is invited.*

In Central America itself it is interesting to note that there seem not to be any community-oriented development associations, unless we include the Settlement Day groups themselves. Thus, one does not find organizations working together to improve such things as water supply, sanitation, and so forth, though there have been some recent efforts in Honduras by Garifuna to persuade the government, through AID, to do some of these things for the coastal villages.†

---

* In December 1978, I attended one of these dances, which was ostensibly given to raise money for the people in the *barrio* in which I had lived in Livingston. I discovered later that in this particular case the persons in charge of the affair absconded with all of the funds, a fact some Garifuna found very distressing, but that others claimed was only "natural." The affair was held in a fairly posh private club with a live band and a bar run by members of the sponsoring group. Matchbooks bearing the name of the development association were distributed gratis throughout the evening. It is possible that the expenses merely came to more than the income, and that the organizers did not make off with any funds after all. However, it was impossible to discover the truth of the matter. What does seem certain is that the home community derived no benefit from the event.

† Personal communication from Dr. Carolyn McCommon and Dr. Fernando Cruz, both of whom have observed and consulted with Garifuna and US Aid personnel.

In Belize, in contrast to Guatemala and Honduras, there has been considerable politicization of the people, but such consciousness of national politics and its potential for achieving power is still relatively weak among the Garifuna in general, even though the leader of the opposition party in Belize has for some time been a Garifuna. It could be argued that their survival over the past two centuries has in part depended on their ability to insulate themselves from the outside world when necessary.

4. Discussion

As I suggested at the outset, it is my contention that the migratory process has been largely responsible for shaping the Garifuna social organization for some time. Not only has it had a profound effect upon household and family structure, but we can also see its effects in religious, cultural, and political matters as well. Throughout the society today, women are more involved than is often the case elsewhere. Although the fiction persists that men are dominant and the primary decision-makers, the ethnographic reality is that women are strong, outspoken, knowledgeable, and effective. Kerns (1983) has shown that it is generally after they reach the age of 50 or so, their childbearing years behind them, that women move into the special status category of "elder" in which they can exert tremendous influence. In Belize, there is even a Garifuna woman who has been elected to the national legislature. In all of the towns and villages when one asks for the most prominent and influential people, women's names will be advanced.

Such women, as grandmothers, form an impressive repository of information concerning all kinds of issues. At the present time, as migration of young women to New York and elsewhere has increased, we are seeing further elaboration of a long-standing pattern in which elder women form the stable core around which the rest of the society revolves. It is also true that older men occupy a respected place in the society as a whole. However, it is ironic that those very men who have been most successful on the outside, having earned money to help support many children and women in various families, are precisely those who, in old age, are likely not be familiar with the affairs of the home community. Since they have spent so much of their time away, they are out of touch and if they go home to retire, they are likely not to be heavily involved in the more intimate and internal Garifuna cultural matters. At the same time, their experience on the outside has probably not prepared them adequately to lead their people *vis-à-vis* the large society either, since they tend to cluster together and apart from others in their new world.

Increased residence in New York by women creates two situations that may have an impact on the preservation of the traditional culture, however. First, since young women will have less opportunity to observe and to learn the dances, songs, food preparations, and other activities, there may be a gradual erosion of the content of this folk culture. In both Dangriga and Los Angeles contestants for Queen of Settlement Day must demonstrate their abilities along these lines – and often fail miserably. However, this group tends to be in their teens, and in the recent past they might have learned as they approached their mature years while living in their mothers' houses. Second, even if they do learn what they must know to carry on tradition, they may move to New York or Los Angeles after their children are grown, thus taking their expertise with them. It seems doubtful they can continue such activities in any meaningful way under the radically different circumstances in the U.S. Isolated events among fragmented communities cannot maintain cultural systems.

4.1. The Future

The hope of the future, I believe, is the young intellectual who leaves the home community to further his or her education and then returns in early maturity, having developed a perspective that combines ethnic pride with a real understanding of the problems facing both the Central American republics *and* the world economy so important to the U.S. as well. In Belize and in Honduras one can already sense a ferment attributable in large part, I believe, to this new breed of migrant. In the years to come I suspect that Garifuna society will persist, its general outlines conforming fairly well to those just described. A few reservations are, however, in order.

Many of the traditions will be increasingly preserved and transmitted in writing and in photographs, rather than purely by mouth and precept. As such, they will tend to become symbols of ethnic pride rather than the basis of the culture itself. As the expatriate component increases, such symbols will be ever more important in preserving the identity of the group. Intermarriage with Americans, especially with black Americans and expatriates from the West Indies and the Caribbean, will occur, and some Garifuna will undoubtedly pass into these other populations and be lost. But at the same time, there will be others who remain with the Garifuna themselves, thus continuing to alter the frequencies of various genes in the Garifuna gene pool.

Since the household and mating patterns of the Garifuna are quite similar to those found in many other segments of the black American population (Stack, 1974), I would expect relatively little change there, with the exceptions that I have noted. The various voluntary associations, again, are not too different from what we find among other immigrants to the U.S. Here again, the societies will probably continue to flourish, and thus help preserve the ethnic identity of the group in this country.

The future is not so clear for the Central American's situation. I believe the present migratory process will have continuing impact there, however. Not only will it continue to provide basic resources for the home villages, but it will provide feedback of another sort as well. The group will increasingly make its "minority voice" felt in the three home countries, in my opinion. The very concept of a minority group, in its sociopolitical sense, is one of the most powerful tools the Garifuna are acquiring. It will be satisfying, for those of us who have known and observed the Garifuna over time, to see them come into their own.

ACKNOWLEDGMENT

Fieldwork in New York City was funded by a grant from the Ford Foundation to the senior author. Grateful acknowledgment is made of this support.

References

Cominsky, S., 1976, Birth rituals and symbolism: A Quiche Maya-Black Carib comparison, in *Ritual and Symbol in Native Central America*, (Philip Young & James Howe, eds.), pp. 105–117, University of Oregon Press.

Davidson, W., 1974, The Carib (Garifuna) of the Central America: A map of their realm and a bibliography of research, *National Studies* (Belize) 2(6):43–51.

González, N. L., 1959*a*, The nonunilineal descent group in the Caribbean and Central America, *A. Anthropol.* 61(4):578–583.

González, N. L., 1959*b*, West Indian characteristics of the Black Carib, *Southwest J. Anthropol.* 15(3):300–307; reprinted in *Peoples and Cultures of the Caribbean* (Michael Horowitz, ed.), Doubleday, Garden City, N.Y. 1971.

González, N. L., 1960, Changes in Black Carib kinship terminology, *Southwest. J. Anthropol.* 16(2):144–159.

González, N. L., 1965, Black Carib adaptation to a Latin urban milieu, *Soc. Econ. Studies* 14(3):272–278.

González, N. L., 1969, *Black Carib Household Structures: A Study of Migration and Modernization*, American Ethnological Society, University of Washington Press, Seattle, translated into Spanish as *La Estructura Del Grupo Familiar Entre Los Caribes Negros: Un estudio de migracion y modernizacion*, Seminario De Integracion Social Guatemalteca, Publicacion No. 39, 1979.

González, N. L., 1970, Towards a definition of matrifocality, in *Afro-American Anthropology: Problems in Theory and Method*, (Norman Whitten, ed.), pp. 231–243, The Free Press, New York.

González, N. L., 1979*a*, Garifuna settlement in New York: A new frontier, *Int. Migration Rev.* 13(2):255–263.

González, N. L., 1979*b*, Sex preference in human figure drawings by Garifuna (Black Carib) children, *Ethnology* 18(4):355–364.

Herskovits, M. J., 1938, Acculturation, in: *The Study of Culture Contact*, J. J. Augustin, Inc., Locust Valley, N.Y.

Kerns, V., 1977, Daughters bring in: Ceremonial and social organization of the Black Carib of Belize, Ph.D. dissertation, University of Illinois, Urbana.

Kerns, V., 1983, *Women and the Ancestors*, University of Illinois Press, Urbana, Illinois.

Munroe, R., 1964, Couvade practices of the Black Carib: A psychological study, Ph.D. dissertation, Harvard.

Sandford, M. S., 1971, Disruption of the mother–child relationship in conjunction with matrifocality: A study of child-keeping among the Carib and Creole of British Honduras, Ph.D. dissertation, Catholic University of America.

Stack, C.B., 1974, *All Our Kin*, Harper and Row, New York.

5

Demographic Patterns of the Garifuna (Black Caribs) of Belize

I. LESTER FIRSCHEIN

1. Introduction

The existence of a balanced polymorphic hemoglobin S gene maintained by the selective advantage of the heterozygote ($Hb^A Hb^S$) genotype within the Black Carib population is a problem that has received the previous attention of this author (Firschein, 1961). The data demonstrated that the sickle cell gene (Hb^S) was maintained at equilibrium values due to the greater fertility of heterozygous mothers. The advantage of the female heterozygote relative to homozygotes in the population was determined to be 1.45:1.* It was suggested that this fertility differential measured the genetic success of female heterozygotes in

---

* It is customary in population genetic analysis where a state of balanced polymorphism is maintained to indicate the average fitness of the heterozygote by the value W if the fitness or relative survival of the normal homozygote is arbitrarily taken as unity. In the Black Carib population, where the average frequency of the heterozygote at equilibrium is 0.263, it can easily be shown that W must equal 1.17. This value does not indicate how or when the equilibrium is brought about. Presumably the selective pressure may operate between the formation of the zygote and the reproductive period. Both the fertility ratio f and the frequency of the heterozygote are subject to large sampling errors. However, the significant difference in fertility between homozygous and heterozygous females happens to be of just the right order of magnitude to account completely for the observed frequency of sickle cell heterozygotes. It must be admitted, however, that it is quite possible that part of the selection may involve differential child mortality, as other workers have indicated (Allison, 1954, 1955; Lehmann and Raper, 1956).

I. LESTER FIRSCHEIN • Department of Anthropology, Hunter College – City University of New York, New York, New York 10021.

response to a single environmental variable, specifically, the presence of *falciparum* malaria.

It appears more appropriate, however, to define the dynamic biology or "life history" of a human population in terms of its overall adaptiveness to environmental pressures. The following report is an outline of the demographic features of the Black Caribs. It attempts to expand discussion of such an outline beyond strictly genetic parameters. This may enable us to characterize the population in terms more explicit than usually derived through a strict genetic interpretation, since it draws upon a wider range of information interrelating culture and biology.

Aside from population adaptiveness in a biological context, I shall attempt to utilize information involving the society's culture, which, in a sense, is the cohesive denominator of a biologically integrated population. Not only must a population have an adaptive biology, but the cultural implementation of this biology must be adaptive as well. Similarly, any biological constraints placed on a human population, adaptive or nonadaptive, must be maintained through behavior or culture. The understanding of human cultural behavior and its evolutionary ramifications must ultimately be based on demographic variables: fertility (natality), fecundity, mortality, family size, and birth spacing.

2. Methods

In 1946 the British Colonial Office held a census of their West Indian Colonies (Colonial Office, 1946, 1949), including British Honduras (Belize). Although prior census enumerations of populations are available for 1881 and 1921 the 1946 census included, for the first time, vital statistics on the racial groups within the various colonies. In addition to the total count of racial groups by sex, age, and dwelling place, two important factors relating to fertility were enumerated:

1. Number of children at present age of mother.
2. Age of mother at birth of first child.

Essentially, the following data are drawn directly from the results of the 1946 census. Additional data on fertility and mortality were made available through the auspices of the Government Registry Office in Belize, where registries were maintained on births and deaths. The data are listed for each year by:

1. Race, birth date, name, name and age of mother, name and age of father (only legal unions were recognized), father's occupation, mother's occupation, and, as of the year 1954, parity of the birth of the child.
2. Race, date of death, name, age, cause of death (if autopsied or otherwise known).

3. Results

3.1. Population Size

The 1946 census recorded the Black Carib population as consisting of 4112 individuals, comprising approximately 7% of the total population of British Honduras. Other major racial stocks were tabulated as follows: black (22,693), "mixed" (18,360), Amerindian (10,030), white (2329), and small groups of East Indians and Chinese. The size of the Black Carib population as recorded by the census was, however, an underestimate. At the time of the census, there were 100 or more young adult males at work on the third lock of the Panama Canal. Additionally, a sizeable number of Black Caribs were erroneously listed as black. Supplementary census information allows a more accurate estimate of the true size of the Black Carib population. For example, in the enumeration of "language spoken," 4715 were listed as fluent in the Black Carib tongue. This figure is larger by some 600 individuals than the census-determined population size. Further study revealed that the entire population of Barranco (322 inhabitants), the southernmost village in the colony, was registered as belonging to the black ethnic group. It is, however, an all Black Carib village. Punta Gorda, the next village to the immediate north, was listed as containing only 245 Black Caribs. It is shown in Table 4 that Black Carib mothers living in Punta Gorda gave birth to 347 children during the 10 years following the census. This number is slightly higher than the number of births that occurred in the Black Carib village of Seine Bight, which contained 505 inhabitants at the time of the census, suggesting that the Punta Gorda Black Carib population was larger than the census enumeration. Carib inhabitants for the villages of Punta Gorda and Barranco account for the additional 600 individuals belonging to the Black Carib language group. In order to correct census figures of 1946, these 600 individuals were distributed at the prevailing percent of occurrence for age group and sex; thus the estimated total size of the Black Carib population was adjusted to 4711 individuals.

Table 1 shows the population size of the Black Caribs of British Honduras for the years 1881, 1921, 1946, and 1956, Although the racial composition of

Table 1. Black Carib Population Size and Mean Annual Increase for Belize

Census year	Population number	Mean annual growth rate
1881	2037	
		0.3
1921	3165	
		0.8
1946	4711	
		3.0
1956	6154	

Table 2. Population Pyramid Extrapolated from 1946 Census with Birth–Death Registration

Age	Number of males	Number of females	Total	Percent total	Cumulative total percent
0–4	491	537	1028	16.70	16.70
5–9	380	420	800	13.00	29.70
10–14	226	285	511	8.3	38.00
15–19	254	324	578	9.39	47.39
20–24	284	315	599	9.73	57.12
25–29	226	281	507	8.24	65.36
30–34	164	212	376	6.11	71.47
35–39	138	195	333	5.41	76.88
40–44	117	160	277	4.50	81.38
45–49	114	156	270	4.39	85.77
50–54	98	144	242	3.93	89.70
55–59	78	127	205	3.33	93.03
60–64	42	74	116	1.88	94.91
65–69	48	70	118	1.92	96.83
70 +	74	120	194	3.15	100.00
Total	2734	3420	6154	100.00	

Table 3. Age and Sex Distribution of the Black Caribs of Belize Based on 1946 Census Data

Age	Number of males	Number of females	Total	Percent total	Cumulative total percent
0–4	252	303	555	11.78	11.78
5–9	268	328	596	12.65	24.43
10–14	288	320	608	12.91	37.34
15–19	230	288	518	10.99	48.33
20–24	169	221	390	8.28	56.61
25–29	144	204	348	7.39	64.00
30–34	121	160	281	5.96	69.96
35–39	121	165	286	6.07	76.03
40–44	117	149	266	5.65	81.68
45–49	90	135	225	4.78	86.46
50–54	56	80	136	2.89	89.35
55–59	64	80	144	3.06	92.41
60–64	64	73	137	2.91	95.32
65–69	45	64	109	2.31	97.63
70 +	46	66	112	2.38	100.00
Total	2075	2636	4711	100.00	

the colony was not given for the census years of 1881 and 1921, the "language spoken" for individuals over the age of 5 was enumerated, and by applying a rough correction based on the expected number of children under the age

of 5, the size of the Black Carib population for these census years was estimated.

A similar estimate was made for the year 1956. Here, the number of births
and deaths since the 1946 census were tabulated; then, by extrapolation from
the corrected 1946 census, a population age pyramid table was constructed for
males and females (Table 2). Census data are fraught with errors of omission,
particularly the underregistration of the younger age groups. In the age structure
(Table 3) based on the census of 1946, there is a constriction at the base corresponding to the first two age categories (0–4 and 5–9 years). This constriction
is shown in Fig. 1. Normal demographic expectations are that the base of the age
pyramid should be much broader than the overlying older age groups. This is the
expected demographic expression of an expanding population, such as the Black
Caribs. When the age structure of the population is calculated for the year 1956
and reconstructed from accurate birth–death data, the younger age groups are
found to compose, as expected, the largest percentage of the population (see

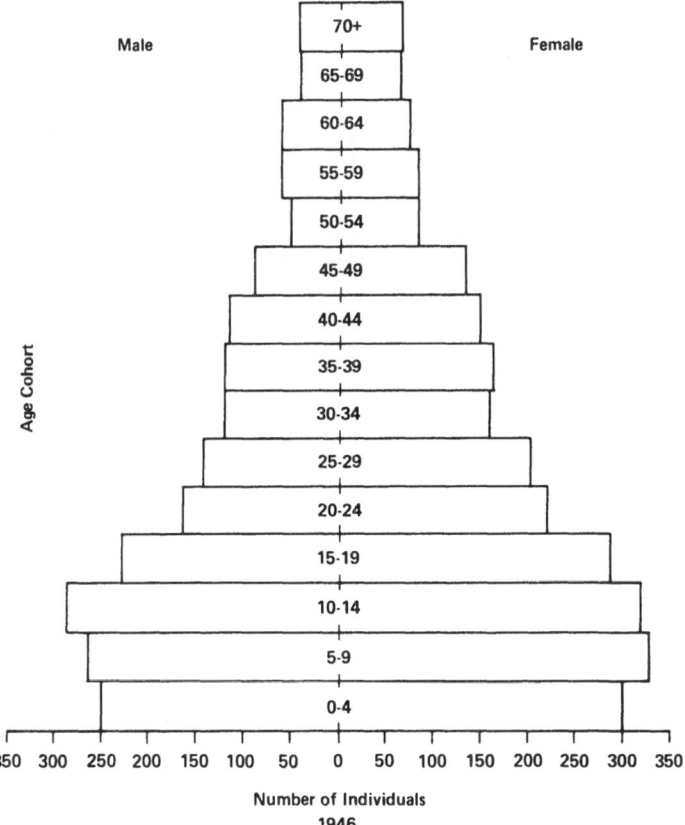

FIGURE 1. Age and sex structure of the Black Caribs of British Honduras, based upon the
1946 census, represented by a population pyramid.

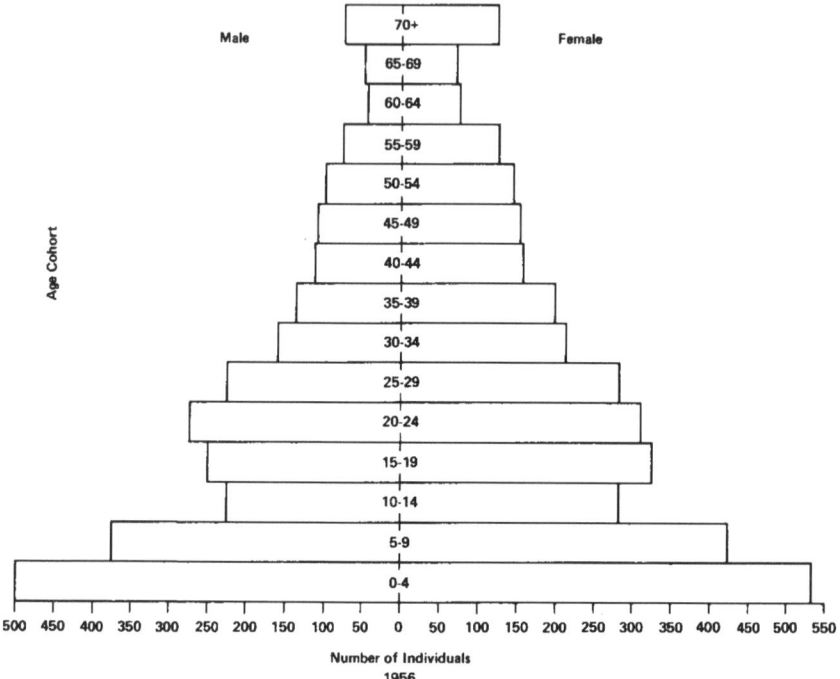

FIGURE 2. Population pyramid of the Black Caribs based on census estimates for 1956.

Fig. 2). However, the effect of underregistration during the 1946 census is reflected in the size estimates for the next two higher age groups.

The mean annual growth rate (MAGR) for the intercensus time periods was calculated on the basis of the following formula:

$$\text{MAGR} = \frac{100(\text{Pop}_2 - \text{Pop}_1)}{\text{Pop}_1(\text{Time}_2 - \text{Time}_1)}$$

Table 1 indicates that the 1946–1955 time interval showed the highest yearly MAGR increase, 3.0%.

3.2. Family Size

The fundamental problem for a meaningful interpretation of demographic change is the assessment of the causes of changing family size through the years. Census data alone cannot indicate changes in family size and, in fact, may lead to erroneous conclusions. For example, a decrease in mortality (due to improved medical care) can mask patterns of lowered fertility and smaller family size. One must realize that family size may involve a decision-making process with an element of cultural change brought about by contact with other cultures.

Table 4. Fertility Rate by Locality, 1946–1956

Village	Number of mothers	Number of births	Rate
Stann Creek	550	1077	1.96
Hopkins	78	176	2.26
Seine Bight	150	333	2.22
Punta Gorda	165	347	2.10
Barranco	60	116	1.93

Table 5. Average Number of Children Born Alive per Mother Based upon the 1946 Census

Ethnic group	All mothers	Mother over 45 years
American Indian	4.74	6.15
White	4.17	5.62
Black	4.32	5.95
Mixed (white–black)	4.62	6.18
Carib	4.17	5.40

Table 6. Fertility Ratio of Ethnic Groups[a]

Ethnic group	Age group of females	Fertility ratio
Carib		
1946	15–44	46.76
1956	15–44	69.13
Amerindian		
1946	15–44	71.04
Black		
1946	15–44	49.27
Mixed		
1946	15–44	59.89

[a] Fertility ratio: number of children age 0–4 per 100 females in age group 15–44.

Therefore, let us first look at data from Black Caribs who live in areas where cultural values and stresses are variable.

In Table 4, fertility rates for five Black Carib villages have been tabulated for the period from 1946 to 1956. Stann Creek and Punta Gorda, the second and third largest towns in Belize, are mixed "creole" (blacks) and Black Carib. Hopkins, Seine Bight, and Barranco are smaller, exclusively Black Carib towns. The fertility rate is lower in the towns with mixed inhabitants and it is these towns that contain the strongest possibility of "change by contact." The low fertility rate for Barranco has quite another explanation and will be dealt with later in the discussion on sex ratio.

Tables 5 and 6 compare the fertility of the Black Caribs with other ethnic

Table 7. Size of Family for Mothers of Completed Fertility

Age cohort	Total number of mothers	Number of mothers with given number of children[a]									
		1	2	3	4	5	6	7	8	9	10+
45–49	101	15 (14.9)	13 (12.9)	17 (16.8)	11 (10.9)	8 (7.9)	8 (7.9)	8 (7.9)	7 (6.9)	3 (3.0)	11 (10.9)
50–54	63	11 (17.5)	6 (9.5)	5 (7.9)	9 (14.3)	7 (11.1)	3 (4.8)	7 (11.1)	6 (9.5)	1 (1.6)	8 (12.7)
55–59	63	7 (11.1)	5 (7.9)	9 (14.3)	9 (14.3)	8 (12.7)	3 (4.8)	6 (9.5)	4 (6.3)	5 (7.9)	7 (11.1)
60–64	63	4 (6.3)	6 (9.5)	7 (11.1)	10 (15.9)	7 (11.1)	7 (11.1)	5 (7.9)	8 (12.7)	4 (6.3)	5 (7.9)
65 +	101	9 (8.9)	7 (6.9)	11 (10.9)	11 (10.9)	12 (11.9)	13 (12.9)	9 (8.9)	7 (6.9)	4 (4.0)	18 (17.8)
Total	391	46 (11.8)	37 (9.5)	49 (12.5)	50 (12.8)	42 (10.7)	34 (8.7)	35 (8.9)	32 (8.2)	17 (4.3)	49 (12.5)

[a] Figures in parentheses are percentages of total number of mothers.

Table 8. Size of Family for Mothers of Incompleted Fertility

Age cohort	Total number of mothers	Number of mothers with given number of children[a]									
		1	2	3	4	5	6	7	8	9	10+
15–19	35	32 (91.4)	3 (8.6)								
20–24	96	52 (54.2)	29 (30.2)	13 (13.5)	2 (2.1)						
25–29	136	44 (32.2)	28 (20.6)	34 (25.0)	12 (8.8)	11 (8.1)	5 (3.7)	2 (1.5)			
30–34	107	27 (25.2)	11 (10.3)	18 (16.8)	15 (14.0)	9 (8.4)	7 (6.5)	8 (7.5)	7 (6.5)	3 (2.8)	2 (1.9)
35–39	122	23 (18.9)	17 (13.9)	10 (8.2)	15 (12.3)	13 (10.7)	14 (11.5)	12 (9.8)	6 (4.9)	7 (5.7)	5 (4.1)
40–44	112	23 (20.5)	12 (10.7)	11 (9.8)	10 (8.9)	9 (8.0)	10 (8.9)	9 (8.0)	11 (9.8)	10 (8.9)	7 (6.3)
Total	608	201 (33.0)	100 (16.4)	86 (14.1)	55 (9.0)	42 (6.9)	36 (5.9)	31 (5.1)	24 (3.9)	20 (3.3)	14 (2.3)

[a] Figures in parentheses are percentages of total number of mothers.

groups in the colony (Colonial Office, 1946, 1949). It is interesting to note that aside from the small group of whites, the Black Caribs had the lowest average number of children born alive per mother. There is, however, a marked increase in the Carib fertility ratio when it is based on the reconstructed 1956 age pyramid (Table 6). The fertility ratio was computed only for the age group of females 15–44 years.

Table 7 gives data on the size of family for 391 Black Carib mothers with completed fertility (over 45 years) at the time of the 1946 census. In order to evaluate trends toward a reduction in family size, one could compare the same classes of data for Black Carib mothers in varying cohort groups of subsequent censuses. However, a more revealing method of comparison uses data from within the same census. Dividing the cohort of mothers with completed fertility into two groups, a mean number of children of 5.01 is obtained for mothers age 45–54 and a mean number of children of 5.84 for mothers over 60 (Table 11). A t-test applied to these data ($t = 2.18$) indicates that there is a significant increase in family size between these two groups of mothers at the 0.025 level. If the prolific mothers in the age bracket 15–44 are considered (Table 8), even though these women have not completed reproduction, the data suggest a reduction in family size that correlates with progressively younger female cohorts. Table 9 indicates one of the factors that may be involved in the reduction of family size. This table plots the age of mother at birth of her first child. Females of completed and incomplete reproductive spans are analyzed separately. It must be realized that within the age class of females who have not

Table 9. Age of Female at First Child (1000 Females from 1946 Census)

Age	Distribution at completed fertility		Distribution at incomplete fertility		Total percent
	Number	Percent	Number	Percent	
10–14	4	1.0	22	3.4	2.6
15	17	4.3	30	4.9	4.7
16	20	5.1	38	6.2	5.8
17	21	5.4	59	9.7	8.0
18	45	11.5	89	14.6	13.4
19	36	9.2	75	12.3	11.1
20	69	17.6	80	13.1	14.9
21	31	7.9	55	9.0	8.6
22	26	6.6	43	7.1	7.0
23	28	7.2	33	5.4	6.1
24	19	4.9	21	3.4	4.0
25–26	28	7.2	28	4.6	5.6
27–29	23	5.9	22	3.6	4.5
30–34	15	3.8	11	1.8	2.6
35–39	8	2.0	2	0.3	1.0
40 +	0	0	1	0.2	0.1

Table 10. Number of Mothers per Age Cohort in Percent

Age	Percent
15–19	13.9
20–24	51.3
25–29	78.2
30–34	77.0
35–39	85.3
40–44	87.6
45 +	91.8

Table 11. Mean Number of Children per Prolific Woman by Age Cohort

Age group of mother	Number of mothers	Mean number of children
15–19	35	1.086
20–24	97	1.660
25–29	136	2.566
30–34	107	3.822
35–39	122	4.459
40–44	112	4.937
45–49	101	4.911
50–54	63	5.175
55–59	63	5.365
60–64	63	5.524
65 +	101	6.040
Total	1000	

completed reproduction, there is a large segment of females who have not begun reproduction, a demographic artifact that can lead to the erroneous conclusion that the percent of mothers who had their first child at a comparatively young age is higher in the 15- to 44-year age groups than for mothers who are over 45 years of age. When Table 10 (which tabulates the number of mothers per 100 females in the population at 5-year age intervals) is examined, it becomes apparent that, if beginning of motherhood is standardized in the age groups of 15–44 years to equal that of females who have completed fertility (among whom 91.8% have borne children), there appears a marked tendency in younger cohorts to delay reproduction until a later age. For example, at age 24, 80.7% of all mothers now over 44 years of age have had at least one child. At age 20–24, mothers comprised only 51.3% of all females in this age bracket at the time of the 1946 census. The data may also be interpreted as a reflection of an apparent increase in sterility within this population, an idea expressed by the Medical Officer assigned to the Stann Creek Hospital. His clinical data on younger women suggest that venereal disease is a major cause of this effect.

Other demographic data on this population are not as conclusive in elucidating the possible causes of trends toward decreased family size. Table 12,

Table 12. Distribution of Parity and Sex at Birth

	Parity[a]										
	1	2	3	4	5	6	7	8	9	10+	Total
1955											
Males	28 (25.9)	19 (17.6)	14 (13.0)	10 (9.3)	12 (11.1)	10 (9.3)	9 (8.3)	3 (2.8)	1 (.9)	2 (1.8)	108
Females	21 (22.8)	14 (15.2)	16 (17.4)	12 (13.0)	14 (15.2)	3 (3.3)	5 (5.4)	2 (2.2)	3 (3.2)	2 (2.2)	92
Total	49 (24.5)	33 (16.5)	30 (15.0)	22 (11.0)	26 (13.0)	13 (6.5)	14 (7.0)	5 (2.5)	4 (2.0)	4 (2.0)	200
1954											
Males	32 (31.6)	16 (15.8)	15 (14.8)	9 (8.9)	12 (11.9)	6 (6.0)	4 (4.0)	5 (4.9)	0 (0.0)	2 (1.9)	101
Females	19 (19.8)	23 (23.9)	16 (16.7)	10 (10.4)	14 (14.6)	5 (5.2)	2 (2.1)	4 (4.2)	2 (2.1)	1 (1.0)	96
Total	51 (25.9)	39 (19.8)	31 (15.7)	19 (9.6)	26 (13.2)	11 (5.6)	6 (3.1)	9 (4.6)	2 (1.0)	3 (1.5)	197

[a] Figures in parentheses are percentages.

which indicates the distribution of birth by parity as determined by the years 1954 and 1955, reveals that 17–18% of the children born during this period were to families possessing five or more children. An analogous parity distribution has been constructed for all births prior to the census of 1946:

Parity	1	2	3	4	5	6	7	8	9	10+
Total	26.8	19.0	14.9	11.2	8.6	7.0	4.8	3.3	2.0	2.9

Children born into families of five or more children constituted some 20% of the total number of children ever born to these women. These data suggest that, on the average, there is little variation in large family sizes, the percentage of first births is low, and rate of first births has not changed significantly over the years. By contrast, the U. S. statistics for the census year 1950 reflect the real demographic effect of reduced family size by indicating a higher percentage of first births (36%) than in previous census years.

Aside from a suspected cohort differential in fertility among the Black

Table 13. A Comparison of Fertility between the Census Population and a Sample with Known Hemoglobin Phenotypes

Size of family	Number of families	Percent of families	Number of children	Percent of children
Census population				
1–3	132	33.0	267	12.6
4–6	126	32.2	614	29.0
7+	133	34.0	1237	58.4
Total	391	100.0	2118	100.0
Hb^A/Hb^S mothers				
1–3	11	22.0	24	6.8
4–6	12	24.0	66	18.8
7+	27	54.0	262	74.4
Total	50	100.0	352	100.0
Hb^A/Hb^A mothers				
1–3	56	38.6	114	16.1
4–6	50	34.5	241	34.0
7+	39	26.9	354	49.9
Total	145	100.0	709	100.0
Combined mothers				
1–3	67	34.4	138	13.0
4–6	62	31.8	307	28.9
7+	66	33.8	616	58.1
Total	195	100.0	1061	100.0

Carib mothers, we can delineate, within mother cohorts, both high- and low-fertility groups (Table 13). Of the 391 mothers with completed fertility surveyed in the 1946 census, one-third may be classified as a group of highly fertile females, who contributed by far the largest component to population growth, some 58% of all births. Table 13 compares the census results with those derived from my genetic survey of abnormal hemoglobins (Firschein, 1961), which included mothers with completed reproduction who had been selected on a random basis. Heterozygous mothers ($Hb^A Hb^S$) appear to have larger family sizes. For the normal homozygote ($Hb^A Hb^A$) mothers, the majority of families are small in size.

3.3. Sex Ratio

One of the most intriguing aspects of the demographic study of the Black Caribs is the unique sex ratio present in this population. Table 14 shows the population sex ratio by age. This table has been constructed from the two population pyramid tables for the years 1946 and 1956. The sex ratio for 1946, the census year, may be validly questioned, especially for the data concerning the low sex ratio recorded for the younger age groups (0–4 and 5–9 years). Generally speaking, census data show a notorious deficiency of the male sex for the age group 0–4 years; the 1946 census of British Honduras is no exception. Table 15 indicates a trend toward male underenumeration for other ethnic groups, such as blacks and the Amerindians. In these ethnic groups the sex

Table 14. Population Sex Ratio Computed from the 1946 and 1956 Population Pyramid

| Age group | Sex ratio | |
	1946	1956
0–4	83.17	91.44
5–9	81.71	90.48
10–14	90.00	79.30
15–19	79.86	78.40
20–24	76.47	90.16
25–29	70.59	80.43
30–34	75.62	77.36
35–39	73.33	70.77
40–44	78.52	73.12
45–49	66.67	73.08
50–54	70.00	68.06
55–59	80.00	61.42
60–64	87.67	56.76
65–69	70.31	68.57
70 +	69.70	61.67
Total	78.72	79.94

Table 15. Sex Ratio of Chidren among Ethnic Groups,
1946 Census

	Sex ratio	
Ethnic group	Age 0–4	Age 5–9
Carib	83.17	81.71
Black	90.79	108.63
American Indian	95.73	105.13
Mixed	98.94	98.99

Table 16. Reproductive Performance of Black Carib Mothers

Genotype of mother	Number of mothers	Mean number of children	f Ratio
Hb^A/Hb^S	89	6.17	$\Big\}1.45^a$
Hb^A/Hb^A	254	4.25	

[a] Significant at the 0.01 level.

ratio for the 0–4 age interval is low, while the sex ratio for the following age category, 5–9, exhibits a normal value. The apparent explanation for this discrepancy is the usual underenumeration of males in the younger age set. On the other hand, the Black Carib data are consistent, the sex ratio being low for both age groups, as well as being commensurate with the actual birth records obtained from official registries. The average sex ratio for both time-set populations was of the order of 79 males for every 100 females.

The data obtained during the hemoglobin study survey (Firschein, 1961) on the reproductive performance of mothers have been used to test the hypothesis that the sex ratio of offspring is related to sickle cell genotypes. Table 16 summarizes the data of the previous study. In this table the f ratio indicates the advantage of the heterozygote mother (Hb^AHb^S) over that of the normal hemoglobin type (Hb^AHb^A) mother. The data suggest that the sex composition of Black Carib families is different, depending upon the presence or absence of an abnormal hemoglobin gene in the mother. The Hb^AHb^A mothers have a low sex ratio, 71 males per 100 females, compared to a normal sex distribution for mothers of the genotype Hb^AHb^S, 108 males per 100 females. Since the difference in the sex ratio of offspring is statistically significant ($\chi^2 = 7.96, P < 0.01$), we must recall the malarial hypothesis in order to explain this incongruity (Firschein, 1961).

The Central American model describes the fitness of the Hb^S gene by suggesting that normal homozygous mothers (Hb^AHb^A) have more pregnancy interruptions than heterozygous mothers (Hb^AHb^S). It is further suggested that this loss of fetal life involves many more male than female fetuses and that this is the basis for the observed new-born sex ratio.

If the new-born sex ratio indicates a deficiency of males for Hb^AHb^A

Table 17. Observed and Expected Numbers of Heterozygotes

Genotype	Number of males		Number of females	
	Observed	Expected	Observed	Expected
$Hb^A Hb^S$	52	54	112	127
$Hb^A Hb^A$	140	138	401	386

mothers compared to $Hb^A Hb^S$ mothers, then the rate of the sickling trait should be higher in males than females in the Black Carib population. We indeed show that the expected value of the sickling trait in males is 28% and in females 25%. The actual values tested in the Black Carib population were 27% for males and 22% for females. The expected sex ratio of the population under iteration was 81:100, higher than the census-obtained values. It should be noted that the observed frequency for heterozygous males and females approximates the equilibrium values calculated. We can test the hypothesis that the Black Carib population is in close agreement to the "iterative" derived value for the sickling gene (Hb^S) by comparing the observed numbers of heterozygotes ($Hb^A Hb^S$) and the expected values at equilibrium by sex (Table 17).

The differences between the population sample and the "iterative" values of males and females at equilibrium (χ^2 for 3 d.f. $= 2.46, P = 0.48$) is not significant and probably due to sample fluctuation. The data reinforce the contention that the selective pressures are operating between the zygote and birth. The concordance between expected and observed values leads to the belief that the Central American model (as constructed on the basis of a sex ratio differential rate of production between $Hb^A Hb^A$ and $Hb^A Hb^S$ mothers) is essentially correct.

The greatest change in the demography of the Black Caribs is in survival rates for the very young, i.e., age group 0–4 years. This dramatic change has been brought about by two innovations instituted at hospital clinics located in Black Carib towns: increasing care for the pregnant mother, which included the distribution of supplementary iron rations and vitamins, and the operation of a childrens' clinic. At this clinic, every child in the village under the age of 2 was examined at least twice a month. Vaccines were administered, such as BCG for tuberculosis, yellow fever, smallpox, and typhoid, and malarial and tuberculosis chemotherapy was included. The mortality rate for many diseases has been drastically reduced, particularly for malaria. These recent health measures and the fact that an increasing proportion of births now take place at the hospital in Stann Creek, where maternity beds are provided as a free service of the government, have changed mortality patterns among the Black Caribs. In the following discussion I will detail some of these demographic changes, particularly the sex ratio at birth and the sex ratio of mortalities.

The most intensive activity of health measures instituted by the Medical Service in order to reduce mortality took place in the Stann Creek District.

Table 18. Births, Deaths, and Survivorship for Selected Year Intervals

	1951–1955	1941–1945	1932–1936
Births			
Total	692	539	581
Male	361	259	269
Female	331	280	312
Percent male	52.168	48.052	46.299
Sex ratio	109.07	92.50	86.22
Deaths, 0–4 years			
Total	107	95	110
Male	60	60	70
Female	47	35	40
Percent male	56.075	63.158	63.636
Sex ratio	127.66	171.43	175.00
Percent dying before fifth year	15.462	17.625	18.933
Percent of males dying before fifth year	16.620	23.166	26.022
Percent of females dying before fifth year	14.199	12.500	12.821
Surviving to fifth year			
Total	585	444	471
Male	301	199	199
Female	284	245	272
Percent male	51.453	44.820	42.251
Sex ratio	105.99	81.23	73.16
Percent surviving to fifth year	84.538	82.375	81.067

Therefore the Registry records of births and deaths for this district were tabulated for three different time periods: 1932–1936; 1941–1945; 1951–1955 (Table 18). In the Stann Creek District, 55% of all deaths occurred in the 0–4-year-old cohort during the 5-year period 1941–1945. In the following 10-year period, 1946–1955, 45% of the total deaths occurring were in the same cohort. The major clue to the suggestion of an improvement in survivorship may be discerned when data on the sex ratio of deaths is analyzed. The earlier years tabulated show a high mortality of males when compared with later years. The sex ratio of death in the 0- to 4-year-old class for 1932–1936 is 175 males dying per 100 females; for 1941–1945, it is 127 males per 100 females. The sex-dependent differential death rate lowers the sex ratio of the survivors and the data are compatible with the sex ratio of the 0- to 4-year-old class constructed for the population age pyramids for the years 1946 and 1956 (Table 14). This is in line with the concept that the extreme age-stratified sex ratio that is observed in the Black Carib population is due to two major components: excessive *in utero* and post natal male deaths.

The differential mortality of the male sex in the age group 0–4 years may be followed in another manner. In the interval 1951–1955, 17% of all males born died before their fifth year of life, and 13% of the females died. However, for the earlier year intervals, the female death rate remained at about 14% of the total number of females born, while the mortality rate for males was higher, i.e., 26% for the interval 1932–1936. The progressive decrease in death from earlier to late years indicates that this value progressively increases as well: 1932–1936, 86:100; 1941–1945, 92:100; and 1951–1955, 109:100. Although in terms of percentages there has been a decrease in the number of male deaths in the 0–4-year-age group, the total mortality rate for the population as a whole has not diminished correspondingly. This may be expressed by examining the percent of all children surviving to their fifth year of life. This figure ranges from 81% for the 1932–1936 interval to 85% for 1952–1955. This seemingly paradoxical situation is based on the fact that the sex ratio at birth was low for the earlier years tabulated. It is necessary, therefore, to disengage the two increments that contribute to the population sex ratio – namely, sex ratio at birth and the sex ratio of mortality – to show that the decline in mortality is real. The increment to population growth in recent years has been with regard to the male sex, and it is the survivorship of the male that has increased almost twofold in the period of 20 years.

Table 19. Life Table Data for Males Based on Birth and Death Certificates, 1946–1956

Age	Expected life span	Expectation of life
Birth	30.33	30.33
0–1 month	36.38	36.38
1 month–1 year	45.65	44.65
1–2	51.17	49.17
2–3	52.89	49.89
3–4	54.33	50.38
4–5	55.62	50.62
5–10	58.80	51.30
10–14	59.10	46.60
15–19	60.84	43.34
20–24	62.50	40.00
25–29	70.90	43.40
30–34	63.78	31.28
35–39	65.24	27.74
40–44	66.38	23.88
45–49	68.70	21.20
50–54	70.96	18.46
55–59	72.76	15.26
60–64	75.07	12.57
65–69	78.08	10.58
70–74	82.00	9.50
75–79	84.38	6.88
80–84	88.25	5.75
85–89	92.00	4.50
90–94	0	0

A life table, based on birth and death certificates, has been constructed in order to show the effect of mortality on males during the period 1946–1955. Table 19 tabulates both the expected life span for particular age intervals as well as the expectation of life (i.e., years of life remaining). It is interesting to note that the average expectation of life remaining for any male at birth is only 30 years even though the life table is based on the prevailing death rates of a period when the mortality of males has greatly improved. However, if the male survives to the fifth year of life, the average years of life remaining is 51 years. If a male lives to early adulthood, then his life span will be in the neighborhood of 70 years. Life expectancy for the adult Black Carib male is actually the highest for any population in British Honduras and for most of Central America as well.

Table 20 has been constructed from data obtained from the 1946 census and indicates the percent of surviving children by age of mother enumerated. It is suggested that the increase of the sex ratio at birth was probably due to the lessened incidence of *in utero* deaths through the mechanism of placental dysfunction caused by the presence of a *Plasmodium* parasite. Births in Stann

Table 20. Percent of Surviving Children by Age of the Mother

Age group of mother	Number of mothers	Children born	Children surviving	Percent surviving
15–19	35	38	27	71.05
20–24	97	161	133	82.61
25–29	136	349	271	77.65
30–34	107	409	294	71.88
35–39	122	544	415	76.29
40–44	112	553	433	78.30
45–49	101	496	371	74.80
50–54	63	326	213	65.34
55–59	63	338	208	61.54
60–64	63	348	222	63.79
65 +	101	610	323	52.95
Total	1000	4172	2910	69.75
45 +				
Total	391	2118	1337	63.13

Table 21. Sex Ratio at Birth by Locality, 1946–1956

Village	Number of births	Proportion of males	Males per 100 females
Stann Creek	1077	50.32	101
Hopkins	176	51.70	107
Seine Bight	333	49.55	98
Punta Gorda	347	44.26	79
Barranco	116	36.79	58

Creek have normalized in terms of the sex ratio since 1946, while the town of Barranco still exhibited the exceedingly low sex ratio, i.e., 58:100 (Table 21). At the time of my survey it was reported by the Medical Officer of the district (personal communication) that the children of Barranco had a higher spleen rate (indicating malarial parasitism) than did Stann Creek inhabitants. Possibly the low sex ratio of Barranco reflected the placental damage on consequent abortion of the fetus. There may be other factors to consider, however, in order to explain the precipitous rise in the sex ratio. Analysis based on the parity and sex birth data available for the years 1954 and 1955 (Table 13) suggests that male births in the first parity far exceed those of females. In a demographically expanding population one would expect the increment of first births to increase over the years due to the recruitment of more females into the primiparous class. This phenomenon would in itself increase the sex ratio of the population. However, when census data for 1946 are analyzed (Table 13) and the parity distribution of births for mothers are enumerated, the number of children born of different parity, especially of parity one to four, has not changed in the years prior to 1946 when compared to those born in 1954 and 1955. Therefore the increase in male births in the later years is independent of parity of birth.

In the random reproductive survey, random samples of mothers were interviewed in the town of Stann Creek in 1956. Mothers with four or more children alive or who had at least reached their sixth birthday before death were tabulated. A little less than one-fourth of the total Black Carib population were included in this sample. For comparative purposes, white families from the U.S. were analyzed in the same manner (Rife and Snyder, 1937). The distribution of family size for these samples is shown in Table 22.

Table 23 indicates the distribution of both populations for the probability P that sex composition within families approaches unity. So that a proper χ^2 can be utilized, the families are grouped into equal classes based on the expectations of the distribution of families in the Black Carib population by sex of progeny at unity. This is necessary to test the proposition that all mothers produce children at a particular sex ratio that can be considered as a reflection of some randomized factor. However, if it can be demonstrated that there is a dichotomy in the

Table 22. Family Size Distributions

Family size	Black Caribs ($N = 171$)	U.S. white ($N = 191$)
4	48	90
5	48	49
6	32	17
7	23	16
8	10	7
9	4	4
10	6	8[a]

[a] Extrapolated from families of 10 or more children.

Table 23. Demographic Patterns of the Black Caribs[a]

♀	♂	P	Carib observed	Expected	White observed	Expected	Cumulative P
N = 4							
4		0.062	6	2.98	7	5.58	1.000
3	1	0.250	15	12.00	19	22.50	0.937
2	2	0.375	16	18.00	37	33.75	0.687
1	3	0.250	9	12.00	22	22.50	0.312
	4	0.062	2	2.98	5	5.58	0.062
N = 5							
5		0.031	3	1.49	3	1.52	1.000
4	1	0.155	11	7.44	7	7.60	0.967
3	2	0.313	13	15.02	16	15.34	0.812
2	3	0.313	9	15.02	14	15.34	0.499
1	4	0.155	10	7.44	8	7.60	0.186
	5	0.031	2	1.49	1	1.52	0.031
N = 6							
6		0.016	3	0.51	2	0.27	1.000
5	1	0.093	8	2.98	1	1.58	0.981
4	2	0.233	4	7.46	3	3.96	0.888
3	3	0.313	8	10.02	5	5.32	0.655
2	4	0.233	6	7.46	3	3.96	0.342
1	5	0.093	2	2.98	2	1.58	0.109
	6	0.016	1	0.51	1	0.27	0.016
N = 7							
7		0.008	0	0.18	0	0.13	1.000
6	1	0.056	1	1.29	1	0.90	0.988
5	2	0.163	7	3.75	1	2.61	0.932
4	3	0.271	8	6.23	3	4.34	0.769
3	4	0.271	3	6.23	6	4.34	0.498
2	5	0.163	4	3.75	3	2.61	0.227
1	6	0.056	0	1.29	2	0.90	0.064
	7	0.008	0	0.18	0	0.13	0.008
N = 8							
8		0.004	0	0.04	0	0.03	1.000
7	1	0.032	3	0.32	0	0.22	0.995
6	2	0.112	2	1.12	0	0.78	0.963
5	3	0.217	2	2.17	1	1.52	0.851
4	4	0.269	2	2.69	2	1.88	0.634
3	5	0.217	0	2.17	3	1.52	0.365
2	6	0.112	1	1.12	1	0.78	0.148
1	7	0.032	0	0.32	0	0.22	0.036
	8	0.004	0	0.04	0	0.03	0.004
N = 9							
9		0.002	0	0.01	0	0.01	1.000
8	1	0.018	0	0.07	0	0.07	0.998
7	2	0.072	0	0.29	0	0.29	0.984

Table 23 (continued)

♀	♂	P	Carib observed	Expected	White observed	Expected	Cumulative P
6	3	0.168	3	0.67	1	0.67	0.912
5	4	0.242	0	0.97	0	0.97	0.744
4	5	0.242	0	0.97	2	0.97	0.502
3	6	0.168	1	0.67	0	0.67	0.260
2	7	0.072	0	0.29	1	0.29	0.092
1	8	0.018	0	0.07	0	0.07	0.020
	9	0.002	0	0.01	0	0.01	0.002
N = 10							
10							
9	1	0.001	0	0.01	0	0.01	1.000
8	2	0.010	0	0.06	0	0.08	0.999
7	3	0.045	0	0.27	0	0.36	0.989
6	4	0.120	2	0.72	1	0.96	0.954
5	5	0.208	1	1.24	1	1.66	0.834
4	6	0.242	3	1.45	2	1.94	0.626
3	7	0.208	0	1.24	2	1.66	0.384
2	8	0.120	0	0.72	2	0.96	0.176
1	9	0.045	0	0.27	0	0.36	0.056
	10	0.010	0	0.06	0	0.08	0.011
		0.001	0	0.01	0	0.01	0.001

[a] Sex ratio of Carib families: whites: females 0.500 males 0.500.

distribution of the sex ratio within families, then we may opt for a genetic (i.e., single gene) explanation of the sex ratio as observed in the Black Carib population. Families with three females, two males; four females, two males; five females, three males; six females, three males; etc., were placed in the class 0.33–0.44% of males. Families with the reverse distribution (i.e., three males, two females; four males, two females; etc.) were included in the class 0.56–0.67% of males (Table 24). There is a very significant difference in the distribution of Black Carib families ($P < 0.001$), while the white families agree with the expectation of sex of progeny distributed at unity ($P > 0.95$). Testing the data at the observed sex ratio within the Black Carib families (76.37:100, or 0.433 males) gives the value $P < 0.05$ (Tables 25, 27).

The data can also be tested according to the distribution of families at the cumulative frequencies of the expected binomial values P for different sized families, at increments of 0.100 (Table 26). The white families tested for the rate of unity (0.500) agree with expectation ($P > 0.98$), while the Black Carib families do not ($P < 0.001$). If the Black Caribs are tested at the observed rate (0.433), then $P = 0.14$. If we examine the distribution of males and females within Black Carib families (Table 25) and test for the significance of the distribution between observed and expected by sex in the same manner, we derive a χ^2 of 169.80 with 7 d.f. ($P < 0.001$) for the Black Carib families, and a χ^2 of 13.34 with 7 d.f. ($P = 0.06–0.07$) for the white families (Table 27).

Table 24. Test for the Significance of the Difference between the Observed and Expected[a] Distribution of Families

Class, % males	Carib		White	
	Observed	Expected	Observed	Expected
0–0.3	61	35.54	42	45.55
0.33–0.44	31	33.85	25	28.48
0.5	29	32.22	46	42.94
0.56–0.67	19	33.85	30	28.48
0.7–1.0	31	35.54	48	45.55
Total	171		191	
x^2		25.90		1.13
d.f. 3				
P		< 0.001		> 0.95

[a] Females 0.500; males 0.500.

The departure from expectation of the observed distribution of Black Carib families, according to the distribution of the sex of progeny within families, suggests that the observed sex ratio production differential between Hb^AHb^A and Hb^AHb^S genotypes in mothers is also reflected in families sampled in the random reproductive survey. There is a particularly marked surplus of families with the lowest percent of males, class 0–0.3 (D^2/expected = 18.239). The same effect is discernible for males and females within families (D^2/expected = 101.506 for females and 16.712 for males). The class 0–0.3% of males contributed more than two-thirds of the total x^2 value in each case. There is also an excess of families in the class denoting a high sex ratio (0.7–1.00). Particularly revealing is the extreme biomodality of the D^2/expected values in the Black Carib data when the percent of male classes are plotted as a histogram. The division of families into high- and low-sex-ratio lines is not significantly marked in the white families analyzed. This suggests that there are probably two distinct sex ratio production rates for mothers of the random survey families. We may artificially apportion the random survey families according to the empirical data derived from the abnormal hemoglobin data (Firschein, 1961, Tables 7, 8). It is possible to test if the dichotomized sex ratio observed with the random survey reflects two distinct classes of families. The binomial formula of expectation P used in this test is as follows: 0.247 of the 171 mothers sampled average a male sex rate of 0.52 (i.e., 108 males per 100 females), which would represent the Hb^AHb^S mothers, and conversely, 0.743 of the mothers sampled average a male sex rate of 0.41 (i.e., 71 males per 100 females). This would represent the Hb^AHb^A mothers in the sample. However, on the basis of the distribution of family size for the two hemoglobin classes of mothers (Firschein, 1961, Table 4) an adjustment had to be calculated into the formula of the binomial distribution

Table 25. Sex Distribution in 171 Families with Four or More Living Children[a]

♀ ♂	P	Cumulative frequency P	Observed	Expected
N = 4				
4	0.103	1.000	6	4.9
3 1	0.315	0.898	15	15.1
2 2	0.360	0.579	16	17.3
1 3	0.184	0.219	9	8.8
4	0.035	0.035	2	1.7
N = 5				
5	0.058	1.000	3	2.8
4 1	0.223	0.937	11	10.7
3 2	0.340	0.114	13	16.3
2 3	0.260	0.374	9	12.5
1 4	0.009	0.114	10	4.8
5	0.015	0.015	2	0.7
N = 6				
6	0.033	1.000	3	1.1
5 1	0.151	0.960	8	4.8
4 2	0.289	0.809	4	9.2
3 3	0.295	0.520	8	9.4
2 4	0.168	0.225	6	5.4
1 5	0.051	0.057	2	1.6
6	0.006	0.006	1	0.2
N = 7				
7	0.019	1.000	0	0.44
6 1	0.100	0.971	1	2.30
5 2	0.228	0.871	7	5.24
4 3	0.292	0.643	8	6.72
3 4	0.223	0.351	3	5.13
2 5	0.101	0.128	4	2.32
1 6	0.024	0.027	0	0.55
7	0.003	0.003	0	0.06

[a] Observed: males 0.433, females 0.567.

because the random reproductive survey consisted of families with four or more children. The adjustment yielded a frequency of 0.186, representing that portion of the sample of $Hb^A Hb^S$ mothers with four, five, or six children, and a frequency of 0.397 for those mothers with seven or more children. The χ^2 test for the goodness of fit between the observed and the expected values is 6.79 ($P <$ 0.08). An examination of the differences between the expected and observed values suggests an alternative hypothesis concerning the distribution of sexes within families. The fact that the class 0–0.3% of males observed was still higher than expected, and the class 0.7–1.00% of males expected was also elevated, means that only a small number of females had families with a low sex

Table 26. Demographic Patterns of the Black Caribs

Cumulative P	Observed	Expected	D	D^2	D^2/expected
Caribs: males 0.433, females 0.567					
0.000	8	6.04	−1.96	3.84	0.636
0.100	15	7.49	−7.51	56.40	7.530
0.200	15	16.51	1.51	2.28	0.138
0.300	12	18.41	6.41	41.09	2.232
0.400	5	3.83	−1.17	1.36	0.355
0.500	24	27.72	3.72	13.84	0.499
0.600	9	8.18	−0.82	0.67	0.082
0.700	15	18.93	3.93	15.44	0.816
0.800	31	31.56	0.56	0.31	0.010
0.900	37	30.88	−7.00	49.00	1.587
					χ^2 13.885
					9 d.f.
					$P = 0.014$
Caribs: males 0.500, females 0.500					
0.000	5	7.52	2.52	6.35	0.844
0.100	13	12.26	−0.74	0.55	0.045
0.200	5	4.42	−0.58	0.34	0.077
0.300	15	22.87	7.87	61.94	2.708
0.400	12	21.26	9.26	85.75	4.033
0.500	0	0.97	0.97	0.94	0.969
0.600	29	32.16	3.16	9.98	0.310
0.700	8	7.20	−0.80	0.64	0.089
0.800	20	25.89	5.89	34.69	1.340
0.900	64	36.20	−27.80	772.84	21.349
					χ^2 31.764
					9 d.f.
					$P < 0.001$
Whites: males 0.500, females 0.500					$P < 0.001$
0.000	10	9.47	−0.53	0.28	0.029
0.100	13	10.92	−2.08	4.33	0.396
0.200	3	3.28	0.28	0.08	0.024
0.300	30	29.64	−0.36	0.13	0.004
0.400	20	19.68	−0.32	0.10	0.005
0.500	2	0.97	−1.03	1.06	1.093
0.600	46	46.89	0.89	0.79	0.017
0.700	3	5.31	2.31	5.34	1.006
0.800	21	22.48	1.48	2.19	0.097
0.900	43	46.17	3.17	10.05	0.218
					χ^2 2.889
					9 d.f.
					$P > 0.98$

Table 27. Test for the Significance of the Difference between the Observed and Expected Distribution of the Sexes within Families

Class, % males	Carib		White	
	Observed	Expected	Observed	Expected
0–0.3				
Male	62	37.10	33	43.86
Female	274	150.43	163	176.27
0.33–0.44				
Male	77	81.26	57	68.77
Female	121	127.35	89	105.72
0.5				
Male	79	84.36	107	100.88
Female	79	84.36	107	100.88
0.56–0.67				
Male	69	127.35	115	105.72
Female	42	81.26	77	68.77
0.7–1.0				
Male	127	150.43	193	176.27
Female	31	37.10	50	43.86
x^2		169.80	13.34	
d.f. 7				
P		< 0.001	0.06–0.07	

ratio, while the majority of the mothers had a normal sex ratio. If we can assume that 75% of the mothers had a normal sex distribution of children (i.e., 52% males), then, in order to characterize the random reproductive survey sample at its initial observed percent of males (0.433), we can give a distribution of 0.17% of males for the remaining 25% of the mothers.*

The expected binomial distribution of sex of progeny within families based on this premise yielded a χ^2 with 3 d.f. of 3.16 ($P = 0.40$). Table 28 summarizes the data tested according to the class of percent of males in families.

There is no biological incongruity to the concept that not all mothers who possess the $Hb^A Hb^A$ genotype are deficient in children of the male sex. If, as suggested, the level of the frequency of the Hb^S gene is related to the intra-uterine fetal–maternal incompatibility due to the presence in the blood stream of the $Hb^A Hb^A$ mother of a *Plasmodium* parasite, one should consider that this may operate in a qualitative manner. The reason why some mothers have a low sex ratio might mean that once a fetal–maternal incompatibility occurred, these mothers lose more progeny by the same process. Other mothers, although

---

* Computation: We have $0.750(0.52) + 0.250X = 0.433$. Thus $X = (0.433 - 0.390)/0.250 = 0.043/0.250 = 0.17$.

Table 28. Analysis of the Sex Distribution in the Random Reproductive Survey, 171 Families

Class percent of males in family	Observed	Expected 0.50	Expected 0.433	Expected 0.247 0.52 / 0.753 0.41		Expected 0.75 0.52 / 0.25 0.17	
0–0.3	61	35.54	52.59	54.70		58.65	
0.33–0.44	31	33.85	38.55	37.61		28.57	
0.5	29	32.22	30.72	29.69		26.04	
0.56–0.67	19	33.85	26.72	26.16		27.28	
0.7–1.00	31	35.54	22.32	22.84		30.46	
x^2 d.f. 3		25.90	8.50	6.79		3.16	
P		<0.001	<0.05	<0.08		$=0.40$	

genetically predisposed for such fetal–maternal interaction, might never have had the opportunity to develop this course of events. Therefore there may be some Hb^AHb^A mothers whose reproductive history is no different, at least in terms of sex of offspring, than for the group of Hb^AHb^S mothers who are unaffected by a fetal–maternal interaction. The critical examination of the distribution of sexes within the families strengthens the viewpoint that the presence or absence of an abnormal hemoglobin gene (Hb^S) in the mother shapes the demographic dimensions of the Black Carib population.

4. Discussion

If the data for mothers belonging to the two different genotypes are summarized, percentages of fertility (as revealed by the 1946 census) are identical, namely:

1. A "high"-fertility group of mothers, who produced 58% of all children in the sample.
2. An "average"-fertility group, who produced 29% of all children in the sample.
3. A "low"-fertility group, who produced 13% of all children in the sample.

Thus, through both the census data and the random survey we can establish that approximately one-third of the females who bear children have large families. This suggests that one of the factors in the changing trends of family size in the Black Carib population may be the result of a change in the frequency of the hemoglobin S gene within this population. It may also be appropriate to speculate on the possible effect of the distribution of genetic factors for sterility or reduced fertility in this particular population. Such genes (if they exist at all) would tend to be at a low level in the Black Carib population, which is presently characterized by large family size. Conversely, if the Black Carib population was to stabilize its population size through reduction in average family size, there might be a gradual accumulation of those genetic factors that control the population level of fecundity. Although selection would still operate negatively on such factors, they would nevertheless remain proportionately higher in the more stable population, where the genetic contributions of both high and low-fertility lines are about equal. Therefore when the Black Carib population assumes new demographic dimensions in terms of family size, the genetic quality related to the fecundity of the population as a whole may also change.

It is reasonable to conclude that we cannot ascribe to all human populations the same genetic capacity for reproduction. From the standpoint of population fitness, all primitive human populations were close to the so-called "species" maximum value of the intrinsic rate of natural increase. This value has been termed the biotic potential, which, in a sense, is the adaptive biological characteristic of human populations that demographers attempt to measure. Although in animal populations natural selection may alter the life history of a species so as to increase its biotic potential, in human populations the situation is more complex. Not only must primitive populations have a high physiological capacity to reproduce, but they must contain social organizations necessary to maintain a high birth rate. A human population may go to extinction rapidly if it loses its adaptive capacity in but one of these areas. The fecundity of a population may be similar for all primitive populations, which usually are not rationally self-limiting. But a shift in fertility may ultimately change the population's potential fecundity at the genetic level. This may be brought about in human populations, not by natural selection per se, but by instituted cultural mores that are newly acquired.

In order to survive, a human population must have an adaptive culture geared to a prevailing adaptive biotic production. Culture, as used in this context, is understood to be that group of social opinions that, directly or indirectly, results in a delicate balance between the social pressures toward bearing children and the biological phenomenon of population growth when weighted against the extractive efficiency of the population within the environment. In reality, the time lag between cognizance of population growth and the necessity to derive operative cultural devices to limit growth is very great. This statement appears to be substantiated by the demographic data on the Black Caribs. With no apparent shift in the trends toward population growth, the Black Caribs are only generations away from a point of mass starvation and consequent population decline. Therefore it is appropriate at this point to examine very briefly the mechanisms that might be responsible for alterations in the biological life potential of human populations.

Operational in the maintenance of equilibrium for human population size is the fact that the reproduction is a reflective act, conditioned by cultural forces. The data on the Black Caribs suggest that the area most responsible for control of population size is the age of mother at birth of her first child. If there is an increase in age at first birth, there is a consequent reduction in the years of exposure to the risk of conception. Other factors being equal, an average increase of 5 years for age at first birth would reduce the total fertility by approximately 20%.

Another facet of population biology that may be altered by socially instituted mores would be increasing the time interval between effective births. In many human societies this has been accomplished by copulation taboos, abortion, or infanticide. This may provide a hiatus of 3 or more years between children. At the moment the data indicate that the Black Carib population is an expanding one. Evidently as part of the cultural makeup of the Black Carib society, there is a conscious wish on the part of the female to beget children; a large family is a socially sanctioned accomplishment. Among Black Carib families, one may find that the spacing of children differs, depending upon the age of the mother at the birth of her first child. In the present generation a young mother exhibits spacing of 3—4 years between births. In the case of mothers who started a family at a relatively later age than average, the spacing of children becomes attenuated. We have recorded in certain families, where the mother started child rearing at the age of 25—30, three consecutive births with little more than a 1-year interval between each birth. So at present the onset of late motherhood may not be an effective *modus operandi* in this population for family size limitation.

References

Allison, A. C., 1954, Protection afforded by the sickle-cell trait against subtertian malarial infection, *Br. Med. J.* 1:290–294.

Allison, A. C., 1955, Notes on sickle-cell polymorphism, *Ann. Hum. Genet.* 19:39–51.

Colonial Office, 1949, Census of population of British Honduras, Government printer, Belize.

Firschein, I. L., 1961, Population dynamics of the sickle-cell trait in the Black Caribs of British Honduras, Central America, *Am. J. Hum. Genet.* 13(2):233–254.

Lehmann, H. and Raper, A. B., 1956, Maintenance of a high sickling rate in an African community, *Br. Med. J.* No. 4988: 333-336.

Rife, B. C. and Snyder, L. H., 1937, The distribution of sex ratios within families in an Ohio city. Studies in human inheritance XVI, *Hum. Biol.* 9(1): 99-103.

6

Past and Present Evidence of Interethnic Mating

Virginia Kerns

1. Introduction

In the last century, a number of Europeans and North Americans traveled through Black Carib settlements in Central America and recorded their impressions of the inhabitants. Despite only fleeting contact, they were struck by the distinctive "manners and customs" of the Black Carib, whom they described, almost without exception, as an "exclusive," endogamous people. A midcentury census from Belize, which enumerated many mixed Caribs, offers a conflicting view: in just 60 years, between their initial entry into Belize in 1802 and the compilation of the 1861 census, Black Caribs had apparently reproduced with a variety of non-Caribs.

Observers in this century have characterized the contemporary Black Carib, like their ancestors of 100 years ago, as a highly endogamous population. According to several ethnographers, Black Caribs rarely mate across ethnic lines. Yet recent census data, collected in several Black Carib communities in Belize and Guatemala, suggest that interethnic unions are not exceptional.

The issue of interethnic mating, to judge from these various sources, has long been a confused one, obscuring a central link between Black Carib culture history and population biology. Without detailed figures on the frequency of reproduction with non-Caribs, the extent to which the Black Caribs were and are a genetically isolated population must remain a matter of conjecture. Neither narrative accounts nor extant population statistics can finally resolve this question. These sources do, however, provide evidence of interethnic mating,

VIRGINIA KERNS • Department of Sociology, Virginia Polytechnic Institute and State University, Blacksburg, Virginia 24061.

which I discuss in the following sections of this chapter, beginning with contemporary accounts and then moving to historical ones. My reading of these
accounts has been colored by my own research experience with Black Caribs,
experience that leads me to suspect that the emphasis on ethnic endogamy has
been somewhat misplaced. Contemporary interethnic mating by the Black
Carib clearly has some "traditional" (18th- and 19th-century) precedent.

2. Twentieth-Century Accounts

Prevailing opinion about the incidence of interethnic mating has shifted
only slightly during this century. Conzemius (1928, p. 123) simply noted in passing
that they "seldom intermarry with other races." Taylor (1951, pp. 38, 40), writing several decades later, similarly described the Black Carib as "a society apart,
whose members rarely intermarry or have any social dealings with the other,
non-Carib communities with which they come in contact." He added that
Miskito Indians were the only group with whom they had "intermarried to any
extent in recent years," and he alluded to his occasional encounters with individuals who claimed mixed Miskito—Carib ancestry. Coelho (1955, pp. 30f.)
also specifically mentioned Black Carib "individuals living in Mosquitia who . . .
are of partly Miskito Indian descent."

More recently, Adams (1957, p. 380), apparently drawing on the accounts
of Guatemalan informants, has characterized legal and extralegal marital unions
by the Black Carib as "tending to be endogamous within the ethnic unit." Firschein
(1961, p. 235) explicitly refers to informants' claims that "only in exceptional
cases will a Black Carib marry outside the group or bear children of the 'creoles'"
in Belize.

Gonzalez (1969, p. 29) takes a different position. Writing about Black
Caribs in Livingston, Guatemala, she states, "Today mixed marriages *do* take
place, upon the Caribs' own admission, and according to my own observations,
predominantly with Negroes . . . . Nevertheless, the Caribs maintain as an ideal
that they never marry with anyone outside their own group."

To judge from Ghidinelli's (1976, p. 75) figures on the parentage of children
born in Livingston, interethnic mating by Black Caribs is not at all uncommon
there. I have converted his data on the parentage of Black Carib children from
percentages to numbers; these are summarized in Table 1.

As Table 1 shows, only Ladinos (who, with Black Caribs, constitute the
majority of the population of Livingston) were specified as parents of the mixed-
Carib children. Negroes were not separately enumerated, although presumably
they might be included among the men listed as "padre desconocido" or among
the women belonging to "otros grupos ethicos." Only 46% of the children were
known to have two Black Carib parents, while 21% were known to have a non-
Carib parent. The remainder, or 33%, had Black Carib mothers but fathers whose
ethnic identity was unknown to the census takers.

Table 1. Parentage of Black Carib and Mixed-Carib Children Born in Livingston, Guatemala, 1972

Paternal ethnic identity	Maternal ethnic identity	Number of children	Percent of children
Black Carib	Black Carib	26	46
Black Carib	Ladino	4	7
Black Carib	Other[a]	5	9
Ladino	Black Carib	3	5
Unknown[b]	Black Carib	19	33
Total		57	100

[a] "Otros grupos etnicos."
[b] "Padre desconocido."

Table 2. Interethnic Unions of Black Caribs in Punta Gorda, Belize, 1965

Male's ethnic identity	Female's ethnic identity	Number of ethnic unions	Percent of ethnic unions
Black Carib	Creole, mixed Creole	3	33
Creole	Black Carib	3	33
Black Carib	Spanish	2	22
East Indian	Black Carib	1	11
Total		9	99

Cosminsky (1976, p. 106) provides data of a different type on interethnic mating in the nearby town of Punta Gorda, Belize. She enumerates interethnic unions, rather than their offspring, specifying the gender of Black Caribs with non-Carib spouses.* I have summarized her data in Table 2.

Table 2 shows that the majority of the interethnic unions formed by Black Caribs in Punta Gorda (six of the nine) were with Creoles. This is in apparent contrast to nearby Livingston, where most mixed-Carib children of known parentage had a Ladino parent. In Punta Gorda, unlike Livingston, the Spanish (as Spanish-speaking Mestizos are called in Belize) are an extremely small minority, about 5% of the population. Creoles, far more numerous, constitute nearly 18% of the population. They form the second largest ethnic group in the town, following the Black Carib with 70% (Cosminsky, 1976, p. 197). In Livingston and Punta Gorda alike, Black Caribs form most interethnic unions with members of the next largest ethnic group: Ladinos in the case of Livingston, Creoles in the case of Punta Gorda.

During my own fieldwork in several Black Carib villages in Belize, I did not

* "Spouse" refers here and throughout the chapter to partners of extralegal as well as legal coresidential unions.

have access to statistics comparable to Ghidinelli's on child-productive inter-ethnic mating. For a number of reasons discussed in Section 3.1, the government of Belize has not consistently collected accurate and detailed census data on ethnicity; and currently, as a matter of policy, it deemphasizes ethnic differences in an attempt to foster national unity and a sense of common identity among the small but highly plural populations (Grant, 1976, p. 8). My own obser-vations, however, and informants' statements as well, convince me that inter-ethnic unions are not unusual. I was personally acquainted with a number of Black Carib men and women in villages and elsewhere who lived with non-Carib spouses. Informants told me of many more cases, particularly men who claimed to have resided with non-Carib women or to have reproduced with them while working in other districts in Belize. These claims are obviously difficult to document.

Whatever their basis in fact, the claims themselves are significant. Neither these men nor any of my other informants described interethnic unions as undesirable or otherwise objectionable, and none expressed personal reluctance to form such a union. Villagers did not state ethnic endogamy as an ideal, in constrast to the town residents, who were Cosminsky's and Firschein's infor-mants in Belize and Gonzalez's informants in Guatemala. Indeed, a number of men and women explicitly denied that ethnicity should be a primary con-sideration in the selection of a spouse. Women spoke of the importance of a man's character and wage-earning abilities. Men stressed an even temperament and fidelity as important qualities in a woman. Both men and women referred to mutual attraction, "love," as ideally the primary criterion in selecting a spouse; and this and the other qualities, they insisted, were not unique to Black Caribs but might also be found in a non-Carib.

Many of the men and women whom I questioned did express a preference for local endogamy, which they explained as a matter of pragmatic and personal choice. Women, in particular, voiced strong reservations about living with "strangers" in other Black Carib communities, and a great many expressed a preference to live near their own kin (Kerns, 1983). Since Black Carib villages in Belize include very few non-Caribs as residents, to practice local endogamy in these communities is to practice ethnic endogamy. In contrast to Punta Gorda, where 30% of the population was non-Carib when Cosminsky collected figures on interethnic unions, less than 1% of the population was non-Carib in the three villages I surveyed. Most of these were adult males, born elsewhere and living in the natal communities of their Black Carib spouses.

Despite differences in ethnic composition between Black Carib towns and villages, the data I collected on interethnic mating in the three villages (Table 3) are generally consistent with those for Punta Gorda. In villages and town alike, the majority of the interethnic unions were with Creoles (66% in Punta Gorda, 60% in the villages), who constitute the largest ethnic group in Belize. The next most numerous in villages and towns (about 20% in both cases) were unions with

Table 3. Interethnic Unions in Three Black Carib Villages, Belize, 1975

Male's ethnic identity	Female's ethnic identity	Number of interethnic unions	Percent of interethnic unions
Creole	Black Carib	3	60
Black Carib	Maya	1	20
Spanish	Black Carib	1	20
Total		5	100

Spanish, who, following Creoles, are the country's next largest ethnic group. Of course, the close correspondence of these figures may simply be a matter of change. Alternatively, it may indicate a rather regular relationship between the proportional ethnic composition of the national (or perhaps regional) population and the proportion of various non-Caribs with whom Black Caribs form unions. Thus, both town- and village-dwelling Black Caribs in Belize most frequently form interethnic unions with Creoles, the largest ethnic group – and this despite their often cited reluctance to do so (e.g., Waddell, 1961, p. 72; Burdon, 1935, p. 224).

Finally, there is the question of the actual incidence of interethnic mating and its relation to the ethnic composition of communities and the practice of local endogamy. The Black Carib population of Belize is concentrated in two towns, Punta Gorda and Dangriga (the former Stann Creek Town), where men and women can find non-Carib spouses within the community. The figures in Tables 2 and 3 suggest that the incidence of interethnic mating is higher in towns than in villages. There were nearly twice as many interethnic unions in Punta Gorda as in the three villages, although the Black Carib population of the town was somewhat smaller (about 1250 in 1965 as compared to a total population slightly under 1450 for the villages in 1975). In Punta Gorda, however, unlike the villages, nearly half of the interethnic unions (four of the nine) were locally endogamous (Cosminsky, 1976, pp. 105f.).

In the villages, in contrast, all of the interethnic unions were locally exogamous. I found that the vast majority of the unions (85%) in the villages were endogamous to both community and ethnic group. Of the minority (15%) of locally exogamous unions, about one-fifth were interethnic. In other words, although local exogamy was quite uncommon, in about one of every five cases in which spouses did come from different communities, one was a non-Carib. Table 4 shows the number and proportion of exogamous and endogamous unions in the three villages. It enumerates only coresidential unions. Although a number of village residents claimed to have extraresidential relationships with non-Caribs in other communities, I have not included these, because of the difficulty of documenting them.

Although I initially thought it likely that interethnic mating and my

Table 4. Endogamous and Exogamous Unions in Three Black Carib Villages, 1975

	Local endogamy		Local exogamy	
	Number of unions	Percent of unions	Number of unions	Percent of unions
Intraethnic unions	146	85	21	12
Interethnic unions	–	–	5	3
Total	146	· 85	26	15

informants' liberal attitudes toward it represented a recent change, I soon gave up this idea. In the course of collecting genealogies, I discovered that several of my elderly informants, born before or shortly after the turn of the century, claimed a non-Carib parent or grandparent. After I returned from the field, I also found documentary evidence of interethnic mating.

These documentary sources of information on the Black Carib fall into two categories: narrative accounts written by travelers to Belize, Guatemala, and Honduras and by government officials in Belize; and population statistics for 19th-century Belize. I will deal separately with these sources in the following two sections, beginning with narrative accounts. Accepted literally, these accounts suggest that the Black Caribs were a strictly endogamous and genetically isolated population during the last century. Population statistics suggest otherwise.

3. Nineteenth-Century Accounts

Nineteenth-century travelers' accounts and government reports that include ethnographic information on the Black Carib vary widely in quality. Most travelers had only fleeting and superficial relations with the Black Carib. A few, notably Thomas Young (1847), were curious and culturally sensitive observers whose contact was more sustained and whose accounts provide more reliable and detailed information.

While many travelers, as transient observers, left cursory and somewhat confused accounts of the Black Carib, officials who resided in Belize were no better informed, to judge from their reports. Belizean authorities had opposed the entry of the earliest Black Carib immigrants in the first decade of the 19th century. Official resistance soon gave way to neglect, as the population settled in remote areas along the southern coast. Given the geographical isolation of Black Carib settlements, at a distance from officialdom, government correspondents apparently drew on hearsay for their occasional accounts of the Black Carib. One official, for example, described the Black Carib as "a mixed race, said to be descended from the Mosquito Indians and African Negroes" (Great Britain, 1870, p. 30).

Most 19th-century accounts agree that, however mixed the Black Caribs' ancestry, they were a strictly endogamous group. Reports of their endogamy cover nearly the entire span of the last century, beginning with Orlando Roberts' account, written after his journey through several Black Carib settlements in 1820 or so. When Roberts visited these settlements, the inhabitants were themselves newcomers to the territory, having arrived less than a generation before from their homeland in St. Vincent. Roberts (1827, p. 273) explicitly stated that a Black Carib was the source of his information on ethnic endogamy: "Louis, one of their headmen, informed me, that they never interfered with the Indians, by intermarriage or otherwise."

Later travelers, who were not so clear about their sources of information, also commented on Black Carib endogamy. John Lloyd Stephens (1841, pp. 12, 28), in one of the most widely read travelers' accounts of the era, noted the prevalence of interethnic mating between whites and (Creole) blacks in Belize. From his account, however, Black Caribs were not party to this "amalgamation," which he found so remarkable. Spending only a day in a Black Carib settlement in southern Belize, he described them as "living apart, as a tribe . . . not mingling their blood with that of their conquerors." Some years later, in 1859, a resident of Belize wrote about the Black Carib population, "They congregate in villages apart and seldom, if ever, intermarry with the negroes" (Burdon, 1935, p. 224).

In the latter part of the century, Helene Sandborn, the daughter of the American coffee magnate, traveled through a Black Carib settlement in Guatemala. She remarked in passing, "The Caribs are especially noticeable for keeping themselves very distinct, and never intermarrying with other tribes" (Sanborn, 1886, p. 30). During the same period, Maudslay and Maudslay (1899, pp. 155, 189) had some contact with Black Caribs both in Belize and Guatemala. They characterized the Black Caribs as "an exclusive people," adding, "it is most curious to note how distinct they have kept from the Creole negroes, no Carib woman ever being known (unless a change has quite recently been made) to cohabit with a negro of another race."

Despite these assertions, there is reason to suspect that ethnic endogamy was not absolute. A careful reading of the accounts suggests that a number of factors produced an image of the Black Carib as a closed, highly endogamous ethnic group. These include their distinctiveness, both culturally and linguistically, from other ethnic groups; pronounced social distance vis-à-vis non-Caribs in certain contexts; and the geographical isolation of their settlements.

It deserves emphasis that none of these factors necessarily prevented sexual relations between individual Black Caribs and non-Caribs; population statistics bear witness to the fact that such relations did occur, resulting in mixed offspring. But certainly these several factors helped to sustain an image of the Black Carib as a closed group. One writer noted, for example, that "they cling tenaciously to their traditions, and neither care to inform an outsider about their private lives" (Charles, 1890, p. 115). Others wrote that "they seem to be an exclusive people, who give one the idea of tolerating the white population of the village rather than being tolerated by them." Maudslay and Maudslay (1899, p. 155) gave as supporting evidence of this view the fact that Black Caribs refused to sell fish to their non-Carib neighbors "until the wants of every Carib household are supplied . . . and not infrequently the whole catch is disposed of to the Caribs and the white people get none of it." Similarly, Sanborn (1886, p. 30) remarked that "they will not sell, at any price, their market goods until every Carib has first been supplied." Unlike the other observers, however, she attributed this pattern of distribution to "very strong family feeling." If the present provides any guidance to the past, she was correct. In many Black Carib villages, the sale of fish is still governed by kinship and personal relationships as well as by commercial considerations (Kerns, 1983).

In other situations, Black Caribs may have deliberately promoted the view that they were very distinct and separate from other groups. Bedford Pim (1863, pp. 295, 312) commented about the Black Carib men in his employ:

> It was amusing to hear the contemptuous way in which they spoke of
> the [Negro] natives, and to see the distant manner which they pre-
> served towards them . . . [Y]ou could not insult a Carib more than by
> hinting at *any* relationship between himself and the African.

Since wage labor was quite competitive, the Black Carib men whom Pim described may well have found it to their advantage to emphasize any differences between themselves and black non-Caribs, given their employer's biased view of the latter. "I am not partial to the negro," he commented; "his sloth and insolence irritate me." The Black Carib, however, he considered "a very different race . . . eminently industrious, thrifty, and intelligent" (Pim, 1863, p. 295).

According to Young (1847, pp. 134f.), in contrast, there was no visible antagonism between the Black Carib and non-Carib men he observed. His account does suggest an element of social distance among the men who attended re-creational "nightly assemblies." Black Carib men took active roles as singers, dancers, and musicians, while Miskito and Sambo men simply looked on. Their fellowship was obviously limited, more a matter of association than coparticipation, but it appears to have been amiable enough.

To casual observers, scenes like those described by Bedford Pim and Thomas Young may have reinforced their image of the Black Caribs as a highly bounded and endogamous group, a view still prevalent among non-Caribs in Belize. Many non-Caribs today, and perhaps those in the past, employ a questionable deductive process that begins with male interethnic relationships and proceeds directly to male–female ones. Social distance between Black Carib and non-Carib males does not, however, and did not preclude interethnic mating.

A final fact that surely contributed to the widespread view of Black Caribs as a closed ethnic unit during the 19th century was a geographical one: the isolation of their settlements. No doubt it was this isolation that led one resident of Belize to note about the Black Caribs' "Their ambition is to be left alone, and live as their forefathers have before them, and if disturbed or annoyed, simply move to another place" (Fowler, 1879, p. 52). Contemporary writers, who likewise draw on casual contact or hearsay, make similar assertions, sometimes linking geographical isolation with ethnic endogamy (e.g., Dobson, 1973, p. 256).

Two other points about 19th-century reports of Black Carib endogamy require brief comment. One is that, despite apparent consensus, there are some significant differences among the accounts. One traveler, Sanborn, characterized the Black Carib as strictly endogamous; but it is clear from her other comments that her contact with them was particularly limited and brief, and that much of her information came from a non-Carib fellow traveler. The other travelers whose accounts I have cited all qualified their statements about endogamy in one way or another. Roberts referred to an informant's claim that Black Caribs did not intermarry with *Indians*. Two other travelers, Maudslay and Maudslay, as well as a resident of Belize who reported on the Black Carib, state that unions with *Negroes* were unknown or very rare; and the Maudslays further restricted this observation specifically to Black Carib women. Finally, Stephens, who was so impressed with the extent of the black—white interbreeding in Belize, implied that Black Caribs, unlike black Creoles, did not form unions with *whites*. At first glance, then, these accounts seem corroborative; a more careful reading reveals fundamental differences among them.

The second point is that Thomas Young (1847), who left the most detailed description of the 19th-century Black Carib, explicitly noted one instance of interethnic mating by early immigrants to the Mosquito Shore. A "very old" informant, who had arrived there as a boy in the company of several other Black Caribs (most of them male), described to Young (1847, pp. 129f.) their reception by the Miskito Indian inhabitants of the area. The old man claimed that

> They were immediately fed, and taken much notice of; they built them-selves houses, made plantations, *intermarried with the natives, and gradually increased in numbers* and importance, till at length they determined, from some cause not now to be ascertained, to remove to Little Rock [emphasis added].

Unlike other travelers, whose contact with the Black Carib was far more limited, Young made no sweeping generalizations about ethnic endogamy. Although he resided on the Mosquito Shore for 3 years (1839–1841) and traveled extensively there, he did not characterize the Black Carib as "exclusive" or strictly endogamous. His silence may represent simple oversight or, alternatively, a more profound insight into Black Carib life. Perhaps Young refrained from commenting on a subject that defined easy summation. Population statistics from 19th-century Belize show the complexity of inter-ethnic mating there.

3.1. Nineteenth-Century Population Statistics

In censuses taken during the last decades of the 19th century in Belize, Black Caribs were separately enumerated. The 1881 census shows that of the colony's total population of 27,452, nearly one-tenth, some 2037, were Black Caribs. The remainder of the population was divided among five other categories: "natives" of the colony, including the native-born "colored," Indians, and mestizos; "Yucatecans"; "Central American Spaniards"; black West Indians; and Europeans (Bristowe and Wright, 1888, pp. 200f.).

There is good reason to exercise caution in using 19th-century census materials from Belize. Census takers there worked under such difficult conditions that errors were inevitable in their reports. Not only was communication problematic, but the population was quite mobile. The seasonal movement of laborers, as well as travel during holiday periods, interfered with accurate census taking. Bristowe and Wright (1888, p. 220) specifically mention these problems in relation to the 1871 and 1881 censuses, observing that

> due allowance must be made for the fact that the census of 1871 was taken during Christmas-time, when the Central District in particular was very full, owing to large numbers of people coming in for the Christmas festivities; and that the census of 1881 was taken in April, at a time when large numbers had left the towns and returned to their labours at cutting wood at Roman and other places out of the colony.[*]

Census takers faced obstacles that made the collection of accurate figures a formidable task. But they compounded the problem of accuracy with ambiguity, by classifying the population into varying ethnic categories from one census to the next. This may indicate their continuing uncertainty about how to construct meaningful categories in Belize, where there were no legal or serious social barriers to interethnic mating, and where, consequently, much of the population was of mixed ancestry. Interethnic unions appear to have been more common than not, to judge from Stephens' (1841, p. 12) observations as well as the returns of the 1861 census. Given such a population, census takers in Belize usually responded by dividing it into a few gross, very arbitrary, categories; witness the category "natives" in the 1881 census, or "colored" and "mixed" in other enumerations, where nonwhite individuals of various ethnic origins were grouped in one catchall category.

In contrast to the usual strategy of "lumping," at least one instance of remarkable ethnic "splitting" occurred in 19th-century census taking in Belize. This was in the census of 1861, at a time when large-scale immigration into the country was underway. Some of this immigration was the result of attempts to import foreign labor in the wake of emancipation, although Belize lagged far behind most other British West Indian territories in this effort. Many of the

---

[*] Bristowe and Wright apparently refer to the Roman River. On the map that forms the frontispiece of his book, Squier (1855) identifies the Roman River as the Rio Aguan, the name used on contemporary maps of Honduras. Young (1847, p. 124) mentions the Roman River as a site of mahogany works where many Black Carib men sought employment as woodcutters.

other new residents were refugees from the Yucatan. Fleeing the War of the Castes, they settled primarily in the northern part of Belize (Dobson, 1973, pp. 294 ff.).

Perhaps in response to this on-going immigration, and the anticipated change to formal colonial status (which Belize was granted in 1862), census takers in 1861 collected very detailed figures on the ethnic composition of the population. They used some 40 highly specific categories, based on ethnic (racial and national) origins. So fine was the classification that one category, "Swiss," contained a single individual. Unfortunately, even this specificity did not entirely dispel the ambiguity that plagued other censuses of the century. Some of the ethnic categories that census takers used in 1861 remain highly ambiguous. The distinction between "Carib and English" and "Anglo-Carib," for example, is not readily apparent.

Table 5 shows the ethnic categories used in the 1861 census and the number of individuals enumerated for each major ethnic group and mixed category.* (Some of the mixed categories appear twice in the table. "Africo-Caribs," for example, are included both as mixed Caribs and mixed Africans.) Of the colony's total population of 25,635, some 1825 people were classified as Black Carib and 560 others as mixed Carib. The last figure attests to the fact that Black Caribs contributed to the mixed population of Belize during the last century.† The census data do indicate that child-productive interethnic mating by Black Caribs was *relatively* less common than by other ethnic groups in Belize at midcentury. The data do *not* indicate that it was exceptional.

In view of these figures, assertions that Black Caribs never mated across ethnic lines, or that they never mated with Europeans (whites) or Africans (Creoles, Negroes) in 19th-century Belize, are unfounded. Table 5 shows that Black Caribs reproduced with all of the other major ethnic groups (except Chinese and East Indians, whose numbers were negligible), and that they did so roughly in order of the other groups' proportional representation in the population. Thus, most mixed Caribs were the offspring of unions between Black Caribs and Indians, who were the largest ethnic group enumerated. These

---

* The primary source for these census data is the Blue Book of Statistics for the Colony of British Honduras (Colonial Office, 1861), which I consulted at the Public Records Office, Kew, England. Bristowe and Wright (1890) and the Colonial Office (1948, p. 225) provide summaries of the 1861 census data, regrouped into very general categories. In Table 5, I have used the original categories, with the exception of European nationalities, which I put into the European (non-Hispanic white) category. It included 880 Anglo-Saxons, 59 French, 46 Germans, 44 Belgians, 26 Portuguese, 13 Dutch, nine Italian–French, seven Italians, seven Anglo-Americans, five Portuguese–French, two Danes, two Anglo-French, and one Swiss, for a total of 1101 Europeans living in Belize in 1861.

† Belize was not exceptional in this regard. Writing about Guatemala, Brigham (1887, p. 421) commented that it was difficult to study race "in a country where there is so much amalgamation." He then listed the names of 15 "crosses," beginning with the well-known "Mestizo" or "Ladino" and proceeding to such types as "Barsino," "Grifo," and "Chaniso."

Table 5. Ethnic Composition of Belize, 1861

Ethnic group	Number	Mixed ethnic group	Number
		Indian and Carib	323
		Carib and Indian	110
		Africo-Carib	97
		Carib and African	15
		Spanish and Carib	10
		Anglo-Carib	3
		Carib and English	2
Black Carib	1825	Total mixed Carib	560
		Indian and Spanish	3765
		Spanish and Indian	3693
		Anglo-Indian	464
		Indian and Carib	323
		Indian and African	252
		Africo-Indian	213
		Carib and Indian	110
		French and Indian	32
Indian	4675	Total mixed Indian	8852
		Anglo-African	2544
		Africo-English	1488
		Africo-Spanish	340
		Indian and African	252
		Africo-Indian	213
		Africo-Carib	97
		Spanish and African	36
		Carib and African	15
African	2528	Total mixed African	4985
		Indian and Spanish	3765
		Spanish and Indian	3693
		Africo-Spanish	340
		Spanish and English	71
		Anglo-Hispanic	51
		Spanish and African	36
		Anglo-Honduranian	16
		French and Spanish	12
		Spanish and Carib	10
Spanish	1713	Total mixed Spanish	7994
		Anglo-African	2544
		Africo-English	1488
		Anglo-Indian	464
		Spanish and English	71
		Anglo-Hispanic	51
		French and Indian	32
		Anglo-Honduranian	16
		French and Spanish	12
		Anglo-Carib	3
		Carib and English	2
European (non-Hispanic white)	1101	Total mixed European	4683
East Indian	9	Total mixed East Indian	0
Chinese	7	Total mixed Chinese	0

Carib–Indians accounted for 433 of the total 560 mixed Caribs, or 77%. There were 112 Carib–Africans, representing 20% of all mixed Caribs. Africans formed the second largest group in Belize in 1861. The remainder of mixed Caribs, 10 Carib–Spanish and five Carib–Europeans, respectively comprised 2% and 1% of the total. The Spanish were the third largest group enumerated in the census, and Europeans the smallest.

The 1861 census also included information on the regional distribution of ethnic groups in Belize. In the past, as today, the majority of the Black Carib population was concentrated in the southern region of the country, where their settlements were located. Most mixed Caribs, however, lived outside the south. Table 6 shows the regional distribution of Black Caribs and mixed Caribs in 1861.

Slightly less than one-quarter of the Black Carib population lived in the central and northern regions of Belize in 1861. Presumably, many of them were men, who routinely left their homes in the south to find seasonal wage work in other areas of the country (Kerns, 1983, p. 33). Most mixed Caribs – some 60% of them – also lived in the central region and the north. Many men today, as I have already mentioned, claim to have reproduced with non-Carib women while working in other areas of the country. Their great-great-grandfathers may have done so as well.

Table 6. Regional Distribution of Black Caribs and Mixed Caribs in Belize, 1861

Region	Ethnic group	Mixed Caribs		Black Caribs	
		Number	Percent	Number	Percent
North	Carib–Indian	140			
	Carib–African	48			
	Carib–Spanish	3			
	Carib-European	0			
	Subtotal	191	34	101	6
Central	Carib–Indian	81			
	Carib–African	56			
	Carib–Spanish	7			
	Carib–European	2			
	Subtotal	146	26	298	16
South	Carib–Indian	212			
	Carib–African	8			
	Carib–Spanish	0			
	Carib–European	3			
	Subtotal	223	40	1426	78
	Total	560	100	1825	100

Table 7. Ratio of Mixed to Nonmixed Individuals for Major Ethnic Groups in Belize, 1861

Ethnic category	Number of mixed individuals	Number of nonmixed individuals	Ratio of mixed to nonmixed
Black Carib	560	1825	0.30
Indian	8852	4675	1.89
African	4985	2528	1.97
European	4683	1101	4.25
Spanish	7994	1713	4.66

While mating with non-Caribs occurred, Table 7 shows that the incidence of child-productive interethnic mating by Black Caribs was far lower than by any of the other major ethnic groups. The figures from Table 5 are used to give in Table 7 the ratio of mixed to nonmixed individuals for each of the major categories.

Table 7 suggests that Black Caribs engaged in relatively less child-productive interethnic mating than did the Indian, Spanish, African, and European residents of Belize. Further, they were the only major ethnic group to produce fewer mixed than nonmixed individuals. Less than one-third as many mixed Caribs as (nonmixed) Black Caribs were enumerated in the 1861 census. In contrast, there were four times as many mixed as nonmixed Spanish and Europeans, and almost twice as many mixed Africans and mixed Indians, respectively, as nonmixed Africans and Indians.

The Black Caribs were highly endogamous *only relative to* these other groups.

4. The Problem of Genetic Isolation

Although population statistics provide evidence of interethnic mating, one extremely murky issue that they cannot resolve is whether the Black Carib population was genetically isolated. The question is, did mixed Caribs in the past ever remain within the ethnic group and contribute to the gene pool by reproducing with nonmixed Black Caribs? Or were they, and any children they produced, categorically excluded from the ethnic group on the basis of their mixed ancestry?

Conflicting answers have been given to these questions with regard to the contemporary population. According to Firschein (1961, p. 235), "individuals and the children of the few mixed marriages that do exist are not considered as belonging to the Black Caribs and generally they live outside the environs of the group." Gonzalez (1969, p. 29) states, in contrast, that "children resulting from mixed [Black Carib and Negro] unions are nearly always raised as Caribs, being abandoned by their Negro parent." Firschein describes the Black Carib as a genetically isolated population, while Gonzalez does not.

My own research with the Black Carib suggests that they are not a genetically isolated population today and were not one in the past. Genealogical evidence, slender as it is, shows that some, but not all, mixed Caribs did in fact reproduce within the ethnic unit and thereby contributed to the gene pool. On the basis of informants' statements and actual genealogies, I can suggest one principle to explain which mixed Caribs have generally remained and reproduced within the group and which have not. This principle was summarized in the following words by a middle-aged Black Carib man, a village resident: "If the mother is Carib, the children are Carib. If the mother is Creole, the children are Creole. Children come through the mother." His point was that children born to Black Carib women and non-Carib men are usually identified and enculturated as Black Carib. In the opposite circumstance, this is less likely, although not unknown by any means.

I cannot claim to have surveyed a wide range of men and women about the validity of this principle. I considered interethnic mating an intriguing but tangential issue at that point in my fieldwork. The fact that I gradually collected a body of information about it probably had as much to do with my informants' as my own interests and directed efforts. Several men and women, on their own initiative, brought cases to my attention. I will briefly describe six of these, involving men and women with whom I was personally acquainted. They illustrate the various circumstances that affect the transmission of Black Carib ethnicity to the mixed offspring of interethnic unions.

The first of my informants to mention mixed ancestry to me was a 60-year-old man whose father was Spanish and mother Black Carib. He grew up in his father's community, a predominantly Creole town; but throughout childhood he made frequent and extended visits with his mother to her natal village. He resides there today, and has on an occasional basis for over 40 years. A fluent Carib-speaker, he alternately identifies himself as Black Carib or "mixed." He has no children.

A younger man, about 32 years old and a resident of the same village, was raised there by his Black Carib mother after her brief union with a Spanish man lapsed. He speaks Carib, is married to a Black Carib woman, and has several children with her. The children are uniformly identified by others as Black Carib. As for their father, he has a somewhat situational ethnic identity, emphaizing either his Black Carib or Spanish parentage when it is to his advantage to do so.

This is in contrast to a 55-year-old woman who identifies herself as Black Carib and only on occasion refers to her "Spanish blood," Her father, who was the offspring of a Spanish–Carib union, married a Black Carib woman, with whom he had several children. All of them identify as Black Caribs and have reproduced with Black Carib spouses. The woman scoffs at the idea that there are any "pure Caribs" today in Belize, citing her own ancestry and others', and, as further evidence, the fact that most Black Caribs are dark-skinned. Mythological and contemporary social reality merge in her comment: "Originally, we were light-skinned," she says, but through interbreeding with "other nations" Black Caribs became darker skinned (cf. Taylor, 1951, p. 39).

An older woman, aged 76, refers to her father occasionally as a "Creole man." She explains that her father's mother was a Creole and her father's father a Black Carib. The old woman's father was born well before the turn of the century, probably sometime after 1870. At the age of 8, her father left the Creole settlement where he had been born and went to live with paternal kin in his father's natal village. He learned to speak fluent Carib and eventually formed a union with the old woman's mother, who was herself a Black Carib. The old woman likewise married a Black Carib man and bore several children by him. She and all of her descendants identify themselves and are identified by others as Black Caribs.

A more recent case of interethnic mating involves a 30-year-old resident of the village, a Black Carib man. Several years ago he married a Mayan women whom he met while living in another district. They have several young children, who are usually identified as "mixed" by both the parents and other people in the village. One can only hazard a guess about their reproductive futures, but were they to remain in the village, it would be unusual if they did not form unions there. The children have learned to speak Carib, largely from their playmates.

Finally, there is the case of a Black Carib man who has resided for over 30 years in the western district, where Black Caribs are few and largely transient. A respected government official, he is married to a Spanish woman and has several children by her. None of them speak Carib, and Black Caribs identify them as "mixed." Speaking about the father, another highly educated Black Carib man asserted that he, too, intends to "marry up" the social ladder by taking a Spanish wife (cf. Cosminsky, 1976).

These cases and others offer support for the idea that, generally speaking, "children come through the mother." They suggest that individuals are likely to speak Carib, identify themselves and be identified as Black Carib, and to reproduce within the ethnic group if their mothers are Black Carib, whatever their fathers appear less likely to do so, except in the circumstance that they grow up among Black Caribs. Even then, they seem usually to be identifed as "mixed" or assigned their mothers' ethnic identities, although they may reproduce within the ethnic group. This was the case with two men, fathers of the female informants I have briefly described.

Another shared feature of both of these cases, and several others as well, is that individuals of mixed parentage are generally identified as mixed, while those of mixed grandparentage (with only one non--Carib grandparent) are not. The two women, for example, acknowledge their mixed ancestry but identify them-

selves and are identified by others as Black Carib. Since genealogical remem-
brance is shallow among Black Caribs, rarely extending further than the third or
fourth ascending generation, even this limited recognition of mixed ancestry
may well die with the women's children.

I suspect that more than women's obvious influence as socializers accounts
for the prevailing pattern in the transmission of ethnicity. Life histories and
demographic data show that Black Carib women tend to spend greater portions
of their adult lives than do men residing in Black Carib communities. The
sex ratios of these settlements are generally skewed, with far more adult
females than adult males in residence. To judge from the accounts of 19th-
century travelers, this was also the case in the past (Stephens, 1841, p. 30; cf.
Burdon, 1935, pp. 223f.). At any rate, men today typically spend years of their
adult lives working and residing in non-Carib areas. Their ethnically mixed
children are less likely than those of Black Carib women to grow up in Black
Carib communities.

The several cases of interethnic mating that I have discussed offer some
insight into the transmission of Black Carib ethnicity, and they suggest that the
Black Carib are not a genetically isolated population today. It is difficult to
reconstruct the 19th-century situation; neither written accounts of the period
nor population statistics provide much help in this matter. The living may be
able to provide some clues. Future researchers would do well to work extensively
with very elderly informants, whose parents and grandparents were born in the
last century, and who might provide genealogical information that would help to
clarify the issue of genetic isolation in the past.

5. Conclusions

In dealing with records that pertain to Black Carib culture history and
population biology, researchers must often untangle apparently conflicting
details before drawing even tentative conclusions. The population statistics
reviewed here clearly support only one general point: that contemporary interethnic mating has historical precedent. Census figures and other records suggest
that there have been many exceptions to any normative rule of ethnic endogamy.
Eighteenth-century accounts from St. Vincent refer to unions of Black Caribs
with captive Carib Indians and runaway African slaves. Both the Caribs and
white planters complained of these with great rancor (Labat, 1970, p. 137;
Anon, 1773, p. 26f). If Thomas Young's (1847, p. 129) elderly informant was
a reliable source, some Black Caribs that immigrated to the Mosquito Shore
also mated with non-Caribs there. The 1861 census of Belize offers the next
evidence of this pattern, followed by contemporary ethnographic reports of
interethnic mating.

This raises a final question: Was the Black Caribs' rapid population growth in Central America, and in St. Vincent as well, due in some measure to their reproducing with non-Caribs? To judge from 18th-century records from St. Vincent, a steady influx of fugitive slaves and captive Carib Indian women augmented the Black Caribs' natural population increase. By 1763 the Black Carib numbered 3000 (Anon, 1773, p. 6). Scarcely 35 years later, before they were deported to Roatan, the population had grown to about 5000.* Less than half of this number survived the forced removal from St. Vincent to Central America.† Once there, however, the population reportedly grew quite rapidly. If this growth were to continue, it was predicted, the Black Carib would "obtain the entire ascendancy" of the area north of Cape Gracias à Dios (Roberts, 1827, p. 154; cf. Young, 1847, pp. 36, 159; Squier, 1855, pp. 208, 212). This has in fact, come to pass. the Black Carib today form the primary population of the long coastal strip between Dangriga, Belize, and Plaplaya, Honduras (Davidson, 1976, p. 86).

However difficult it is to grasp the statistical reality of Black Carib mating patterns, both in the past and at present, we can at least be wary of stereotypes that oversimplify that reality. It seems that a number of factors have helped to produce and sustain a widely accepted view of the Black Carib as a strictly endogamous group. Black Caribs have often been willing accomplices to this, to judge from many ethnographic accounts; and the conception remains current among non-Caribs in Belize. It also persists in outsiders' accounts of the country. Waddell (1961, p. 72) remarks in passing that "the Caribs themselves are resistant to intermarriage with 'creoles.'" Dobson (1973, p. 245) sums up prevailing views when she asserts that, "Few of [the Black Carib] have chosen to marry outside their race or to leave the coastal settlements where the majority make their living from farming and fishing." These words might have come from a 19th-century pen, and they are probably as misleading a description of the Black Carib of 100 years ago as they are of those today.

ACKNOWLEDGMENTS

This paper is based in part on fieldwork carried out in Belize from October 1974 to October 1975. I am grateful to the Fulbright-Hays Commission for a doctoral dissertation fellowship and to the Wenner-Gren Foundation for a grant-in-aid (#3058), which made my research possible. I wish to thank Ruth Kerns for her bibliographic help, which added some new pieces to the puzzle.

* This is the figure given by Taylor (1951, p. 26). According to Gonzalez (1983), historians have estimated that as few as 2000 or as many as 5000 Black Caribs were deported.

† Gonzalez (unpublished manuscript) cites archival evidence that 4195 Black Caribs were evacuated in July, 1796, from St. Vincent to the island of Baliseau. Nearly half had died by March, 1797, when the deportation to Roatan began. Only 2026 arrived there.

References

Adams, Richard N., 1957, Cultural Surveys of Panama—Nicaragua—Guatemala—El Salvador—Honduras, Pan American Sanitary Bureau, Scientific Publications, no. 33, Washington, D.C.

Anon, 1773, *Authentic Papers Relative to the Expedition Against the Charibbs and the Sale of Lands in the Island of St. Vincent*, J. Almon, London.

Brigham, W. 1887, *Guatemala, Land of the Quetzal*, Charles Scribner's Sons, New York.

Bristowe, L., and Wright, P., 1888, *The Handbook of British Honduras*, Blackwood and Sons, Edinburgh.

Bristowe, L., and Wright, P., 1890, *The Handbook of British Honduras*, Blackwood and Sons, Edinburgh.

Burdon, J. A., 1935, *Archives of British Honduras*, Vol. III, Sifton Praed, London.

Charles, C., 1890, *Honduras: The Land of Great Depths*, Rand McNally, New York.

Coelho, R., 1955, The Black Carib of Honduras: A study in acculturation, Ph.D. dissertation, Northwestern University.

Colonial Office, 1861, Blue Book of Statistics for the Colony of British Honduras, C. O. 128/42.

Colonial Office, 1948, Report of the British Guiana and British Honduras Settlement Commission, His Majesty's Stationery Office, London.

Conzemius, E., 1928, Ethnographical notes on the Black Carib (Garif), *Am. Anthropol.* 30(2):183—205.

Cosminsky, S., 1976, Carib—Creole relations in a Belizean community, in *Frontier Adaptations in Lower Central America* (Mary W. Helms and Franklin O. Loveland, eds.), pp. 95—114, Institute for the Study of Human Issues, Philadelphia.

Davidson, W. V., 1976, Black Carib (Garifuna) habitats in Central America, in *Frontier Adaptations in Lower Central America* (Mary W. Helms and Franklin O. Loveland, eds.), pp. 85—94, Institute for the Study of Human Affairs, Philadelphia.

Dobson, N., 1973, *History of Belize*, Longman, London.

Firschein, I. L., 1961, Population dynamics of the sickle-cell trait in the Black Caribs of British Honduras, Central America, *Am. J. Hum. Genet.* 13(2):233—254.

Fowler, H., 1879, *A Narrative of a Journey across the Unexplored Portion of British Honduras with a Short Sketch of the History and Resources of the Colony*, Government Press, Belize.

Ghidinelli, A., 1976, La Familia entre los Caribes Negros, Ladinos y Kekchies de Livingston, *Guatemala Indigena* 11(3—4):1—315.

Gonzalez, N., 1969, *Black Carib Household Structure*, University of Washington Press, Seattle.

Grant, C., 1976, *The Making of Modern Belize*, Cambridge University Press, Cambridge.

Great Britain, 1870, Reports on the present state of Her Majesty's colonial possessions, Part 1 — West Indies, *Br. Sessional Papers* XLIX:17—35.

Kerns, V., 1983, *Women and the ancestors: Black Carib Kinship and Ritual*, University of Illinois Press, Urbana.

Labat, J.-B., 1970, *The Memoirs of Père Labat, 1693–1705* (Translated and abridged by John Eaden) Frank Cass, London.

Maudslay, A. C., and Maudslay, A. P., 1899, *A Glimpse at Guatemala*, John Murray, London.

Pim, B., 1863, *The Gate of the Pacific*, Lovell Reeve, London.

Roberts, O., 1827, *Narrative of Voyages and Excursions on the East Coast and in the Interior of Central America*, Constable, Edinburgh.

Sanborn, H., 1886, *A Winter in Central America and Mexico*, Lee and Shepard, Boston.

Squier, E. G., 1855, *Notes on Central America*, Harper, New York.

Stephens, J. L., 1841, *Incidents of Travel in Central America, Chiapas, and Yucatan*, Vol. 1, Harper, New York.

Taylor, D., 1951, *The Black Carib of British Honduras*, Viking Fund Publications in Anthropology, no. 17, Wenner-Gren Foundation, New York.

Waddell, D. A. G., 1961, *British Honduras, A Historical and Contemporary Survey*, Oxford University Press, London.

Young T., 1847, *Narrative of a Residence on the Mosquito Shore*, Smith, Elder and Company, London.

7

Ethnicity and Mating Patterns in Punta Gorda, Belize

SHEILA COSMINSKY and EMORY WHIPPLE

1. Introduction

The town of Punta Gorda in southern Belize is composed of people from a variety of backgrounds. The majority (approximately 70%) are Garifuna* (Black Caribs); the next largest group are Creoles (18%); the remainder includes Spaniards, East Indians, Chinese, Mayans, and others. Carr and Thorpe (1961) report that little interethnic friction exists and that intermarriage among the various peoples is common in Punta Gorda. On the other hand, Taylor (1951, p. 38) reports that the Garifuna rarely intermarry or have any social dealings with the non-Garifuna communities. The validity of these claims will be investigated in terms of data obtained in Punta Gorda. If intermarriage is common, how are ethnic boundaries maintained? If there is little friction, how is interaction structured among these ethnic groups to allow for their persistence without conflict?

The purpose of this chapter is to analyze the degree to which ethnicity is salient in social relations, especially mating and marital patterns. We will first examine the sociocultural indicators that define an ethnic identity for members and for nonmembers (Cohen, 1978, p. 386) and how these are manifested in stereotypes that each group holds about themselves and others. We will then

---

* The term Garifuna is used for both singular and plural, and also to refer to the language. Although according to Hadel's (1975) dictionary the plural is Garinagu, we never heard it used in Punta Gorda. Whether that means its use is disappearing or it is just not used with English, as Garifuna is used, we cannot say.

SHEILA COSMINSKY • Department of Anthropology, Rutgers University, Camden, New Jersey 08102. EMORY WHIPPLE • Department of Anthropology, Indiana University — Purdue University at Fort Wayne, Fort Wayne, Indiana 46805.

focus on the patterns of social interaction in a behavioral frame of reference, examining the rules facilitating or hindering interaction in different social situations. In this chapter we are thus following Barth, who holds that maintaining ethnic boundaries implies "not only criteria and signals for identification but also a structuring of interaction which allows for the persistence of cultural differences" (Barth, 1969).

2. Setting and Background

Punta Gorda is the administrative center of the Toledo District and is located on the southern coast of Belize. In 1970, the population of the town was 2083 (Belize, 1970), an increase from 1789 reported in the 1960 census. The only breakdown of ethnic groups found in the census is in a Table entitled "Working Population by Ethnic Origin and Type of Workers," which lists the following categories: Negro or Black, East Indian, Chinese, Syrian/Lebanese, White, Mixed, Other Races, Not Stated. Presumably, the category "Negro or Black" includes some Creoles and the Garifuna, while other Creoles as well as Spanish would be included in the "Mixed" category, and the Mayan Indians would be under "Other Races." This mixture of racial and ethnic labels does not match the "emic" categories used by the local populations and does not list Garifuna separately; consequently it is not useful for our purposes. The lack of further information on ethnic groups in the census is a reflection of the official government policy of deemphasizing ethnicity and emphasizing Belizean unity (Howard, 1980). The terms used by the people in Punta Gorda to designate the different groups are Carib or Garifuna, Creole, Spanish (sometimes also called "Latins"), Indians or Mayas, Chinese (or Chinee), and East Indians (usually called "coolies"). Using a sample of 1574 names from the Malaria Health Survey, together with information from officials and personal knowledge, we put the population of Punta Gorda in 1965 as 69.6% Garifuna, 17.5% Creoles, 5.1% Spanish, 5.7% East Indian, 1.1% Chinese, and 1.0% others.

The Garifuna are descended from African refugees and Red or Island Carib Indians who inhabited St. Vincent's Island and Dominica (Taylor, 1951). In 1796, they were deported to the Bay Islands and Roatan after an uprising against the English. From there they dispersed to the mainland coast of Honduras, Guatemala, and Belize. This arrival is celebrated and reenacted annually by the Garifuna in Belize on Garifuna Settlement Day, November 19. Celebrations are also held in Los Angeles and New York among Garifuna migrants. In one such celebration in Los Angeles in 1978, special emphasis was placed on children learning and performing Garifuna dances and songs, to preserve these traditions and thus maintain their Garifuna identity. The celebration of Garifuna history plays an important role in reinforcing Garifuna identity and unity. Recently, this day has become an official national holiday in Belize, a reflection of changing political attitudes. Hadel (1972) describes the celebration as "Caribs celebrating the fact of being Carib."

The term Creole usually refers to native-born English- or Creole-speaking blacks with or without European admixture. Taylor (1951, p. 38) says the term Creole applies to any native-born inhabitant of English speech, irrespective of race. Grant (1976, p. 14) says that the term probably meant native-born descendants of British settlers originally, but has developed into a concept with racial and cultural connotations. Creole culture is a non-Indian and non-Mestizo way of life and a set of values derived, with local adaptation, from the Anglo-Saxon countries, Africa, and the West Indies. The African elements of Creole culture are subordinated to the British. The few British expatriates and the group of local whites, who are dwindling, "form an integral part of the Creole complex, although racially they would be excluded from it" (Grant, 1976, p. 14). This amalgam of African and British culture has produced distinctive food preferences, social patterns, the Creole language, and other ethnic markers.

The term Spanish refers to people whose native language is Spanish, irrespective of race. Most often these are of mixed Indian—Hispanic or Spanish origin, from Mexico, Guatemala, or other parts of Belize.

The Mayan Indians are either Mopan- or Kekchi-speakers. They are primarily subsistence agriculturalists living in the inland villages several miles outside of Punta Gorda; they come to town for the market, hospital, and official business.

East Indians were brought into the colony as indentured laborers, some of them working on the estates and plantations in the Toledo District. Today, most of them are independent rice farmers who live outside of Punta Gorda. A few live in town working as civil servants and wage laborers. They are heavily Creolized and are differentiated mainly by dietary patterns, physical features, and possibly family organization.

The dominance of the Creoles and subordinate status of the Garifuna that exists in Belize today should be viewed in national and historical perspective. Garifuna were being admitted into Belize in 1802, although under restrictions. They had to have a permit from the Superintendant before they could be allowed in, "this race being considered most dangerous" (Burdon, 1931, p. 13). Such remarks reveal the early development of stereotypes and prejudicial attitudes that still persist. Nevertheless, the first group of 150 who settled at Stann Creek, Dangriga, proved to be so industrious and well-behaved that others were admitted (Burdon, 1931, p. 166). For the most part, the Garifuna stayed by themselves, fished, and farmed. Increasingly, some of the men became wage laborers working in mahogany camps and on sugar plantations, providing a cheap labor supply. During this period, they also became preferred laborers, partly because of their mobility and their industriousness. Gonzalez (1969, p. 29) argues that increasing economic competition and resentment of the preferred labor status of the Garifuna contributed to the present situation in which the Garifuna are set apart as being "different" and "inferior" to other black groups in the area. Sanford (1975) suggests that this prejudice against the Garifuna stems from the status consciousness of the Creoles at that time, who were trying to cast off their black ancestry and the social disability it entailed, and to whom the Garifuna represented the epitome of what they despised in themselves.

According to Palacio (1975) wage labor was reinforced by the deliberate policy of not granting freehold ownership titles to Garifuna but rather leasing them even though they had been occupying the land for cultivation of subsistence crops. Bolland (1977) argues that this policy was meant to convert the Garifuna from a largely self-sufficient peasantry into a labor supply for the mahogany gangs, and later for the sugar estates. The history of the ethnic stereotypes and relations is described by Gullick (1976) and Whipple (1979).

After the U. S. Civil War, over 66 immigrants from the southern U. S. came and settled in Toledo District and established large sugar plantations, nutmeg plantations, and mahogany camps. Other people, including East Indians, Creoles, and Spanish workers, moved into the area for work. By 1882, Punta Gorda became the capital of the district, with a population of 500. As the town grew, merchants, civil servants, and government officials moved in. These were usually Creoles or Englishmen. The controlling positions in civil service and commerce were filled by persons of light complexion. The town is still controlled economically and politically by non-Garifuna, who are relatively light-skinned. Belize City, the former capital, was the Creole center. Therefore, Creoles were trained by the British for various civil servant positions and became administrative officers throughout the country. Their commercial dominance reflects the success of outsiders, who did not have local kinship and personal obligations. They were also better off economically and had more capital for commercial enterprises. These historical conditions have reinforced and contributed to present-day ethnic stereotypes.

3. Cultural and Social Differentiation

The primary features differentiating ethnic groups mentioned by informants are language, occupation, diet, dress, physical characteristics, religion, attitudes, and values. Table 1 summarizes the Garifuna conceptions of the different ethnic groups. The Creole perceptions are similar but differ with respect to character traits and attitudes. The Garifuna see themselves as sincere, steady, friendly, hard-working, and clannish, but as having difficulty working with others unless with kin; and perceive the Creole as insincere, acting superior, proud, and vain. In contrast, the Creole views the Garifuna as ambitious (the men lazy, but the women hard-working), eager for knowledge, clannish, dishonest with non-Garifuna, rough, open, expressive, superstitious, African, "tribal," and as a person who "steals," "smells," "brags," and "does not marry." Marital status is incorporated in the ethnic stereotypes held by the Creole, but not by the Garifuna.

Table 1. Garifuna Conceptions of Group Differences

Criteria	Garifuna	Creole	Spanish	East Indian	Indian
Language	Garifuna	Creole, English	Spanish	English	Mayan (Mopan) Kekchi (Maya)
Occupation	Fisherman, farmer	Merchant, civil servant	Merchant, laborer	Farmer	Farmer
House	Thatch roof	Zinc roof	Zinc roof	Both thatch and zinc	Thatch roof
Diet	Plantain, fish, cassava	Rice and beans	Rice and beans	Rice, roti, yellow ginger	Corn, tortillas, beans, "grass"
Dress	No shoes, careless	Better, more expensive shoes	Shoes	–	Long skirts, native blouses, no shoes
Religion	Catholic	Anglican, Methodist	Catholic	Methodist, some Catholic	Catholic
Physical features	Darker skin	Lighter skin	Fair skin, straight hair	Dark skin, dark straight hair	Indian features of black straight hair, and slanted eyes
Character, values, and attitudes	Sincere, steady, hospitable, friendly, works hard, loud, clannish, doesn't work with others unless kinsmen	Insincere, feels and acts superior, works hard, proud, vain	Sincere, steady	Insincere, beggars, not good friends, clannish	Sincere, wild, shy, drinks a lot, can be dangerous

3.1. Language

The most emphasized diacritical feature is primary language, according to both Creole and Garifuna informants. The Garifuna language is a version of Island Carib, with French, Spanish, and English influences (Taylor, 1951). Although Garifuna is the primary language of the Garifuna and is spoken by them in most public and private conversations, 89% also speak English. This was according to the 1960 census, and it is presumably higher today. The Garifuna language is an important symbol of identity and history. Parents will scold their children for speaking Creole, which they regard as "bad" or "broken" English, and older Garifuna do not speak Creole.

Many Garifuna are also competent in Spanish, especially those who were born or have kinsmen in Honduras or Guatemala. Some have worked for the United Fruit company in Guatemala and learned Spanish at that time. Several Garifuna can also speak one or both of the Mayan languages (Mopan and Kekchi), which they learned while teaching in neighboring Indian villages. The high degree of multilingualism and facility for languages is regarded as a native ability or racial trait of the Garifuna and is one of the few Garifuna characteristics praised by the Creoles and non-Garifuna.

On the other hand, Creoles use language as a reason for not associating with Garifuna. A few Creole informants said they did not know when they were being talked about by Garifuna because they could not understand the language.

Creoles speak Creole and English. Creole is not considered a separate official language, and the census only mentions English. Some Creoles speak Spanish as their primary language, either because they were born in Guatemala or because their mothers were Spanish. According to the 1960 census, a higher percentage of Punta Gorda residents over 15 years of age spoke Spanish as their primary language (24%) than spoke English (14%), while 60% spoke Garifuna. Yet there is a higher percentage of Creoles than Spanish in Punta Gorda, indicating that some people who are considered Creoles speak Spanish as their primary language. Some of these people switch ethnic identification according to the situation and to whom they are speaking.

Children of interethnic marriages or unions usually speak the language of the mother, unless raised by a father who is separated from the mother.

3.2. Occupation

One of the most frequent ethnic stereotypes believed by both Garifuna and Creoles is that Garifuna males are fishermen and the females work the land, whereas Creole males tend to be in government or commercial jobs. Some Creoles and also some Garifuna women said that the Garifuna male is lazy or "takes it easy" while the Garifuna woman works hard; the Garifuna men admit that they waste too much time. Today, there are actually few fishermen. In 1964, of approximately 224 Garifuna males on the voters list (British Honduras,

1964), 19 listed their occupation as fishermen (8.4%) and 14 as farmer or planter. In 1974, only 10 Garifuna males listed themselves as fishermen and 10 as farmers (Belize, 1974). In 1964, of 125 Creole males, six listed fishermen and 12 listed farmer, whereas in 1974 none said fishermen. The above occupational listing may refer to full-time, larger scale Creole fishermen, whereas many Garifuna who fish do so part-time. Those who fish usually work in the early morning hours and are free the rest of the day. This different working pattern may have contributed to the Creole image of the Garifuna male as lazy.

The number of men fishing fluctuates with the price of fish and the availability of wage labor and other jobs. Also, if the wind is not right, few men in hand- or oil-powered draft can safely put out to sea. Since the amount of money earned by small-scale, part-time fishing is relatively small, this is more a subsistence or a supplementary activity than a money-making one. For this reason, fishermen have low status in the eyes of younger Garifuna. Males do not want to become fishermen and females state that they do not want to marry one. The low status of the fishermen probably is contributing to their numerical decline. However, there are also fewer fish now within paddling distance of Punta Gorda. The fishing grounds are being steadily depleted, especially since the use of outboard motors. Lundberg (1978) reports a similar situation in Barranco, where the decline in fish began noticeably about 10 years ago due to a variety of factors. One of these is Guatemalan commercial trawlers (Ladino fishermen) from Livingston and Puerto Barrios operating illegally in Belizean waters. Lundberg also suspects that the use of gill nets and seines, which has allowed an increase in catch from the littoral zones, has upset the previous equilibrium between the reproduction and harvesting of the fish that had previously existed in the area; it is also contributing to the decline of the fish.

Most Garifuna farming is carried on in the St. Vincent Block, also called the "Carib Reserve," an area of 960 acres behind the town. Any Garifuna not of alien parentage and born in Punta Gorda has a share in the land, for which each head of family pays a nominal tax. According to Bolland (1977), the establishment of reserves was created by the Crown Lands Ordinance of 1872 and was a move to dispossess the Garifuna from the lands and deprive them of the opportunity of holding lands by freehold title. Women, primarily older ones, do most of the tending of the fields and harvesting, while the males clear the land. Rice is the primary crop, both for consumption and market, with cassava as secondary. Plantains, beans, pineapples, and other crops are also grown. However, the number farming is small and many households do not apply for reserve land. The lack of male labor due to the migration for wage labor is another factor contributing to the decline in farming. The few Creoles who engage in agriculture have larger farms, outside of town, and hire laborers to work the land, in contrast to the subsistence-scale cultivation of the Garifuna. The patterns of land tenure are thus different — the Garifuna holding small shares of reserve land and the Creoles owning title to large shares of private land.

Most agricultural produce, meat, and large fish are sold in the local market by small-scale Garifuna and Spanish vendors. Some Mayan vendors come from the inland villages to sell corn, rice, beans, and other agricultural produce. The participation of the Mayans selling produce in Punta Gorda is a recent development related to their increased role in cash crop farming (Howard 1980), and has implications for their relations with the Garifuna.

The store and canteen owners are mainly non-Garifuna. Of 19 merchants in Punta Gorda, nine were Creole, three Spanish, three Chinese, two Garifuna, one Syrian, and one Mayan. There are a couple of very small Garifuna shops, but some informants said that Garifuna refuse to patronize their own merchants to any great extent because they cannot afford to extend credit. Any Garifuna who gets ahead is forced or pressured to redistribute and "share the wealth." This has contributed to the economic success of outsiders, who do not have local social obligations.

Some Garifuna are engaged in service occupations, such as carpenters and tailors. Most males are wage laborers, often at seasonal jobs and therefore are frequently unemployed. Most have migrated at some time to other parts of the country or to the U.S., especially Los Angeles and New York, for various jobs. Several Garifuna women have worked as domestic servants for non-Garifuna families in Guatemala and Belize City or have migrated for work in the U.S.

The Garifuna have long provided many of Belize's teachers, especially in the rural Mayan villages. Many high-status positions and civil service jobs had previously been closed to Garifuna, and partly for this reason they entered the teaching profession. Education was valued and teaching was one path of employment open to them. Most of the schools in the Indian villages have been established by the Catholic Church. The Garifuna are employed as teachers in these schools since they are also Catholic, and there are few qualified Indians. In addition, teachers from other ethnic groups did not want to live under the poor and isolated conditions in the Indian villages. The Garifuna teacher is respected by the Mayans. Garifuna, however, have rarely been appointed to administrative positions in the schools in the larger towns or in Belize City. These are usually filled by priests, nuns, Americans, or Creoles. As more higher paying positions, especially civil service, and new roles open up, fewer Garifuna are staying in the teaching profession.

Relatively few opportunities for wage labor exist either in town or in the district for any ethnic group. This changed briefly during the last couple of years while offshore oil drilling was being carried on off the coast of Punta Gorda and provided jobs for local males. These oil companies, however, have now pulled out. People who want jobs or advancement migrate either temporarily or permanently. Some Garifuna initially start in the teaching profession and then move into a civil service job, while others work at a variety of wage labor jobs. This migratory labor has had a disruptive effect on the traditional culture, especially in the psychosocial realm, according to Palacio (1975), as new acculturated features are integrated. Palacio suggests that the ability of the Garifuna to subsume and adapt to these shocks and disruptions from the economic conditions without losing their cultural identity is a manifestion of their resilience.

3.3. Religion

According to the stereotypes, the Garifuna are Catholic and the Creoles Methodist or Anglican. The Creoles also mention that the Garifuna are superstitious, referring to some of their traditional beliefs. In actuality, 94% of Punta Gorda residents are Catholic (1970 census; Belize, 1970), which is an increase from 86% in the 1960 census (British Honduras, 1960). Almost all the Garifuna and Spanish in town are Catholic. The Creoles are divided; the permanent-resident Creoles tend to be Catholic, whereas the temporary-resident ones are Methodist or Anglican. Creoles who are of mixed Creole–Spanish ancestry or who are from Guatemala are also Catholic. The Methodist Church is the next largest, composed mainly of Creoles and East Indians (6% in 1960 and 4% in 1970). The number of Anglicans has sharply declined, from 90 reported in 1960 to 19 in 1970. There is also a Nazarene Church in Punta Gorda, which seems to be growing and includes members of various ethnic groups. In 1975, the Nazarene service emphasized Spanish with a bilingual English–Spanish service, whereas in 1965 they had sung hymns in Garifuna. This may reflect an increase in Spanish-speakers in their congregation.

Many Garifuna maintain elements of their "traditional" beliefs in addition to their Catholicism. These beliefs focus around dreams, spirits, ancestors, certain ceremonies such as the *dogo*, and the Garifuna religious specialist, the *buiai* (Taylor, 1951). Not all Garifuna believe in these or have attended a *dogo* ceremony, but they know about these beliefs, which do serve as symbols of Garifuna identity for many Garifuna. These beliefs and practices are distinguished from those of *obeah*, de Laurence magic, or what one informant called "voodoo tricks," beliefs that are widespread and shared by members of all ethnic groups. Among some Creoles, the Garifuna has a reputation for curing and a Creole may go to a Garifuna for this purpose.

A close relationship exists between education and religion in Belize. The schools are denominational, although government-supported. In Punta Gorda, one primary school is Catholic and the other Methodist. Most of the students in the Catholic school are Garifuna, although some are Spanish or Creole. The teachers are nuns and the assistant teachers are Garifuna. The Methodist school has primarily Creole and East Indian students and teachers, with a few Garifuna students. The population of the Methodist school is variable, since many of the children are part of the temporary-resident Creole population.

A secondary school, St. Peter's Claver College, opened in Punta Gorda in 1960. Some teachers are Papal Volunteers from the U.S., and several are Belizeans, including some from Punta Gorda. Previously, if a student wanted a secondary education, he or she had to go to Belize City or to Stann Creek. The new secondary school is increasing the educational opportunities for many who could not afford to go to high school in another town. Several students come from Guatemala and Honduras to learn English, thinking there are more opportunities for them in Belize.

Children in the secondary school seem to get along together, even though there is some ethnic slur-name calling, such as "stingy Chinee," "big-time Creole," "ugly Carib fisherman," and "dumb Indian." Nevertheless, the class feeling as potential graduates seems to override ethnic prejudice. Teachers, even Garifuna teachers, however, tend to give preferential treatment to light-skinned children and openly insult some Garifuna children. Although we lack statistical data, Garifuna seem to be punished more often for minor infractions with harder punishments, and more Garifuna are expelled or drop out of school. Despite these problems, the school does offer increased educational and thus potential economic opportunities for the Garifuna.

3.4. Physical

Most informants mentioned that there are physical differences between the different ethnic groups, but had difficulty specifying what these are. Several Garifuna and Creoles said that the Creoles have fairer skin color; others point out that many Creoles are darker than some Garifuna and some Garifuna are fairer than some Creoles. Some Creoles said that the Garifuna had higher and broader cheekbones, due to their Indian ancestry; others stressed the African ancestry of the Garifuna. In general, Creoles consider the Garifuna as "black" regardless of actual skin color, and emphasize their own English heritage as the "son of the Baymen," whereas the Garifuna tend to emphasize their own Carib Indian ancestry (which some informants said was a "white race"). Both groups play down their own African ancestry and emphasize the "Africanness" of the other.

3.5. Surnames

Surname provides a useful ethnic indicator, although it was mentioned by only a couple of informants. The surnames of most Garifuna are Hispanic, such as Lopez, Enriquez, and Martinez, or names purported to be originally Garifuna, such as Arzu and Parchu. Names like Lambey are said by some informants to derive from the French and St. Vincent. A few Garifuna have English-derived names, such as Nicholas, but these are different from the local Creole names, which are usually English names such as Johnson and Foster. The East Indians usually have names of Indian background, such as Singh, Bahadur, or Ranguy, or names of English background, such as Williams. The Spanish have surnames of Spanish origin, most of which are different from the Garifuna names in Punta Gorda. Chinese and Mayans also have distinctive surnames. In cases of mixed offspring, the surname might be misleading. For example, a child with a Garifuna mother and a Creole father might have a Creole name but be identified as a Garifuna. Although there are a few cases of names overlapping ethnic groups and a few cases of intermarriage, names generally provide a clue to ethnic identity for the majority of people in Punta Gorda.

Other sociocultural features that serve as ethnic markers, such as house-type, dress, and diet, have been discussed elsewhere (Cosminsky, 1966, 1976, 1977). These seem to be decreasing in importance today as differentiating features, and thus will not be dealt with in this chapter.

4. Ethnic Relations

Endogamy is the stated ideal for all groups in Punta Gorda. The reasons given are often based on the stereotypes and prejudices discussed earlier. Informants made such comments as, "one should not mix blood," "the Garifuna way of life is too different and too difficult," or "Creole men treat their women better than Garifuna men do." Endogamy is the dominant practice, supported by strong family and social pressures. Although we do not have statistical data at this point, interethnic formal marriages are relatively infrequent, whereas mixed casual unions occur more frequently. Carr and Thorpe's (1961) statement that intermarriage is common in Punta Gorda is not supported by our data, if they are referring to formal legal marriages. If they are using the term loosely to include casual and conjugal unions, there is more validity to the statement. In general, those who deviate from the norm usually marry someone from outside the town. In nine of 10 formal intermarriages of which we are aware, one of the partners had come from outside the town. The one exception involved a Creole male from one of the local elite families and a Garifuna girl, to which there was much opposition on both sides. In contrast to the formal legal marriages, in the several unmarried interethnic unions we knew, both parties were either born in Punta Gorda or had lived there for a long time. Evidence of casual unions was partly based on "outside" children, since these unions are more temporary, more concealed, and more difficult to obtain information about.

Interethnic unions tend to follow certain patterns. These are:

1. Temporary-resident male Creoles have sexual relations only with Creoles and occasionally East Indians. Some believe that East Indian females are good lovers and are also considered potential marriage partners. They also say that these women do not get as fat after pregnancy as Creole or Garifuna women, they have beautiful voices, and keep good homes. Temporary-resident Creole females do not have such relations with non-Creoles. They complain that there are not enough "high-class" men in Punta Gorda.

2. Permanent-resident Creoles, both male and female, are more open in their liaisons. Creole women, however, will seldom have anything to do with

non-Creole men, and when it does occur, the relation tends to end up in formal marriage.

3. Some informants said that a Garifuna male will marry a Creole or Spanish girl (he will marry up), but rarely will a Creole male marry a Garifuna girl. On the other hand, a Creole male will have sexual liaisons as lovers with a Garifuna woman, sometimes resulting in "outside" children, but will rarely marry them. These patterns are illustrated as follows:

Garifuna male—Creole female: civil and religious marriage
Garifuna female—Creole male: casual or conjugal union

4. Unions between Garifuna and East Indians are rare. The Garifuna scorn the East Indians from outside of town, and those who live in town look down on the Garifuna.

These generalizations made by informants are supported by the limited available data. Of 10 intermarried couples, five involved Garifuna males, one involved a female who was one-half East Indian and one-half Garifuna, and only one involved a Creole male and a Garifuna female. On the other hand, of six unmarried unions we knew of, four involved Garifuna females and only one a Garifuna male.

The interethnic mating patterns in Livingston, Guatemala, provide some interesting contrasts. Ghidinelli (1976) has analyzed these patterns and hypothesizes that people of different ethnic groups do not form mixed pairs because (1) the ideal pattern of a partner disagrees with the stereotype that they have of the other culture, and (2) one of the couple has to sacrifice social status to the one of inferior station. In Livingston, the main groups are Garifuna and Ladino (same as Spanish in Belize), rather than Creole. Ghidinelli reports that sexual relations and marriages between Ladino men and Garifuna women are more frequent than those between Ladino women and Garifuna males. He emphasizes the stereotype of sexuality of the Garifuna as important in these relations. To a Ladino male, a Garifuna female is made for sex. If he has relations with her, he is "macho." If a Ladino female, however, has relations with a Garifuna male, the pressure of a double standard is invoked, and she is called a "negrera" and "the whore of whores" (*lo mas puta de los putas*) (Ghidinelli, 1976, p. 285). In 1972–1973, of 28 marriages by Ladino men, only one was with a Garifuna woman. There were none between Garifuna men and Ladino women. The rare cases that occur are outside Livingston, such as in Puerto Barrios or Guatemala City. Of 107 births in 1972, 68 had parents of the same ethnic group, 21 whose fathers were "unknown," and three had Ladino fathers and Garifuna mothers. Of 70 children baptized with a Ladino father, only four had Garifuna mothers.

There seems to be less interethnic mating and more tension in Livingston than in Punta Gorda. This may be a reflection of the lower status of the Garifuna in Guatemala than in Belize and of the Spanish historical influence in contrast

Table 2. Sex Ratios by Age, Punta Gorda, 1970[a]

Age (yr)	Males	Females	Sex ratio
0–4	176	211	0.834
5–9	180	199	0.904
10–14	143	159	0.899
15–19	96	134	0.716
20–24	47	48	0.979
25–29	31	46	0.67
30–34	30	33	0.909
35–39	16	51	0.313
40–44	29	49	0.591
45–49	33	44	0.75
50–54	33	44	0.75
55–59	24	33	0.727
60–64	29	35	0.828
65–69	20	19	1.05
70 +	37	54	0.68
Total	924	1159	0.797

[a] Based on Belize, 1970.

to the British–Creole influence. Further research in this area is necessary to understand the reasons for these different patterns.

The desire for children, especially light-skinned children, the acceptance of outside children, and an excess of Garifuna females tend to promote liaisons across ethnic lines in Punta Gorda.

Both Garifuna men and women consider it important to have many children, resulting in outside children from various liaisons. Women do not hide the fact that a child is an outside child, and there is no stigma attached. The value of machismo will usually pressure one of the woman's lovers to claim paternity. If the child has a chance to go to high school, the mother will seek out the biological father and shame him into paying tuition. In addition, the priest insists on using the name of the biological father for a child when he registers the child for high school. The people thus consider it important to know who is the biological father of a child, regardless of the type of union and status of the child.

Skin color may be one consideration for a woman's choice of mates. This criterion seems to be more prevalent among the younger Garifuna females, in contrast to older women, and may reflect the increasing "creolization" or adoption of Creole values. A woman who has a fair-skinned child receives praise and status, and knows that her child will have it easier in school and future job opportunities. Consequently, the child will be able to take care of his or her mother and family in the future. Having a fair child is also beneficial to a woman's husband or mate. He may claim it as his regardless of actual paternity. But if the child is darker than himself, he may assume that it is an outside child and the woman is reprimanded. Garifuna males are considered by Creoles to father black children, regardless of actual skin color, and therefore a Creole woman does not want to take the risk.

Few economic opportunities exist in Punta Gorda for Garifuna males, and migration is thus necessary to obtain wage labor. Young Creole males, especially those from the elite families, do not need to migrate for jobs as much as do the Garifuna males. Thus there are a greater proportion of young Creole males than Garifuna males staying in town.

The sex ratio according to age is shown in Table 2. Within the age range of women of reproductive age, 15–45 years old, there are 249 males to 361 females, giving a sex ratio of 0.689. The discrepancy is particularly striking in the 35–39 year old group, with 51 females to 16 males. Unfortunately, these figures do not differentiate according to ethnic group. Nevertheless, we feel the existing data suggest that the shortage of males and excess of females is related to the frequency of consanguineal households (Gonzales, 1969) and matri-extended households (Munroe, 1964), to the frequency of casual unions rather than formal marriage, and promotes interethnic mating since the Garifuna males migrate more often than the Creole males.

The recent establishment of a British army post outside Punta Gorda has probably contributed to gene flow. We do not know the extent of miscegenation that has occurred as a result of the presence of the soldiers and hope to obtain data on this in the near future. According to a few informants, some Garifuna girls like the British as possible mates because of their fair skin. The British soldiers, however, prefer to have social and sexual relations with Creole girls and East Indians, but not with Garifuna girls.

In July 1978, a battalion of Gurkha soldiers replaced the British soldiers. We expect that the amount of miscegenation will be less than with the British soldiers, due to the difference in value systems and cultural background of the Gurkhas. The types of relations, however, that are occurring between the Gurkhas and the local ethnic groups have not yet been investigated and remain an area for future research.

Attitudes toward offspring of mixed ancestry seem to be largely an individual matter. In general, if one parent is Garifuna, the offspring are regarded as Garifuna. However, if an offspring of mixed ancestry is raised by the non-Garifuna parent, he may be identified with the ethnic group of that parent. By contrast, if one parent is Creole and the other non-Garifuna and non-Creole (e.g., Spanish, East Indian, Chinese), the offspring are regarded as Creole. How individuals identify themselves is a more complex matter and depends on the situation and to whom he or she is reacting or talking. This variation is related Consequently, which group a person regards as higher status may depend upon to the ambiguity of the ethnic stratification hierarchy. This hierarchy differs in the Garifuna and Creole viewpoints:

Garifuna view	Creole view
Spanish	Creole
Creole	Spanish
Garifuna	East Indian
East Indian	Garifuna
Indian	Indian

the group with which he or she identifies, and this is relative to whom he or she is speaking. Skin color and primary language are two key variables. Individuals who are intermediate in skin color or language competency may sometimes control the choice of identity by referring to themselves as one or the other. This is also the case of offspring of Creole–Spanish unions. Some of these people in Punta Gorda identify themselves as Creole there, but switch when they go to Guatemala to being Spanish.

Ethnic stratification tends to coincide with economic stratification. Punta Gorda has two classes: an upper class of merchants and government officials and civil servants, who are non-Garifuna, mostly permanent-resident Creoles, and a lower class made up of the rest of the population. Within the elite there are ties of marriage, kinship, and freindship. Although much individual variation exists, there is virtually no middle class. The teachers tend to form a separate clique and one might view them as an incipient middle class. The few Garifuna who are either storeowners or civil servants may form an elite within the Garifuna community, but they are not part of the upper class of Punta Gorda.

The color–class system as proposed by Smith (1966) does exist in Punta Gorda, although less rigidly than on the national level. Within the Creole community and the nation as a whole, a fair skin means high social and economic position. According to Smith, in most of the British West Indies, social stratification is based on twin factors of the hierarchical ranking of color and occupation. Occupational mobility keeps the system open to a limited degree. The emphasis, however, lies on the value placed by all groups on color differences.

In Punta Gorda, most of the elite have light skin, although there are some Creoles in the local elite with relatively darker skin. On the other hand, there are no Garifuna in this group, regardless of skin color. It should be remembered, however, that in the mind of most Creoles, the Garifuna are "black," or darker than themselves, no matter what the actual skin pigmentation is, so that the color–class system still holds in the psychological dimension.

Another feature of the status system that Smith (1956) considers important is that ethnic groups that do not fit readily into the color–class hierarchy, such as the Chinese and East Indians, are able to infiltrate at all levels and to take over functions where a relative lack of status consciousness is an advantage, particularly in the retail and distributive trades. Although there are a few Chinese in these trades in town, the majority are Creoles, who are very status conscious. In fact, it is these trades that have been their pathway to achieving and maintaining a higher status. In this respect, Punta Gorda differs from some other parts of the Caribbean.

Ethnic conflicts, like class conflicts, result from the unequal distribution of, and competition for, scarce resources (Van den Berghe, 1975, p. 73). We suggest that the relatively low degree of conflict observed, at least openly, among ethnic groups in Punta Gorda is due to the lack of economic competition within the town, together with the migration of the ambitious and discontented. Tensions and prejudices are manifested in stereotypes, remarks, and social distance patterns of the majority of the townspeople. The attitude, however, seems to be one of "live and let live" rather than of hostility.

The economic stratification system that places non-Garifuna in economic control of Punta Gorda is maintained by the political control that this group has. Nevertheless, politics is an increasingly important sphere of joint participation and ethnic relations. The People's United Party (PUP) is the party in power nationally. In Punta Gorda, it is composed mainly of Garifuna and some of the elite Creoles. Most other Creoles and Spanish in town tend to support the opposition party, formerly the National Independent Party, now the United Democratic Party (UDP), as do a good number of Garifuna, especially the civil servants and upwardly mobile. The political parties cross-cut ethnic lines, and some Garifuna who were previously very strong PUP supporters have recently switched to the opposition party. Dances, social clubs, and other activities are often organized along party lines.

The Town Board is the local governing body and is composed of seven members elected for 3 years. In 1974, all were PUP members, and the majority were Garifuna. the Mayor of the town was a Creole and a PUP member. Much of the local political and economic power was concentrated in this family. The District Officer is usually a Creole, although occasionally a Garifuna has held the office. The other civil servants and clerks are from various ethnic groups. In Punta Gorda, ethnicity seems to be decreasing as a basis for political action. Political affiliation and interest cross-cut ethnic segments and in many situations override ethnic allegiances.

5. Summary and Conclusions

The stereotypes and symbols of ethnic differences use various criteria, which differ with the context and the individual. An individual may also use different models to accommodate divergences from the stereotype. An element of choice is open to the individual concerning the way he or she defines the social situation and which criteria and which ties he or she will manipulate.

Endogamy is the stated ideal and predominant practice by all ethnic groups. Nevertheless, interethnic mating does occur, more frequently in the form of conjugal and casual unions than in civil or religious marriages. As discussed in Section 4, such relations tend to occur according to rules or patterns. The ideal of endogamy and the different ethnic stereotypes serve to maintain ethnic boundaries and ethnic identity. At the same time, several factors are promoting interethnic mating. These include the desire for children, the acceptance of outside children, the value placed on light skin (mainly held by younger women), the color–class hierarchy, increasing economic competition, migration, and an excess of females.

ACKNOWLEDGMENTS

Fieldwork was conducted in Punta Gorda by Sheila Cosminsky in the summer of 1965 under the auspices of the Brandeis University Summer Field School Program through a National Science Foundation Grant, and in January 1975, and by Emory Whipple in 1969 and 1974–1976.

References

Barth, F., 1969, *Ethnic Groups and Boundaries,* p. 19, Little Brown, Boston.

Belize, 1970, Abstract of Statistics, Vol. 1, Belmopan, Government Printer.

Belize, 1974, Voter Registration List for Toledo South, Government Printer.

Bolland, O. N., 1977, *The Formation of a Colonial Society,* Johns Hopkins, Baltimore.

British Honduras, 1960, Census of British Honduras, Jamaica Tabulation Center, Department of Statistics, Jamaica.

British Honduras, 1964, List of Voters for Toledo South Electoral Division for 1965, Belize City, Government Printing Office.

Brockmann, C. T., 1977, Ethnic and racial relations in Northern Belize, *Ethnicity* 4:246–262.

Burdon, Sir J. A., 1931, *Archives of British Honduras,* Vols. I, II, Sifton Praed, London.

Carr, D., and Thorpe, J., 1961, *From the Cam to the Cays,* Putnam, London.

Cohen, R., 1978, Ethnicity: Problems and Focus in Anthropology, *Ann. Rev. Anthrop.* 7:379–403.

Conzemius, E., 1928, Ethnographic notes on the Black Carib, *Am. Anthropol.* 30:183–205.

Cosminsky, S., 1966, Interethnic relations in Punta Gorda, British Honduras, unpublished Ms., Brandeis University.

Cosminsky, S., 1976, Carib–Creole relations in a Belizean community, in *Frontier Adaptations in Lower Central America* (M. Helms and F. Loveland, eds.), pp. 95–114, Institute for the Study of Human Issues, Philadelphia.

Cosminsky, S., 1977, Interethnic relations in a southern Belizean community, *Ethnicity* 4:226–245.

Ghidinelli, A., 1976, La Familia entre los Caribes Negros, Ladinos y Kekchies de Livingston, *Guatemala Indigena* 11(3–4):1–315.

Gonzalez, N. S., 1969, *Black Carib Household Structure,* University of Washington Press, Seattle.

Grant, C. H., 1976, *The Making of Modern Belize,* Cambridge University Press, Cambridge.

Gullick, C. J. M. R., 1976, *Exile from Saint Vincent: The Development of Black Carib Culture in Central America up to 1945*, Malta, Progress Press.

Hadel, R. S. J., 1975, *Dictionary of Central American Carib*, Belize, Belize Institute of Social Research and Action and St. John's College.

Howard, M., 1980, Ethnicity and economic integration in Southern Belize, *Ethnicity* 7:119–136.

Lundberg, P., 1978, Barranco: A sketch of a Belizean Garifuna (Black Carib) habitat, M.S. Thesis, Department of Geography, University of California, Riverside.

Munroe, R., 1964, Couvade practices of the Black Carib: A psychological and social structural study, Ph.D. dissertation, Harvard University.

Palacio, J., 1975, Problems in the maintenance of the Garifuna (Black Carib) culture in Belize, Presented at the American Anthropological Association, San Francisco.

Sanford, M., 1971, Disruption of the mother–child relationship in conjunction with matrifocality, Ph.D. dissertation, Catholic University.

Sanford, M., 1975, From the bottom looking up in a developing country, Presented at the American Anthropological Association, San Francisco.

Smith, R., 1956, *The Negro Family in British Guiana*, Routledge and Kegan, London.

Taylor, D., 1951, *The Black Caribs of British Honduras*, Viking Fund Publications in Anthropology, no. 17, Wenner-Gren Foundation, New York.

Van den Berghe, P. L., 1967, *Race and Racism*, Wiley, New York.

Whipple, E., 1979, Modernization and music among the Garifuna of Punta Gorda, Belize, Ph.D. Dissertation, Indiana University.

PART II

MORPHOLOGICAL SECTION

8

Nutrition and Growth in Early Childhood among the Garifuna and Creole of Belize

CAROL JENKINS

1. Introduction

The presence of nutritional stress and growth retardation among the children of Central America and the Caribbean has been well documented (Bengoa, 1975; Gueri, 1981; McIntosh, 1980). Although Mestizos, or people of mixed European and Amerindian stocks, and indigenous Amerindian peoples make up the majority of Central America's inhabitants, descendants of African-derived populations may be found in communities along the Caribbean coast, stretching from Panama to Belize. In Belize, people of African descent comprised approximately 64% of the total population in 1976 (Belize, 1976). They are divided into two distinct ethnic groups, the Garifuna, or Black Carib, and the Creole. As the majority, with 56% of the total population, the Creole enjoys relatively higher status in social, political, and economic spheres than does the Garifuna (Sanford, 1974; Cosminsky, 1977; Kerns, 1977; Chibnik, 1975). Although there appears to be less congruency between ethnic and socioeconomic status in Belize than in other nations — for example, Guyana (Despres, 1975) or Guatemala (Newman, 1977) — class distinctions are growing. Differential access to wealth and resources remains largely conditioned by historical and occupational factors related to cultural heritage. These differences are reflected in the health status of children, especially between birth and 5 years of age.

During early childhood growth is very rapid, particularly during the first

CAROL JENKINS • Institute of Medical Research, P.O. Box 378, Madang, Papua New Guinea.

year, requiring adequate nutrition and health care if normal growth is to be preserved. Also during this period, future growth and development may be significantly influenced by repeated or long-endured episodes of nutritional stress. Unless adequate nutritional status is acquired and sufficient catchup growth takes place, severely undernourished children may be left stunted, never fully realizing their genetic potential (Graham and Adrianzen, 1972; Johnston, 1978).

Many children succumb to the combined insults of malnutrition and infection which together account for the greatest number of deaths in this age group (Scrimshaw *et al.*, 1968). Diarrheal diseases, in particular, are significantly implicated in the high infant and early childhood mortality rates throughout the Caribbean and Central America (Puffer *et al.*, 1971; Sinha, 1979). The diminution in breastfeeding, the increasing use of starchy weaning foods, and the use of contaminated infant feeding bottles are often cited as responsible agents in this process (Jelliffe, 1968; Raphael, 1979). Other behavioral factors may also contribute to childhood nutritional status. For example, the hierarchy of resort in health care practices is a factor that may either aid or hinder the recovery of an ailing child. Among some ethnic groups, widespread knowledge of herbal teas in the treatment of diarrhea may help prevent dehydration. On the other hand, when a doctor is not consulted until the last resort and dehydration is prolonged, recovery may be severely hampered.

2. Methods

2.1. Research Design

The research reported here was conducted in Belize during 1979. Two principal objectives were pursued. First was to assess the frequency of early childhood malnutrition in two administrative districts, one coastal and the other inland. The coastal district, Stann Creek, is mainly inhabited by the Garifuna and secondarily by the Creole, while the inland district, Cayo, is composed primarily of Creole and Mestizo communities.

A second research objective was to determine which of a series of bio-cultural factors significantly contributed to poor nutritional status in the survey communities. For this reason children whose growth is poor are compared to those whose growth is clearly above average along a series of selected demographic, dietary, and health-related variables. This information was obtained through structured interviews with the children's mothers.

2.2. Research Techniques

Children attending public health clinics for the purpose of immunization were measured and their mothers interviewed. Anthropometrics included weight, stature, head circumference, mid-upper arm circumference, and triceps skinfold. Weight was recorded to the nearest ounce on a Triner double-beam scale which was frequently recalibrated. Among children under 3 years old, length was measured in the supine position on a custom-made board and recorded to the nearest millimeter. The height of older children was measured with a standard anthropometer. Head circumference was measured with a flexible steel tape at the point of greatest circumference directly above the brow ridge and recorded to the nearest $\frac{1}{2}$ cm. Upper arm circumference was taken with a steel tape at a point midway between olecranon and acromion and recorded to the nearest $\frac{1}{2}$ cm. Triceps skinfold was measured at the midpoint of the upper arm, over the triceps, with a Lange skinfold caliper and recorded to the nearest millimeter. Measurements were always taken on the left arm. Shoes were removed before weight or stature was measured and, generally, children wore very light clothing. Adjustments were made whenever heavy belts or unusually heavy clothing was encountered.

Mothers were interviewed regarding their own reproductive histories and the health and feeding histories of their children. In addition, a smaller sample of 24-hr diet recalls for children aged 1–6 years was collected and representative portions weighed at table. A triple-beam Ohaus balance was used to obtain average weights of locally produced food items, such as fruits and breads. Recipes were obtained for composite foods.

2.3. Sample Size and Location

The sample is composed of 198 Creole children and 188 Garifuna children from about 2 weeks to $5\frac{1}{2}$ years of age. Their mothers included 142 Creole and 135 Garifuna. Ethnic affiliation was based on self-identification. Children's birth dates were always known and interviews were conducted in either English or Spanish. Survey locations included two administrative towns, San Ignacio and Dangriga, the nation's capitol, Belmopan, and 15 villages.

2.4. Methods of Analysis

Dietary intakes were converted to nutrient values with the aid of *Food Composition Tables for Use in the English-Speaking Caribbean* (Caribbean Food and Nutrition Institute, 1974) and, when necessary, the U. S. Department of Agriculture Handbook No. 456, *Nutritive Value of American Foods* (Adams, 1975). Recommended dietary allowances were taken from *Recommended Dietary Allowances for the Caribbean* (Caribbean Food and Nutrition Institute, 1976). Percentages of attained recommended dietary allowances for energy, protein, and iron were calculated for each child.

Malnutrition was assessed using several different measures: weight-for-age, height-for-age, weight-for-height, and arm circumference. Since local standards for healthy Caribbean children are not available, the U. S. National Center for

Health Statistics growth standards were utilized as reference values (National Center for Health Statistics, 1976).

Among children older than 6 months, an arm circumference below 13.5 cm approximates 80% of expected reference values (Burgess and Burgess, 1969; Frisancho, 1974). This limit yields a measure of moderate to severe malnutrition (Anderson, 1979).

While weight reflects the recent nutritional status of a child, stature reflects past nutritional circumstances. Following the recommended scheme of Seone and Latham (1971), children were classified as stunted, i.e., exhibiting past chronic malnutrition, whose weight-for-age and height-for-age were below the fifth centile of reference values but whose weight-for-height was normal. Those with normal (i.e., above the fifth centile) height-for-age but who had low weight-for-age and weight-for-height were considered to exhibit current short-term malnutrition. Finally, those with values below the fifth reference centile on all three measures were designated as exhibiting current on-going malnutrition of long duration. Children in all three categories were grouped into a classification labeled "poor growth," while those whose values reached the U. S. 75th centile or above were grouped under the label of "better-than-average growth." A step-wise discriminant function was performed (Biomedical Data Program 7M) utilizing these two groups of children in order to ascertain which of a variety of factors would successfully discriminate between them. Only those factors with a probability of at least 0.01 were considered significant for the present study.

3. Results

3.1. Comparative Growth of Creole and Garifuna Children

Tables 1 and 2 present the means and standard deviations for weight and height in Creole and Garifuna children, sexes combined, birth to 5.5 years old. Birth weights were obtained from clinic records. Figure 1 presents weight-for-age curves for Creole and Garifuna children compared to those of other children of African ancestry, both in Africa and the Western hemisphere. The relatively low position of Afro-Belizeans is evident. By the age of 5 years, Garifuna children are surpassed in weight by all available comparable samples. Creole children in Belize are heavier than Garifuna children at all ages after birth.

Figure 2 shows stature-for-age curves among children of African ancestry. While Garifuna and Creole children do not exhibit significantly different average statures, both are considerably below the values for well-off African children. By the age of 5, Afro-Belizeans are shorter than the tropical forest-dwelling Bush Negroes of Surinam (Eveleth and Tanner, 1976).

As can be seen in Fig. 3, both Garifuna and Creole children exhibit retarded growth in head circumference relative to the U. S. standards, approximating the fifth centile at 3 years of age. These data suggest that Garifuna

Table 1. Means and Standard Deviations for Weight

	Weight, kg					
	Creole			Garifuna		
Age,[a] months	N	X	S.D.	N	X	S.D.
Birth	102	3.26	0.51	270	3.42	0.58
0.5–3	12	4.86	1.04	13	4.80	0.76
3–6	12	7.33	0.82	19	6.33	0.78
6–12	28	7.92	1.58	26	7.56	1.14
12–18	19	9.44	1.61	26	8.31	1.61
18–30	35	10.77	1.71	35	10.81	1.70
30–42	35	13.29	1.72	26	12.78	1.45
42–54	28	14.15	3.22	27	14.01	1.94
54–66	15	15.82	2.04	9	14.48	2.29

[a] Sexes combined.

Table 2. Means and Standard Deviations for Stature

	Stature, cm					
	Creole			Garifuna		
Age,[a] months	N	X	S.D.	N	X	S.D.
0.5–3	13	57.44	3.58	13	55.88	3.29
3–6	12	64.98	2.15	19	62.80	3.10
6–12	28	68.82	5.25	26	68.06	4.29
12–18	21	75.80	5.02	26	71.87	5.20
18–30	34	82.85	4.42	36	81.54	4.52
30–42	38	91.03	5.43	26	89.97	5.11
42–54	31	96.55	5.95	27	96.02	4.95
54–66	16	99.95	6.48	9	99.89	5.98

[a] Sexes combined.

children experience greater interference with normal growth between 6 months and 2 years, after which a period of accelerated growth takes place, enabling them to catch up with their Creole peers.

Upper arm circumference and triceps skinfold curves are presented in Fig. 4 and compared to values for well-off and slum-dwelling children in Ibadan, Nigeria (Eveleth and Tanner, 1976). While Afro-Belizeans fall directly between the socioeconomic extremes in Ibadan, Creole children consistently exhibit greater arm circumferences and thicker skinfolds than do the Garifuna, at all ages after 3 months.

3.2. Nutritional Status

Garifuna children experience significantly greater malnutrition than do Creole children. Among children older than 6 months, 23, or 15.3% of the

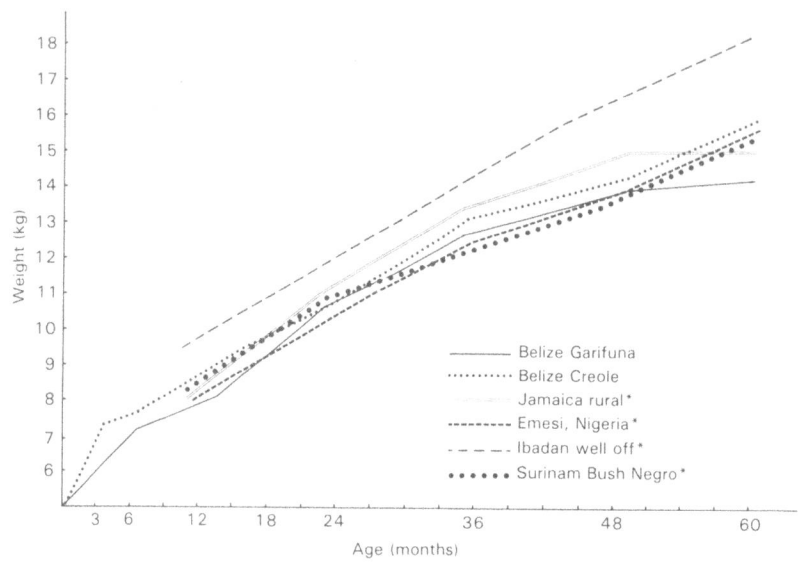

FIGURE 1. Weight-for-age among children of African ancestry, birth to 5 years, sexes combined. (* From Eveleth and Tanner, 1976.)

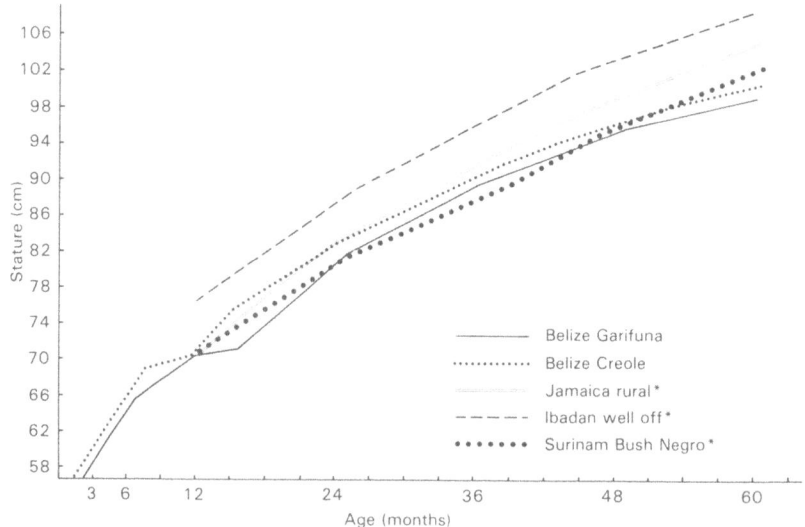

FIGURE 2. Stature-for-age among children of African ancestry, birth to 5 years, sexes combined. (* From Eveleth and Tanner, 1976.)

Garifuna children had arm circumferences below 13.5 cm, while only 10, or 6%, of the Creole children exhibited the same. These differences are statistically significant $(\chi^2 = 4.03, P > 0.01 < 0.05)$. Rates of malnutrition of varying

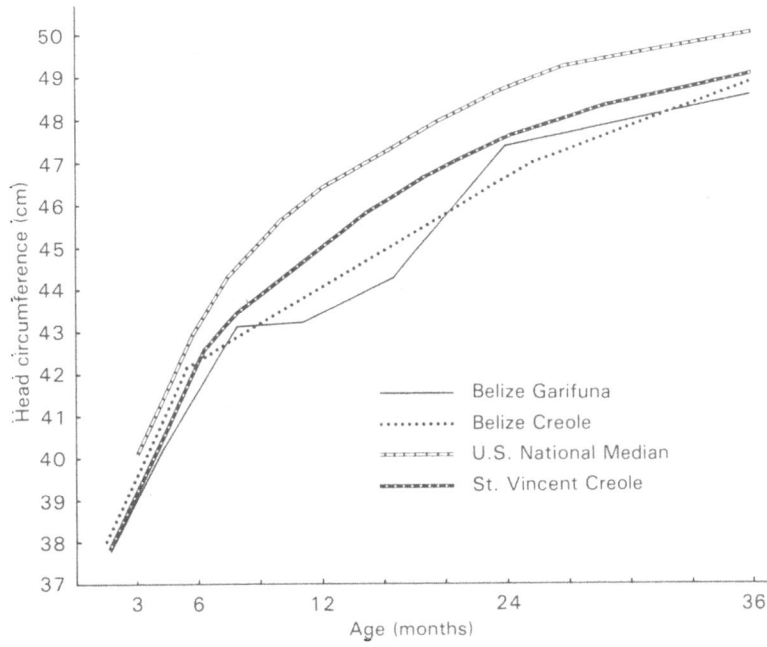

FIGURE 3. Head circumference by age among children, birth to 3 years, sexes combined. (St. Vincent Creole from Antrobus, 1971.)

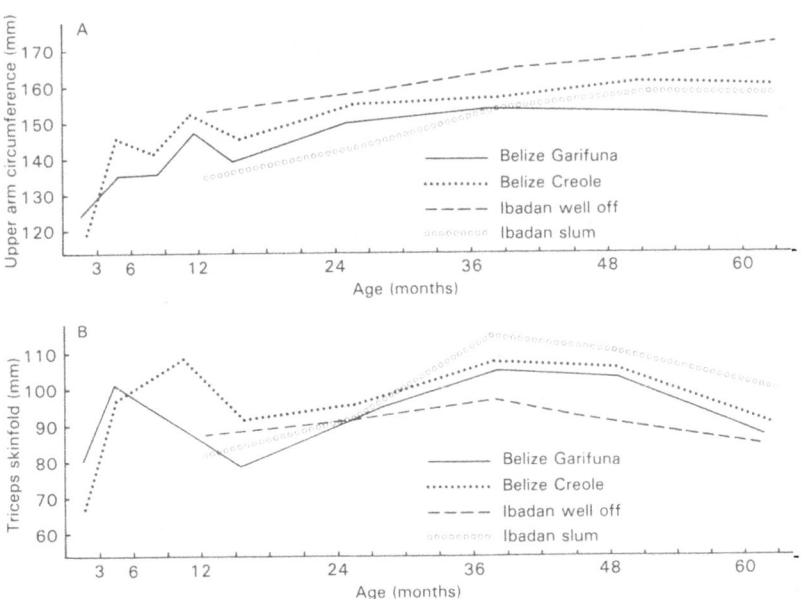

FIGURE 4. (A) Arm circumference and (B) triceps skinfold among children of African ancestry, birth to 5 years. (Ibadan from Eveleth and Tanner, 1976.)

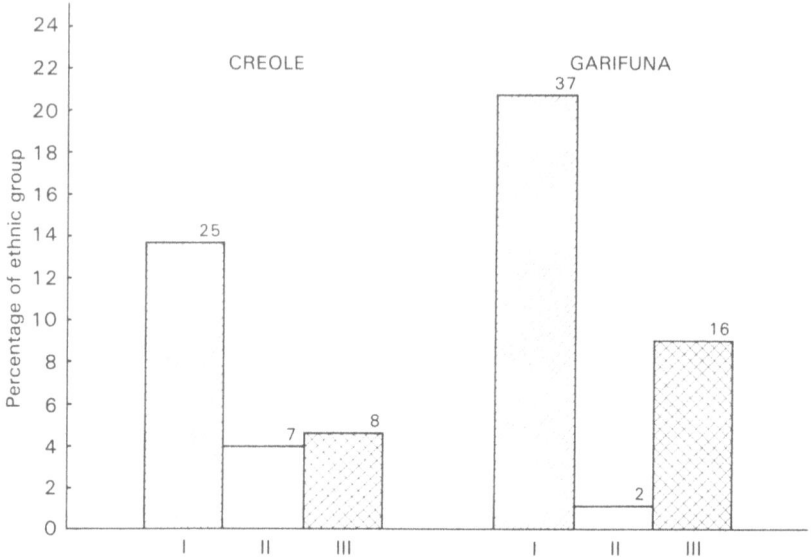

FIGURE 5. Duration of malnutrition by ethnic group. I, Past chronic; II, current short-term; III, current long-term.

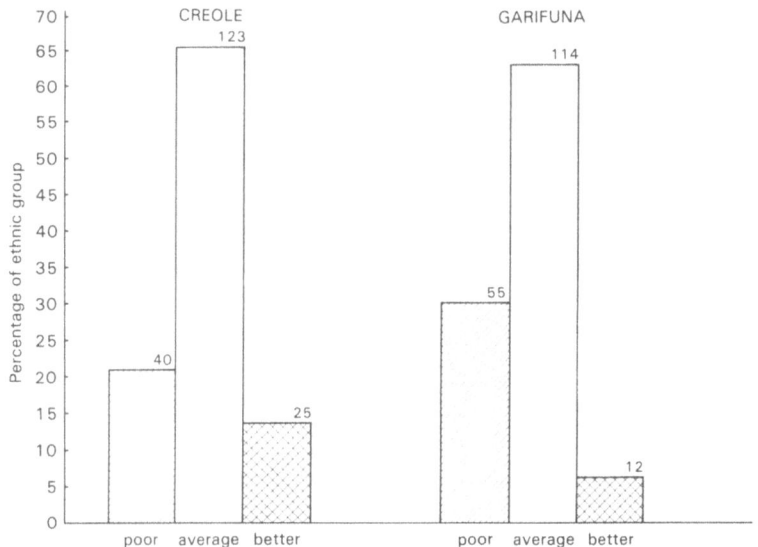

FIGURE 6. Poor, average, and better-than-average growth by ethnic group.

duration are presented in Fig. 5. These data suggest that Garifuna children endure longer periods of chronic and continuing nutritional stress. However, the rate of current short-term malnutrition is greater among Creole children, which suggests that these children more often return to a positive nutritional status after episodes of illness. These results are summarized in Fig. 6, which shows the percentages of children in each ethnic group with poor, average, and better-than-average growth. Garifuna children are represented significantly more often among those with poor growth ($\chi^2 = 4.13$, $P > 0.01 < 0.05$), while Creoles are more often among the better-than-average children ($\chi^2 = 4.65$, $P > 0.01 < 0.05$).

3.3. Biocultural Factors

Three biocultural factors accurately discriminate between the poor and better-than-average growth classes in 71% of cases. These factors include the frequency and severity of diarrhea, the age at introduction to solid foods, and the number of children in the household. Among poor growers, over three times as many Garifuna children ($N = 18$) compared to Creole children ($N = 5$) had been hospitalized with diarrhea, and over twice as many Garifuna children experienced chronic diarrhea, untreated by doctors (15 versus 7). It may be significant that Creole women more often reported the use of herbal teas in treatment for diarrhea than did Garifuna women. Among the better-than-average growth children, only one Garifuna child and no Creole child had ever been hospitalized with severe diarrhea.

Since, when the entire sample is considered, the association between the frequency of diarrhea and the number of months breastfed is highly significant ($P = 0.0001$), differences in breastfeeding patterns between ethnic groups were examined. While 27% of the Creole women had adopted bottle feeding exclusively, only 16% of the Garifuna women had done the same. Garifuna children were more often breastfed for periods of time extending beyond a year. Among those hospitalized with diarrhea, 2% had been breastfed, while 14% had been fed exclusively by bottle.

The age at introduction to solid foods also appears to influence the frequency of malnutrition, whereas the age at introduction to semisolids does not. Considering only children over 6 months old, the average age at first solids for better growers was 0.8 year, while the average age for poor growers was 1.8 years. Ethnic differences in the age at introduction to semisolid or solid foods are not significant, but the types of semisolids or solids most frequently mentioned differ by ethnic affiliation. Table 3 shows the percentages of responses for the most frequently mentioned solid and semisolid foods by ethnic group. These data suggest that Creole children far more frequently skip semisolid foods altogether and are weaned onto the family diet, a pattern that appears to ensure greater variety of foods and better nutrition. (For a more detailed discussion of the Belizean diet, see Jenkins, 1982b.)

Results of the 24-hr recalls for children between 1 and 6 years old are presented for the purpose of ethnic and socioeconomic comparisons and should not be construed to represent average intakes in these population segments.

Table 3. Percentages of Most Frequent Responses Concerning Weaning Foods by Ethnic Group

First semisolids			First solids		
	Creole %	Garifuna %		Creole %	Garifuna %
Cassava gruel	0	18.1	"Irish" potatoes	31.0	24.0
Cornstarch gruel	5.1	3.9	Family diet	27.0	14.0
Infant cereals	31.9	37.0	Fish	9.4	16.3
Custard	11.7	14.3	Eggs	15.0	13.5
Skipped to solids	37.9	13.6	Rice	11.0	11.0

Daily and seasonal variation in children's diets are great, and 24-hr recalls are subject to the effects of reporter error. Nonetheless, the results indicate a generally lower range of nutrient adequacy in the diets of Garifuna children compared to Creole children. Both samples were drawn almost entirely from urban residents. None of the children was either breastfeeding or ill at the time of the survey. An attempt was made to control for socioeconomic status by ranking the families according to primary occupational level. Results are summarized in Table 4. Although the variation within and among groups of children is very large, socioeconomic rank clearly influences dietary adequacy. In both ethnic groups, higher ranking children more often attain recommended dietary allowances. Of the 10 children who did receive 100% or more of their energy requirements, eight were Creole and two were Garifuna.

Because energy levels are generally low and infections frequent, the protein intakes reported in Table 4 may be misleading. Actual bioavailability of protein is likely to be far lower than intakes indicate since protein is appropriated as energy when caloric intake is deficient and its utilization increased during episodes of infection. Therefore, where infection levels are lower and energy intakes greater, as among Creole children, dietary protein is more readily available for physiological maintenance and growth. Of 29 children reportedly receiving 100% or more of their protein needs, 17 were Creole and two were Garifuna. Of six children at the lower range of protein adequacy, i.e., 80% or less of recommended dietary allowance, two were Creole and four were Garifuna.

Iron adequacy also varies considerably within and between groups and is subject to inhibited bioavailability due to the presence of a variety of dietary factors, including phytates, tannic acid, ascorbic acid, and the phosvitin in egg yolks (White, 1975; Monsen, 1980). In general, iron deficiency appears to be less frequent among the Creole than among the Garifuna. Of 11 children receiving 100% or more recommended iron allowances, nine were Creole and two were Garifuna. In the lower range, of those receiving 80% or less of recommended iron allowances, seven were Creole, while 12 were Garifuna.

Demographic factors are also likely to play a part in determining the

Table 4. Medians and Ranges of Percentage Attained Recommended Dietary Allowance of Energy, Protein, and Iron by Socioeconomic Rank and Ethnic Group

Socioeconomic rank	Creole							Garifuna						
		Energy		Protein		Iron			Energy		Protein		Iron	
	N	Median	Range	Median	Range	Median	Range	N	Median	Range	Median	Range	Median	Range
Professional in nuclear family	2	101	61–141	189	94–284	87	73–101	1	103	–	138	–	211	–
Wage earner in nuclear family	14	87	40–186	156	81–207	100	22–286	7	69	54–86	139	89–173	65	51–125
Extended family dependency	5	66	57–87	110	78–149	94	61–202	10	65	43–124	140	45–234	78	42–124
Subsistence food Producers	1	68	–	62	–	94	–	1	39	–	66	–	30	–

nutritional status of children. While the average number of pregnancies does not differ by ethnic group, i.e., 4.3 pregnancies for both Creole and Garifuna women, the average number of dead children does differ significantly ($P = 0.005$). Considering completed pregnancies only and omitting stillbirths, we find that 14 out of every 100 Garifuna children died within 5 years after birth, while the comparable rate among Creoles was eight per 100. The number of children in the households of poor growers averaged 4.5, while among those with better-than-average growth the mean was 3.6 children.

4. Discussion

Clinic-based samples, such as those discussed in the present study, are likely to underestimate the true prevalence of malnutrition in the community at large. Nonetheless, this type of research can yield a useful approximation of the relative prevalence of different degrees of malnutrition in the populations examined. The Creole and Garifuna of Belize represent an excellent example of genetically similar ethnic groups living in the same geographical area under different socioeconomic conditions. These conditions are reflected in the health status of the most vulnerable age group, children from birth to 5 years old. Specific demographic, dietary, and health care factors are significant in determining the nutritional status of Belizean children (Jenkins, 1982*a*). Garifuna children suffer from malnutrition at greater rates than do Creole children, who, like their parents, enjoy the benefits of generally higher social and economic status.

References

Adams, C. F., 1975, Nutritive Value of American Foods, Agriculture Handbook no. 456, U. S. Department of Agriculture, Washington, D.C.

Anderson, M. A., 1979, Comparison of anthropometric measures of nutritional status in preschool children in five developing countries, *Am. J. Clin. Nutr.* **32**:2339–2345.

Antrobus, A. C. K., 1971, Child growth and related factors in a rural community in St. Vincent, *Environ. Child Health* **1971**(December):187–209.

Belize, 1976, *Belize, New Nation in Central America*, Government of Belize, Belmopan.

Bengoa, J., 1975, Prevention of protein–calorie malnutrition, in *Protein–Calorie Malnutrition* (R. E. Olson, ed.), pp. 435–452, Academic, New York.

Burgess, H. J. L., and Burgess, A. P., 1969, The arm circumference as a public health index of protein–calorie malnutrition of early childhood (II) A modified standard for mid-upper arm circumference in young children, *J. Trop. Pediatr.* **15**:189–192.

Caribbean Food and Nutrition Institute, 1974, *Food Composition Tables for Use in the English-Speaking Caribbean*, Caribbean Food and Nutrition Institute, Kingston, Jamaica.

Caribbean Food and Nutrition Institute, 1976, *Recommended Dietary Allowances for the Caribbean*, Caribbean Food and Nutrition Institute, Kingston, Jamaica.

Chibnik, M. S., 1975, Economic strategies of small farmers in Stann Creek District, British Honduras, Ph.D. dissertation, Columbia University.

Cosminsky, S., 1977, Interethnic relations in a Southern Belizean community, *Ethnicity* 4: 226–245.

Despres, L., 1975, Ethnicity and resource competition in Guyana society, in *Ethnicity and Resource Competition in Rural Societies* (L. Despres, ed.), pp. 87–118, Mouton, The Hague.

Eveleth, P. B., and Tanner, J. M., 1976, *Worldwide Variation in Human Growth*, Cambridge University Press, London.

Frisancho, A. R., 1974, Triceps skin fold and upper arm muscle size norms for assessment of nutritional status, *Am. J. Clin. Nutr.* 27:1052–1058.

Graham, G. G. and Adriazen, B. T., 1971, Growth, inheritance and environment, *Ped. Res.* 5:691–697.

Gueri, Miguel, 1981, Childhood malnutrition in the Carribean, *Bull. Pan Am. Health Organ.* 15(2):160–167.

Jelliffe, D. B., 1968, *Infant Nutrition in the Subtropics and Tropics,* 2nd ed., World Health Organization Monograph Series no. 29, World Health Organization, Geneva.

Jenkins, Carol, 1982a, Factors in the aetiology of poor growth in Belize, *CAJANUS* 15 (3):172–184.

Jenkins, Carol, 1982b, A report on contemporary Belizean foodways, *Belizean Studies* 10: 2–9.

Johnston, F. E., 1978, Somatic growth of the infant and preschool child, in *Human Growth,* Vol. 2, *Postnatal Growth* (F. Falkner and J. M. Tanner, eds.), pp. 91–116, Plenum, New York.

Kerns, V. 1977, Daughters bring in: Ceremonial and Social Organization of the Black Carib of Belize, Ph.D. dissertation, University of Illinois at Urbana–Champaign.

McIntosh, C., 1980, Food and nutrition problems associated with natural disasters, *Cajanus* 13(1):18–27.

Monsen, E., 1980, Simplified method for calculating available dietary iron, *Food Nutr. News* 51(4):1–4.

National Center for Health Statistics, 1976, NCHS Growth Charts, Monthly Vital Statistics Report, Vol. 25, No. 3, Suppl. (HRA)76–1120, Health Resources Administration, Rockville, Maryland.

Newman, M. T., 1977, Ecology and nutritional stress, in *Culture, Disease and Healing* (D. Landy, ed.), pp. 319–326, MacMillan, New York.

Puffer, R. Serrano, C. V., and Dillon, A., 1971, *The Inter-American Investigation of Mortality in Childhood*, Pan-American Health Organization, Washington, D.C.

Raphael, D. (ed), 1979, *Breastfeeding and Food Policy in a Hungry World*, Academic, New York.

Sanford, M., 1974, Revitalization movements as indicators of completed acculturation, *Comparative Studies Soc. History* 16(4):504–518.

Scrimshaw, N., Taylor, C., and Gordon, J., 1968, *Interactions of Nutrition and Infection*, World Health Organization Monograph Series no. 57, World Health Organization, Geneva.

Seone, N., and Latham, M. C., 1971, Nutritional anthropometry in the identification of malnutrition in childhood, *J. Trop. Pediatr.* 17:98.

Sinha, D., 1979, Oral rehydiation in diarrhael diseases: A simple solution to a complex problem, *Cajanus* 12(3):138–149.

White, H., 1975, Dietary iron and anemia, *Nutr. M. D.* 2(1, November):1–2.

9

Skin Color of the
Garifuna of Belize

PAMELA J. BYARD, FRANCIS C. LEES, and
JOHN H. RELETHFORD

1. Introduction

This chapter reviews the results of a survey of skin reflectometry among the Garifuna of Belize conducted in 1976. The survey sought to answer several broad questions about skin color in the Garifuna. The first question concerns the physical distinctiveness of the Garifuna in relation to neighboring groups of African extraction, known locally as Creoles. According to Gonzalez, Garifuna differ little, if any, in appearance from other dark-skinned people in the area, yet "Most non-Caribs who have lived in the area for any length of time insist that they can distinguish Caribs merely by looking at them. Some claim that the Carib is slightly lighter in color . . ." (Gonzalez, 1969, p. 25). Demonstration of significant differences in pigmentation between Garifuna and Creoles will support this contention of distinctive physical appearance.

A second area of interest concerns skin color variability within the population, due to sex, age, and local differences. Sex and age variation in skin reflectance readings have been reported by many authors (de Diaz Ungria, 1965; Harrison *et al.*, 1967; Harrison and Salzano, 1966; Kahlon, 1976), and consideration of intrapopulation variability in both Garifuna and Creoles is necessary when comparing the overall means for the two populations.

PAMELA J. BYARD • Department of Anthropology, University of Kansas, Lawrence, Kansas 66045; present address: Department of Anthropology, Case Western Reserve University, Cleveland, Ohio 44106. FRANCIS C. LEES and JOHN H. RELETHFORD • Department of Anthropology, State University of New York at Albany, Albany, New York 12222; present address for Dr. Relethford: Department of Anthropology, State University of New York at Oneonta, Oneonta, New York 13820.

Finally, we wish to estimate admixture proportions of various ancestral groups to the present-day Garifuna based on skin color measurements and compare these estimates to those derived by Crawford from serological markers (see Chapters 16, 18, and 19). While it is generally agreed that the Garifuna are an admixed population of primarily West African origin, with lesser contributions by other groups, such as Island Carib, Red Carib Indian, or possibly European (Taylor, 1951), reconstruction of the population history and resultant genetic composition of these people can expect little verification from ethnohistorical sources, which are vague and contradictory in this respect. It is interesting to note, however, that many early descriptions of the Black Caribs include skin color as an indicator of the genetic affiliation of the population. For instance, Young described the early Black Caribs as "some being coal black, others again nearly as yellow as saffron" (Young, 1847, p. 123). Bard also described extensive variability in skin color among Black Caribs in the mid-19th century: "Most are pure Indians, not large, but muscular, with a ruddy skin, and long straight hair ... Another portion are dark, with curly hair, and betraying unmistakably a large infusion of Negro blood ..." (Bard, 1855, p. 317).

This chapter will relate differences in pigmentation between two groups of Garifuna and between the Garifuna as a whole and Creoles to differences in admixture proportions. Our objectives might be accomplished using any number of biological characters (morphology, dentition, serology, etc.), but the repeated references to skin color in ethnological and historical sources makes it especially interesting to assess physical heterogeneity within and among Garifuna and Creole populations with respect to present-day skin color variation. Finally, comparisons among admixture estimates based on serological and skin colorimetry variables will provide an opportunity to test methods suggested by Lees and Relethford (1978) to estimate admixture proportions from skin color data.

2. Materials and Methods

Eight hundred and forty-seven Belizeans were measured for skin color at Dangriga (Stann Creek), Punta Gorda, and Belize City. Of these, 548 were classified as Garifuna by native assistants and 227 were classified as Creole. The remaining 72 belonged to other ethnicities. The two abridged spectrophotometers most common in field studies of human skin color were used. One is the British-made E.E.L., the other the American-made Photovolt Model 601. Together, they can assess the percentage reflectance of an opaque surface at 15 different wavelengths, ranging from 420 to 685 nm.

Measurements were taken at four body sites: upper inner arm, outer forearm, back of hand, and forehead. Only the upper inner arm measures are used in this chapter, as this site is least influenced by the environment (Livingstone, 1969). All measures were taken in accordance with standard techniques (Weiner and Lourie, 1969).

Interpopulational differences were evaluated by t-tests. While violation of the assumptions of normal distribution and homogeneous variance was observed for some of the variables, the parametric t-test was used because of its generally robust nature (Sokal and Rohlf, 1969). Conclusions based on univariate t-tests over many variables may be erroneous because of inflation of type I error [the experimentwise error rate $\alpha' = 1 - (1 - \alpha)^k = 1 - 0.91^{15} = 0.54$ using 15 variables at $\alpha = 0.05$ (Harris, 1975)]. The appropriate test for equality of means over all variables taken simultaneously is Hotelling's T^2, which was computed using computer program BMDP3D [version of July 7, 1975 (Dixon, 1975)]. Since this test excludes cases with missing values, only complete cases, totaling 308 Garifuna and 175 Creoles, were used. In addition, a stepwise discriminant analysis was performed on these data to determine the usefulness of skin color variables in the classification of individuals as Garifuna or Creole, using all significant discriminant variables.

To evaluate intrapopulation variability among the Garifuna, univariate t-tests and Hotelling's multivariate T^2 tests were performed on subdivisions of the population according to location for Dangriga and Punta Gorda; the number of Garifuna measured in Belize City was too small for analysis. Creole samples from locations other than Belize City were too small to allow comparisons of Creole groups by location.

To assess age trends in pigmentation, the Garifuna sample was partitioned into 5-year age cohorts. Due to the small size of some of the subsamples and severe departures from normality, the Kruskal–Wallis test, a nonparametric equivalent of analysis of variance, was used to compare different age cohorts. The Creole sample was not suitable for analysis of age trends, since it consists primarily of school-age children.

To estimate admixture proportions, mean skin reflectance values for African, Amerindian, and European populations were selected from the literature. While we wished to make maximal use of the data for the Belizean groups by estimating admixture based on both Photovolt and E.E.L. instruments, finding comparable data on possible ancestral representatives presented several problems. To the best of our knowledge, only two other studies use all filters for both machines (Lees et al., 1978, 1979), and many published sources use less than the full complement of filters for either machine. To complicate matters, the E.E.L. instrument has been used primarily on Old World populations and the Photovolt on New World populations. In addition, there are no Amerindian populations measured with all nine E.E.L. filters and only one study (Conway and Baker, 1972) using all six Photovolt filters on nonhybrid American Indians. Direct comparability between the two machines is not possible, due to their different filter characteristics. Garrard et al. (1967) reported linear regression formulas for some of the filters in an attempt to overcome this obstacle. Recently, multiple regression formulas for all 15 filters for use with dark- and light-skinned populations were derived (Lees and Byard, 1978; Lees et

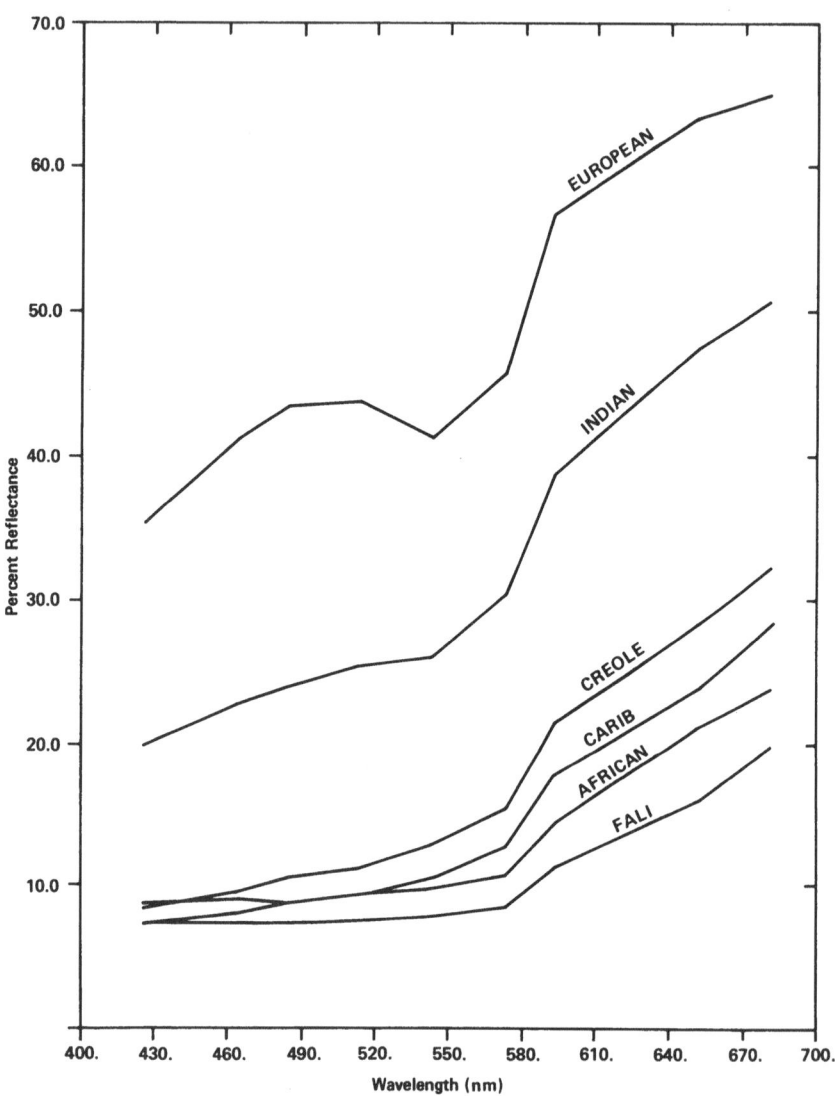

FIGURE 1. Mean reflectance for selected world populations, E.E.L. filters.

al., 1979). Unfortunately, no such formulas exist for American Indian populations.

Comparison of Garifuna and Creole mean reflectances with those of African groups (Fig. 1) shows that the hybrid group means fall below those of a composite "African" group at lower wavelengths. For this reason, a darker West African group, such as the Fali Tinguelin (Rigters-Aris, 1973*b*), seems to be a better choice as representative of the African parent. It does not seem likely that the hybrid groups would have become darker than their African parents, especially with the suspected contribution of Indians and Europeans to their gene pools. In addition, a West African group is more representative of the escaped plantation slaves that first formed the Black Caribs (Taylor, 1951) than a composite of groups from all parts of Africa. The Fali were measured on the E.E.L. machine, and the Photovolt values were estimated using the multiple regression equations of Lees and Byard (1978). As shown in Fig. 1, the Garifuna mean is slightly lower than that of the Fali for the E.E.L. 601 filter. In this case, admixture estimation would have little meaning, and has not been attempted for the Garifuna on that scale.

The E.E.L. means for 12 European populations were taken from reports by Barnicot (1958), Tiwari (1963), Harrison and Owen (1964), Ojikutu (1965), Wasserman and Heyl (1968), Hulse (1973), Rigters-Aris (1973a,b), and Lees et al. (1978).

The lack of conversion formulas for Amerindian data, coupled with the rarity of E.E.L. studies in the New World, limits the number of admixture estimates that can be made for African—Indian hybrids like the Garifuna on E.E.L. filters. The only published E.E.L. data on Amerindians known to us are those of Weiner et al. (1963) on the Aguarana Indians of Peru. These data are further limited in that only the 601, 605, and 609 filters were used in Brazil, and the 605 and 609 filters in Peru. Because of this, admixture estimates could be computed for only two filters. In addition to the untransformed 605 and 609 scales, the "antilog" transformation of the 609 filter ($10^{R609-100)/100}$) was used, as suggested by Harrison and Owen (1964).

The availability of complete Photovolt data sets for African, European, and Indian populations allows calculation of triracial admixture estimates using techniques that cannot be applied to the limited E.E.L. data. Conway and Baker (1972) have published data for four subgroups of Quechua Indians (male and female, urban and rural) on all six Photovolt filters. A total of 17 European and nine African population or subpopulation means on Photovolt filters were taken from the literature (Barnicot, 1958; Leguebe, 1961; Das and Mukherjee, 1963; Tiwari, 1963; Harrison and Owen, 1964; Ojikutu, 1965; Rijn-Tournel, 1965; Huizinga, 1968; Wasserman and Heyl, 1968; Conway and Baker, 1972; Hulse, 1973; Rigters-Aris, 1973a,b; Lees et al., 1978, 1979). Multiple conversion formulas for light-skinned populations (Lees and Byard, 1978; Lees et al., 1979) were used when necessary to convert from E.E.L. to Photovolt readings. The major disadvantage of the Photovolt data is that scaling tests have not been applied to any Photovolt scales. Using hybrids of known composition, Harrison and Owen (1964) and Lees and Relethford (1978) tested the E.E.L. scales for scale linearity and accuracy of admixture estimation, respectively, but the validity of the various Photovolt filters for this purpose is unknown. The Photovolt estimates are thus experimental, but a comparison with E.E.L. estimates should give some indication of their worth.

Two assumptions must be made in order to compare meaningfully measures taken from a variety of studies: first, that variation due to machine differences is nonsignificant, and second, that variation due to multiple observers is non-significant. While the claim for direct comparability has been made for different Photovolt instruments (Post *et al.*, 1976), such claim has not been made for the E.E.L. For at least one sample, however, interobserver error on the same machine has been shown to be nonsignificant for all filters of both machines (Lees *et al.*, 1978).

In addition, admixture studies assume that the parental populations are represented adequately by the samples selected. This assumption cannot be tested today for hybrids formed long ago, and, given the limited nature of comparative skin color data, we are forced to rely on the samples available. Obviously, we are not implying that the Garifuna are made up of Fali Tinguelin, Europeans, and South American Indians, yet the homogeneity within major world groupings for skin color may make exact location of parental groups less crucial than for other characters.

Wherever possible, several different methods were used to derive biracial and triracial admixture estimates for Garifuna and Creoles. For E.E.L. data, only biracial estimates were possible. These involve application of Bernstein's m (1931) to population means for the available raw and transformed variables. For the Creoles, who are primarily African and European, an unweighted mean $\bar{m}$ was computed using the three variables (log 601, 605, and "antilog" 609) chosen for accurate interpopulation scaling by Harrison and Owen (1964). For the Garifuna, only the 605 and 609 filters were available because of the limited comparative material for Amerindian populations.

Several additional estimates of m could be computed for the Photovolt data. These include an unweighted mean $\bar{m}$ over all filters, single estimates of m computed from the first canonical variate resulting from discriminant analysis of African, European, and Indian group means, and values of m computed directly from distance measures, both Euclidean and Mahalanobis D^2 (Mahalanobis, 1936). As used here, Euclidean distance is a mean squared difference of standardized variates (Sokal, 1961). While deficient in many respects, Euclidean distances can be calculated directly from sample statistics. The Mahalanobis D^2 is considered a superior measure, but requires the original variates for calculation. For both measures, the procedure used was to treat the sample means taken from the literature as individual variates belonging to three samples: African, Indian, and European. These three groups were used to define the discriminant space. Garifuna and Creole means were then assigned positions in the discriminant space defined on worldwide variation in skin color. The distance measures were used to compute admixture estimates using variants of the methods suggested by Pollitzer (1964) and Cavalli-Sforza and Bodmer (1971). These methods and their application to hybrids of known ancestry are discussed in detail elsewhere (Lees and Relethford, 1978).

Table 1. Descriptive Statistics and t-Tests for Garifuna and Creoles[a]

Filter	Garifuna				Creoles					
	N	$x(\%R)$	$s(\%R)$	CV, %	N	$x(\%R)$	$s(\%R)$	CV, %	t	d.f.
Photovolt										
Blue	547	9.0	1.5	17.0	216	9.9	2.2	22.4	5.75*	299
Tri-blue	547	6.7	1.2	18.5	216	9.9	1.9	25.2	5.42*	292
Green	547	9.0	2.0	22.0	216	10.3	2.9	28.6	6.17*	294
Tri-green	547	11.4	2.5	22.3	216	13.1	3.7	28.0	6.35*	300
Tri-amber	547	13.9	3.1	22.1	216	16.1	4.5	28.0	6.60*	297
Red	547	25.6	4.1	16.1	216	28.6	5.8	20.3	6.81*	306
E.E.L.										
601	309	7.2	1.5	20.6	175	8.1	1.9	23.9	5.02*	292
602	309	8.1	1.7	21.6	175	9.2	2.5	26.7	5.40*	274
603	309	8.8	2.0	22.3	175	10.2	3.0	29.5	5.42*	260
604	309	9.4	2.1	22.6	175	10.8	3.2	29.5	4.98*	264
605	309	10.7	2.4	22.3	175	12.4	3.7	29.6	5.63*	259
606	308	12.8	2.9	22.4	175	14.8	4.3	28.8	5.73*	264
607	308	17.9	3.8	21.0	175	20.7	5.5	26.7	6.01*	267
608	308	24.0	4.7	19.6	175	27.6	6.5	23.6	6.53*	279
609	308	28.4	4.6	16.3	175	31.7	6.8	21.4	5.76*	267

[a] t-tests are based on separate (versus pooled) variance estimates, since the null hypothesis of homogeneous variance was rejected for each variable (Dixon, 1975, p. 125). Critical value of t for $\alpha = 0.05$ and d.f. $= 120$ is 1.96. The d.f. values are approximate (Dixon, 1975, p. 125). *$P < 0.05$. **$P < 0.01$. ***$P < 0.001$.

3. Results

After deletion of 12 bivariate outliers, basic univariate statistics were computed for Garifuna and Creoles, and are reported in Table 1. For every wavelength, Creoles are both lighter and more variable than Garifuna. As shown in Table 1, the differences between population means are significant for every filter ($P < 0.05$). The null hypothesis of homogeneous variance is also rejected for

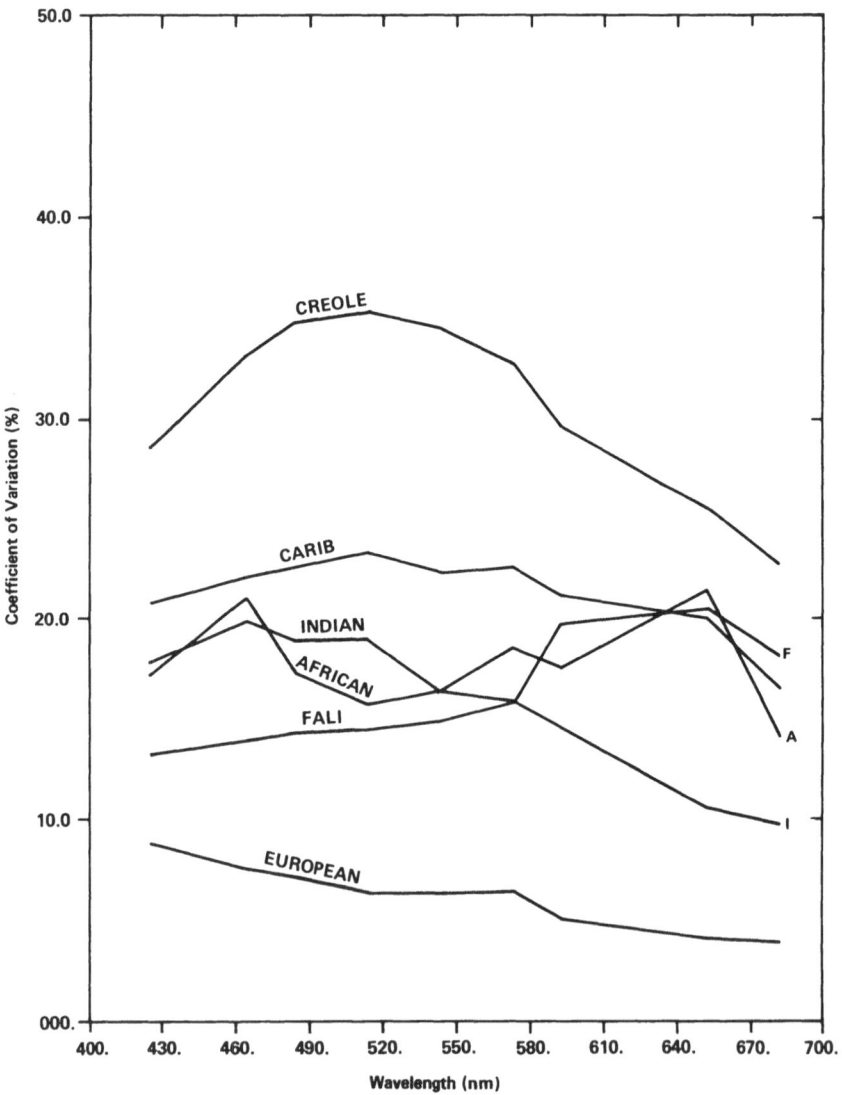

FIGURE 2. Coefficients of variation for selected world populations, E.E.L. filters.

every filter, supporting the hypothesis that Creoles are more heterogeneous in skin coloration than Garifuna. Comparison with coefficients of variation from world samples (Fig. 2) reveals that both groups exhibit high variability, most likely because of their hybrid nature. The coefficients of variation for the Creoles are the highest reported for any population in the literature.

The computed value of T^2 is highly significant, indicating that the two population means are different over all variables ($T^2 = 89.7; P < 0.001$). Since Garifuna means are consistently lower than Creole means, our results contradict some of the the ethnographic literature, which claims that Garifuna seem lighter than Creoles, but provide a possible explanation for the ability of natives to distinguish between the two groups. In an attempt to replicate this ability statistically, stepwise discriminant analysis between the two groups correctly classified 65% of cases as Garifuna or Creole, using the Photovolt tri-amber and the E.E.L. 609 filters together. Since 50% correct classification would be expected by chance, the 65% figure indicates that skin color alone does not account for the ability of native observers to assign individuals to the correct ethnic group with nearly 100% accuracy.

Means, standard deviations, and coefficients of variation for Garifuna males and females are reported in Table 2, along with the results of t-tests for equality of male and female mean reflectances. The same set of statistics for Creoles is reported in Table 3. Garifuna females are significantly lighter than males at nine of the 15 wavelengths, and the T^2 ($T^2 = 29.67; P < 0.05$) value indicates that the difference is significant when all variables are tested simultaneously. For Creoles, female means are higher than male means at all wavelengths, but the differences are not statistically significant in the univariate tests. It may be that the extreme variability of Creoles due to other factors obscures the differences between sexes. Alternatively, lack of significance for the t-tests may be due to the smaller sample sizes for Creoles. Sex differences in Creoles do reach highly significant levels when all variables are considered simultaneously ($T^2 = 35.04; P < 0.01$).

There is some confounding of sex effects and age trends in the Garifuna. Mean reflectance for both sexes rises throughout adolescence, reaching a peak at 26–30 years for females and 31–35 for males. Males and females differ little before puberty and after age 35, but females tend to be lighter in adolescence and early adulthood. Age trends among Garifuna are similar for all filters. Figure 3 illustrates these trends for the Photovolt green filter. The E.E.L. filters have a slightly less regular pattern, perhaps due to the small sizes of some of the age cohorts measured on the E.E.L. The Kruskal–Wallis test statistic for differences among age cohorts is significant ($P < 0.05$) for all filters, but there is little evidence of a linear age effect for this sample.

As shown in Table 4, Garifuna residing in Punta Gorda are consistently lighter than those in Dangriga. The difference is highly significant for every Photovolt filter, but reaches significance for only two E.E.L. filters (606 and

Table 2. Sex Differences, Garifuna[a]

Filter	Males				Females				t	d.f.
	N	x(%R)	s(%R)	CV, %	N	x(%R)	s(%R)	CV, %		
Photovolt										
Blue	165	8.73	1.47	16.84	382	9.07	1.55	17.09	−2.43*	327
Tri-blue	165	6.56	1.18	17.99	382	6.70	1.25	18.66	−1.23	329
Green	165	8.60	1.81	21.05	382	9.12	2.02	22.15	−2.97**	347
Tri-green	165	10.92	2.28	20.88	382	11.58	2.62	22.63	−2.96**	354
Tri-amber	165	13.28	2.85	21.46	382	14.21	3.14	22.10	−3.38***	341
Red	165	24.85	3.82	15.37	382	25.98	4.23	16.28	−3.08*	342
E.E.L.										
601	100	7.23	1.51	20.89	209	7.20	1.47	20.42	0.17	190
602	100	7.97	1.76	22.08	209	8.12	1.73	21.31	−0.71	192
603	100	8.66	1.97	22.75	209	8.86	1.96	22.12	−0.85	194
604	100	9.24	2.14	23.16	209	9.50	1.12	22.32	−1.00	194
605	100	10.30	2.18	21.17	209	10.83	2.45	22.62	−1.92	217
606	99	12.25	2.66	21.71	209	13.00	2.92	22.46	−2.22*	210
607	99	17.14	3.42	19.95	209	18.22	3.86	21.19	−2.47*	215
608	99	23.25	4.17	17.94	209	24.31	4.92	20.24	−1.96*	224
609	99	27.64	4.21	15.23	209	28.77	4.78	16.61	−2.12*	216

[a] See footnote to Table 1.

Table 3. Sex Differences, Creoles[a]

Filter	Males				Females					
	N	x(%R)	s(%R)	CV,%	N	x(%R)	s(%R)	CV,%	t	d.f.
Photovolt										
Blue	86	9.66	2.37	24.53	130	9.07	2.11	20.93	-1.33	167
Tri-blue	86	7.23	1.94	26.83	130	6.70	1.81	24.07	-1.09	173
Green	86	9.91	3.06	30.88	130	9.12	2.85	26.99	-1.59	173
Tri-green	86	12.54	3.81	30.38	130	11.58	2.62	26.17	-1.84	173
Tri-amber	86	15.56	4.81	30.91	130	14.21	4.29	25.98	-1.48	168
Red	86	27.87	6.09	21.85	130	25.98	5.56	19.14	-1.44	171
E.E.L.										
601	70	7.89	2.13	27.00	105	7.20	1.78	21.81	-0.87	130
602	70	9.01	2.51	27.86	105	8.12	2.43	26.05	-0.83	145
603	70	10.06	3.23	32.11	105	8.86	2.85	27.89	-0.35	135
604	70	10.49	3.38	32.25	105	9.50	3.04	27.72	-0.88	137
605	70	12.07	3.88	32.15	105	10.83	3.52	27.94	-0.92	138
606	70	14.49	4.62	31.88	105	13.00	4.03	26.76	-0.83	134
607	70	20.31	5.76	28.66	105	18.22	5.36	25.60	-0.74	141
608	70	27.25	7.07	25.94	105	24.31	6.13	21.99	-0.61	133
609	70	31.36	7.31	23.31	105	28.77	6.45	20.18	-0.56	135

[a] See footnote to Table 1.

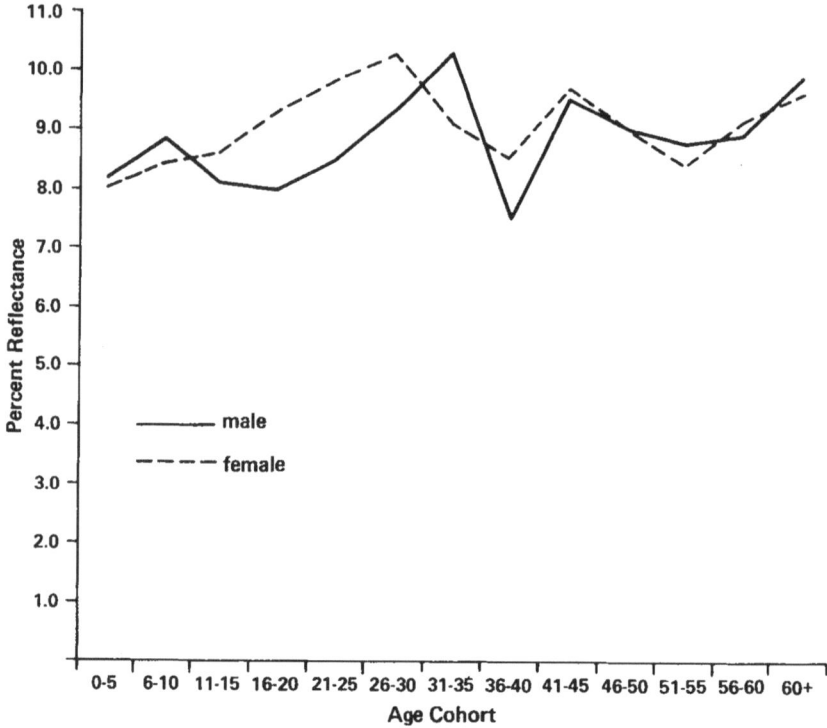

FIGURE 3. Age trends in mean reflectance, Photovolt green filter (650 nm).

609). Hotelling's T^2 is also highly significant ($T^2 = 52.44; P < 0.001$). Failure to reject the null hypotheses of equal means for individual E.E.L. filters may be due to the smaller sample sizes on that machine. Since significant sex and age cohort differences have been demonstrated, it is possible that the differences between the two towns are due to different sex or age compositions of the samples. To test the null hypothesis of equal proportions of males and females at both locations, Yates' corrected χ^2 statistic was computed (Table 5). The χ^2 fails to suggest rejection of the null hypothesis. The null hypothesis of equal sampling of age cohorts at the two locations can be rejected, however (Table 6). This is not unexpected, because fieldwork in Dangriga was conducted in both school and clinic settings, while in Punta Gorda only the local health clinic was visited. This caused a disproportionate increase in the 11–15-year-old category in Dangriga. In an attempt to determine whether locational differences exist beyond those caused by unequal sampling of age cohorts, a comparison between the Dangriga clinic sample alone and Punta Gorda was made. Significant differences remain, with the Punta Gorda mean reflectances again consistently higher ($P < 0.05$ for nine of the 15 variables; $T^2 = 34.84; P < 0.01$). These results

Table 4. Locational Differences, Garifuna[a]

Filter	Dangriga				Punta Gorda					
	N	X̄(%R)	s(%R)	CV,%	N	X̄(%R)	s(%R)	CV,%	t	d.f.
Photovolt										
Blue	316	8.67	1.40	16.15	230	9.38	1.60	17.06	5.33***	454
Tri-blue	316	6.49	1.13	17.41	230	6.90	1.33	19.28	3.79***	443
Green	316	8.61	1.83	21.25	230	9.45	2.07	21.90	4.88***	456
Tri-green	316	10.95	2.37	21.64	230	11.97	2.65	22.14	4.67***	460
Tri-amber	316	13.39	2.87	21.43	230	14.67	3.23	22.02	4.77***	458
Red	316	24.92	3.96	15.89	230	26.64	4.19	15.73	4.84***	477
E.E.L.										
601	226	7.18	1.57	21.87	82	7.31	1.20	16.42	0.78	188
602	226	8.06	1.81	22.46	82	8.11	1.55	19.11	0.25	166
603	226	8.71	2.01	23.08	82	9.02	1.83	20.29	1.29	157
604	226	9.31	2.14	22.99	82	9.70	2.10	21.65	1.40	146
605	226	10.51	2.37	22.55	82	11.05	2.39	21.63	1.77	143
606	225	12.55	2.82	22.47	82	13.36	2.91	21.78	2.18*	140
607	225	17.67	3.71	21.00	82	18.43	3.85	20.89	1.55	139
608	225	23.80	4.47	18.78	82	24.78	4.72	19.05	1.63	137
609	225	28.07	4.54	16.71	82	29.35	4.80	16.35	2.10*	137

Hotelling's $T^2 = 52.44$***

[a] See footnote to Table 1.

Table 5. Sex Composition by Location, Garifuna

	Male	Female	Total
Dangriga	104	212	316
Punta Gorda	61	169	230
Total	165	381	546

$\chi^2 = 2.283$ d.f. $= 1$ $P = 0.1308$

indicate that differences between the two local groups are due to factors other than age or sex distribution of the samples.

Various admixture estimates, using the methods described above, are given in Table 7, along with serological estimates provided by Devor and Crawford (see Chapter 19). The limited variety of estimates for E.E.L. data gives results reasonably congruent among themselves and with the blood group estimates. Biracial estimates for E.E.L. readings suggest that 75–80% of the Garifuna gene pool is derived from African ancestors and 20–25% from Amerindians, which agrees roughly with the biracial estimates based on blood markers. The Creole E.E.L. estimates of African parentage (90–95%) are higher than the biracial serological estimates of about 80%. The remaining European contribution to the Creole gene pool is estimated at 5–10% based on E.E.L. readings and 20% based on blood markers.

For the Photovolt data, a wider variety of biracial and triracial estimates could be derived. The biracial estimates are fairly consistent and similar to serological estimates. The greatest variation occurs with the distance-based estimates, perhaps revealing the differences between Euclidean distance and Mahalanobis D^2. The use of distance for biracial estimates (m_d) assumes that the distances between parents and hybrid are linear (Cavalli-Sforza and Bodmer, 1971). Lees and Relethford (1978) suggest an index of linearity that will equal 1.0 for perfect linearity. In the present study, the index of linearity ranges from 0.78 for the Euclidean distances to between 0.88 and 0.91 for Mahalanobis D^2 values. This suggests that the m_d estimates derived from Mahalanobis D^2 may be more appropriate.

Triracial estimates for the Garifuna nicely bracket the serological estimate based on gamma globulins, but both triracial skin color estimates for the Creoles overestimate Indian admixture and underestimate the European proportion. This is probably because the effects of Indian and European admixture on pigmentation in a predominantly African population are similar. Thus, for populations not differing greatly in melanin concentration, skin color is probably not as precise a genetic marker as gamma globulins. Admixture estimates based upon skin color, then, are useful for determining very dark versus "light" ancestry, but may not be as accurate as sensitive marker genes for estimating specific non-African components.

Table 6. Frequency Table, Age Cohort by Location, Garifuna

Location	1–5	6–10	11–15	16–20	21–25	26–30	31–35	36–40	41–45	46–50	51–55	56–60	>60
Dangriga	7	21	104	26	12	7	11	7	16	10	18	17	60
Punta Gorda	9	32	46	30	12	2	4	8	11	8	12	15	41

$\chi^2 = 24.465$ d.f. $= 12$ $P = 0.0176$

Table 7. Admixture Estimates for Garifuna and Creoles Based on Skin Reflectance Data[a]

Method	Garifuna			Creoles		
	Percent African	Percent Indian	Percent European	Percent African	Percent Indian	Percent European
E.E.L.						
$\bar{m}$	—	—	—	91	—	9
$\bar{m}$ (transformed variables)	—	—	—	95	—	5
$\bar{m}$ (605, 609)[b]	76	24	—	—	—	—
$\bar{m}$ (605, Alog609)[b]	79	21	—	—	—	—
Photovolt						
$\bar{m}$	74	26	—	90	—	10
$\bar{m}$ (transformed variables)	75	25	—	89	—	11
m (canonical variate #1)	73	27	—	77	—	23
m_d (Euclidean)	63	37	—	75	—	25
m_d (Mahalanobis)	71	29	—	73	—	27
$1/d^2$ (Euclidean)	74	26	—	90	—	10
$1/d^2$ (Euclidean)	67	24	9	56	33	12
$1/d^2$ (Mahalanobis)	85	15	—	88	—	12
$1/d^2$ (Mahalanobis)	80	14	6	66	24	10
Average biracial	74	26	—	85	—	15
Serological biracial[c]	78	22	—	80	—	20
Average triracial	73	19	8	61	28	11
Serological triracial[d]	76	20	4	72	8	20

[a] African parent is Fali Tinguelin.
[b] Indian parent is Caingang, Guarani, and Aguarana.
[c] Biracial serological estimate based on eight loci and 26 alleles (Crawford, 1977).
[d] Triracial serological estimate based on gamma globulins (M. H. Crawford, personal communication).

4. Discussion

In light of the present research, ethnographic claims regarding Garifuna—Creole differences are supported. Biological dissimilarity, assessed by skin colorimetry, parallels cultural distinctions, but assignment of individuals to the two groups based on skin color alone is not as accurate as the process used by natives in their social interactions. Obviously, other physical or cultural factors must be aiding their powers of discrimination. Our results do not support claims of lighter coloration for the Garifuna, but do support claims in the literature of high variability in skin color for both groups.

Our investigation of differences within the two populations reveals that in general females are lighter than males. While many authors have noted sex differences in skin color similar to our findings (Weiner *et al.*, 1964; Harrison and Salzano, 1966; Mazess, 1967), few have provided real insight into the causes for these differences, other than to speculate about differences in exposure to sunlight or in endocrine functioning. Because it hardly makes sense to hypothesize that different amounts of light-skinned ancestry in males and females is responsible, we leave the sex-related effect unexplained and combine sexes for interpopulational analysis.

There is some confounding of sex effects and age trends in the Garifuna. Females tend to be slightly darker than males before puberty and after menopause, but are lighter in early adulthood. A similar interaction between puberty and a darkening of skin color has been reported in a sample of Irish schoolchildren (Relethford *et al.*, 1980). Overall, the results of both studies appear to support hypotheses of a pigmentation—endocrine relationship. The underlying mechanisms are still to be discovered, however.

The difference in mean reflectance between the Dangriga and Punta Gorda Garifuna can best be attributed to a larger component of Indian admixture in the Punta Gorda group. The variability in skin-reflectance-based admixture estimates and their inability to distinguish adequately between Indian and European contributions precludes testing this hypothesis with skin color data. In addition, such a test of skin color differences using skin-color-based estimates seems circular. Triracial serological admixture estimates computed separately for the two localities (Chapter 18) indicate that the Indian component is about 8% larger in the Punta Gorda sample than in Dangriga. This may be partially offset by the slightly larger amount of European admixture in the Dangriga population. Biracial estimates seem to support the idea that the difference in pigmentation is due to a smaller African component in Punta Gorda. It seems unlikely that the two populations have diverged in pigmentation due to evolutionary forces during their relatively short period of isolation in similar environments.

The differences between Garifuna and Creoles also seem to be related to different admixture proportions. The Garifuna are primarily African—Indian hybrids, while Creoles are African with a substantial European component. The combined non-African component is slightly greater in Creoles than in Garifuna, contributing to their lighter pigmentation.

Comparison of admixture estimates computed by different methods indicates that most reflectance-based techniques give results in agreement with serological estimates. Photovolt estimates are similar to E.E.L. values, implying that Photovolt scales are usuable for admixture studies, even though they have not been tested on hybrids of known composition. This will be helpful in other studies because many hybrid groups and their likely ancestors have been measured only with the Photovolt machine. Of the many estimation techniques applied to the Photovolt data, those based on Euclidean distance and Pollitzer's proportional distance technique give less consistent and hence possibly less reliable figures than the others. Triracial reflectance-based estimates for the Garifuna are in close agreement with serological estimates, but those for Creoles give very different estimates of Indian versus European admixture.

While the overall agreement of admixture estimates based on skin color and genetic markers is a good sign for skin color studies, it is difficult to be certain of "correct" parental proportions regardless of the character used. In addition to the assumptions required for admixture estimation with serological data, skin color studies must assume a simple genetic model of several independent loci, where each locus has an equal and additive effect on melanin production. This assumption ignores the possible environmental, sexual, developmental, and cultural factors involved in skin color variation. In addition, skin color studies are lacking for cetain key populations or consist of data that are incomplete or not directly comparable to other populations. However, the greater interpopulational compared to intrapopulational variation in skin color and the use of measures designed to minimize environmental influence are advantages that balance some of the problems involved in skin-color-based studies.

ACKNOWLEDGMENTS

We gratefully acknowledge the support of the Research Foundation of the State University of New York, Grant #010-7363A, and Sigma Xi, the Scientific Research Society of North America. The UCLA Health Sciences Computing Facility is also acknowledged for providing computer programs BMDP3D and BMDP7M with the support of National Institutes of Health Special Research Resources Grant RR-3. A special thanks is extended to the people of Belize, without whose cooperation this research would not have been possible, and to M. H. Crawford for providing serological admixture estimates.

References

Bard, S. A., 1855, *Waikna: Adventures on the Mosquito Shore*, J. Blackwood, New York.
Barnicot, N. A., 1958, Reflectometry of the skin in Southern Nigerians and in some mulattoes, *Hum. Biol.* 30:150–160.

Bernstein, F., 1931, Die geographische verteilung der blutgruppen und ihre anthropologische bedeutung, Comitato Italiano per lo Studio die Problemi della Populazione, Instituto Poligrafico dello Stato, pp. 227–243, Rome.

Cavalli-Sforza, L. L., and Bodmer, W. F., 1971, *The Genetics of Human Populations*, W. H. Freeman, San Francisco.

Conway, D. L., and Baker, P. T., 1972, Skin reflectance of Quechua Indians: The effects of genetic admixture, sex and age, *Am. J. Phys. Anthropol.* **36**:267–282.

Crawford, M. H., 1977, paper presented at the 76th annual meeting of the American Anthropological Association, Houston, Texas.

Das, S. R., and Mukherjee, D. P., 1963, A spectrophotometric skin colour survey among four Indian castes and tribes, *Z. Morphol. Anthropol.* **54**:190–200.

De Diaz Ungria, A. G., 1965, La pigmentation de la piel en las indigenas Guahibos, in *Homenage a Juan Comas*, Vol. II (A. Caso *et al.*, eds.), pp. 63–82, Editorial Libros de Mexico, Mexico.

Dixon, W. J. (ed.), 1975, *BMDP Biomedical Computer Programs*, University of California Press, Berkeley.

Garrard, G., Harrison, G. A., and Owen, J. J. T., 1967, Comparative spectrophotometry of skin colour with E.E.L. and Photovolt instruments, *Am. J. Phys. Anthropol.* **27**: 389–396.

Gonzalez, N. L., 1969, *Black Carib Household Structure. A Study of Migration and Modernization*, University of Washington Press, Seattle.

Harris, R. J., 1975, *A Primer of Multivariate Statistics*, Academic, New York.

Harrison, G. A., and Owen, J. J. T., 1964, Studies of the inheritance of skin colour, *Ann. Hum. Genet.* **28**:27–37.

Harrison, G. A., and Salzano, F. M., 1966, The skin color of the Caingang and Guarani Indians of Brazil, *Hum. Biol.* **38**:104–111.

Harrison, G. A., Owen, J. J. T., da Rocha, F. J., and Salzano, F. M., 1967, Skin colour in southern Brazilian populations, *Hum. Biol.* **39**:21–31.

Huizinga, J., 1968, Human biological observations on some African populations of the Thorn savanna belt. I and II., *Proc. Kon. Ned. Akad. Wet. Ser. C Biol. Med. Sci.* **C71**: 356–390.

Hulse, F. S., 1973, Skin color in Northumberland, in *Genetic Variation in Britain* (D. F. Roberts and E. Sunderland, eds.), pp. 245–257, Taylor and Francis, London.

Kahlon, D. P. S., 1976, Age variation in skin color: A study in Sikh immigrants in Britain, *Hum. Biol.* **48**:419–428.

Lees, F. C., and Byard, P. J., 1978, Skin colorimetry in Belize: I. Conversion formulae, *Am. J. Phys. Anthropol.* **48**:515–522.

Lees, F. C., and Relethford, J. H., 1978, Admixture estimation using skin reflectance data, *Am. J. Phys. Anthropol.* **49**:505–510.

Lees, F. C., Byard, P. J., and Relethford, J. H., 1978, Interobserver error in human skin colorimetry, *Am. J. Phys. Anthropol.* **49**:35–38.

Lees, F. C., Byard, P. J., and Relethford, J. H., 1979, New conversion formulae for light-skinned populations using Photovolt and EEL reflectometers, *Am. J. Phys. Anthropol.* **51**(3):403–408.

Leguebe, A., 1961, Contribution a l'étude de la pigmentation chez l'homme, *Bull. Inst. Roy. Soc. Nat. Belg.* **37**:1–29.

Livingstone, F. B., 1969, Polygenic models for the evolution of skin color differences, *Hum. Biol.* **41**:480–493.

Mahalanobis, P. C., 1936, On the generalized distance in statistics, *Proc. Natl. Inst. Sci. Ind.* **2**:49–55.

Mazess, R. B., 1967, Skin color in Bahamian Negroes, *Hum. Biol.* **39**:145–154.

Ojikutu, V. R. O., 1965, Die rolle von hautpigment und schweibdrusen in der klimaanpassung des menschen, *Homo* **16**:77–95.

Pollitzer, W. S., 1964, Analysis of a tri-racial isolate, *Hum. Biol.* **36**:362–373.

Post, P. W., Krauss, A. N., Waldman, S., and Auld, P. A. M., 1976, Skin reflectance of newborn infants from 25 to 44 weeks gestational age, *Hum. Biol.* **48**:541–557.

Relethford, J. H., Lees, F. C., and Byard, P. J., 1980, Sex and age variation in skin color of Irish children, unpublished ms.

Rigters-Aris, C. A. E., 1973*a*, A reflectometric study of the skin in Dutch families, *J. Hum. Evol.* **2**:123–136.

Rigters-Aris, C. A. E., 1973*b*, Réflectometric cutanée des Fali (Cameroun), *Proc. Kon. Ned. Akad. Wet. Ser. C Biol. Med. Sci.* **C76**:500–511.

Rijn-Tournel, J. V., 1965, Pigmentation de la peau de Belge et d'Africains, *Bull. Soc. Belge Anthropol. Prehist.* **76**:79–96.

Sokal, R. R., 1961, Distance as a measure of taxonomic similarity, *Syst. Zool.* **10**:70–79.

Sokal, R. R., and Rohlf, F. J., 1969, *Biometry*, W. H. Freeman, San Francisco.

Taylor, D. M., 1951, *The Black Carib of British Honduras*, Viking Fund Publications in Anthropology no. 17, Wenner-Gren Foundation, New York.

Tiwari, S. C., 1963, Studies of crossing between Indians and Europeans, *Ann. Hum. Genet.* **26**:219–227.

Wasserman, H. P., and Heyl, T., 1968, Quantitative data on skin pigmentation in South African races, *S. Afr. Med. J.* **42**:98–101.

Weiner, J. S., and Lourie, J. A., 1969, *Human Biology: A Guide to Field Methods*, IBP Handbook No. 9, Blackwell, Oxford.

Weiner, J. S., Sebag-Montefiore, N. C., and Peterson, J. N., 1963, A note on the skin color of Aguarana Indians of Peru, *Hum. Biol.* **35**:470–473.

Weiner, J. S., Harrison, G. A., Singer, R., and Jopp, W., 1964, Skin color in Southern Africa, *Hum. Biol.* **36**:294–307.

Young, T., 1847, *Narrative of a Residence on the Mosquito Shore*, Smith, Elder and Co., London.

10

Dental Variation in Black Carib Populations

D. H. O'ROURKE, R. M. BAUME, J. H. MIELKE, and M. H. CRAWFORD

1. Introduction

Many recent studies have demonstrated that tooth size and morphology may be used to assess population affinities among groups that have experienced varying degrees of microdifferentiation (Bailit *et al.*, 1968; Bailit, 1975; Baume and Crawford, 1978; Boyd, 1972; Crawford *et al.*, 1975; Friedlaender, 1975; O'Rourke, 1976*a,b*; O'Rourke and Crawford, 1976, 1980; Sofaer *et al.*, 1972). While the dental traits themselves may be evolutionarily somewhat more conservative than simpler genetic polymorphisms, their relative ease of collection, permanence, and traditional importance in macroevolutionary studies make them an important and appropriate data base from which to evaluate trends in microevolution.

The purpose of the present study is twofold. First, discrete dental traits and odontometrics are used to evaluate population differences in three related Belizean ethnic groups; two of these are Black Carib and one is Creole. Second, the Belizean groups are compared to four Mexican populations of known admixture to determine if patterns of differentiation, explainable in terms of hybridization for the Mexican populations, are similar and uniform in the Belizean groups.

D. H. O'ROURKE • Department of Anthropology, University of Utah, Salt Lake City, Utah 84112. R. M. BAUME • School of Dental Medicine, The University of Connecticut Health Center, Farmington, Connecticut 06032. J. H. MIELKE and M. H. CRAWFORD • Laboratory of Biological Anthropology, University of Kansas, Lawrence, Kansas 66045.

2. Materials

The data used in this study come from stone dental casts collected at two locations in Belize (Dangriga and Punta Gorda) during the summer of 1976. The Mexican material, reported earlier (O'Rourke and Crawford, 1976, 1980), was collected during the summers of 1971 and 1974. The demographic and genetic structure of these populations is well documented (Crawford, 1976).

Tooth size determinations were made using Helois dial calipers accurate to 0.1 mm for all teeth through the first molars. For this analysis, only dimensions from the right side of the jaws were used. Both mesiodistal and buccolingual diameters were measured for each tooth, with the first molar contributing an anterior as well as a posterior width.

For the anterior dentition, the mesiodistal dimension is defined as the maximum length of the tooth parallel to the occlusal and labial surfaces. Due to the complexities of the morphology of the posterior dentition (PMs–M1), however, the mesiodistal dimension for these teeth is defined as the maximum length along the main sulcus of the tooth, in order to reflect the functional role of tooth morphology in mastication.

The buccolingual diameter is defined as the maximum width of the tooth perpendicular to the mesiodistal dimension. For the first molars, the two buccolingual dimensions are taken to be the maximum width of the mesial and distal bulges perpendicular to the mesiodistal measurement.

In addition to odontometric variation, each cast was scored for seven discontinuous traits. These included shoveling of central and lateral incisors, incisor rotation, canine ridges, molar cusp patterns and numbers, Carabelli's cusp, and protostylid. Each of the traits was scored for varying degrees of expression using rank-order measurement scales, with the higher scores indicating the more pronounced expression of the trait. Table 1 indicates the scoring techniques that were employed.

3. Results

3.1. Discontinuous Traits

To assess relationships between the Mexican and Belizean populations based on dental variables, the nonparametric Kruskal–Wallis test was applied to the discrete dental data in order to test the null hypothesis that there were no significant differences between any of the groups. As Table 2 illustrates, the null hypothesis was rarely rejected.

For example, results of the comparison of Punta Gorda and Dangriga Caribs for each discrete variable indicate that only two variables were found to occur in significantly different frequencies in the two groups — rotation of the maxillary and mandibular lateral incisors. With only two out of 16 variables

Table 1. Methods for Scoring Discrete Dental Traits[a]

Trait	Scoring technique
Shoveling I^1, I^2	Three degrees of expression on central incisors: marked, moderate trace, absence
Rotation I^1, I^2, I_1, I_2	Three degrees of expression on incisors: winging, straight, counterwinging
Canine ridges C^1, C_1	Four degrees of expression on canines: absence of ridges, marginal ridges, medial ridge, both marginal and medial ridges
Maxillary cusp number M^1, M^2	Four type classification system on first and second molars: $4+$, $4-$, $3+$, $3-$
Mandibular cusp pattern M_1, M_2	Four type classification system on first and second molars: Y5, Y4, $+5$, $+4$
Carabelli's cusp M^1, M^2	Five degrees of expression on first molar: absence, pit, groove, nonfree tip, free tip
Protostylid M_1, M_2	Five degrees of expression on first molar: pit, groove, nonfree tip, free tip, absence

[a] See Baume and Crawford (1978) for more complete discussion of scoring techniques and references to the original methodologies.

showing significant differences between the two Carib groups, it would appear that there is relatively little differentiation between the two populations with respect to discrete dental variables.

In comparing the Creole samples from the two geographical locations, the picture of homogeneity is even more strongly presented. Here (Table 2) no variable is present in significantly different frequencies between the two populations. Clearly, these two samples represent a very homogeneous sample despite having been collected in two separate locations.

If geographical distinctions show little evidence of differentiation, ethnicity demonstrates even less. Interpopulation ethnic comparisons show that there are no significant differences between Caribs and Creoles (Table 2).

Given the relative homogeneity of the samples, the ethnic comparison was repeated with the combined geographical locations. Table 2 shows that when this is done, no variables differentiate the ethnic designations.

3.2. Odontometrics

The picture of homogeneity of the Belizean groups obtained from the analysis of discrete dental traits is repeated, at least in part, when odontometrics are considered. Here the data are subdivided into three groups: Dangriga Caribs, Punta Gorda Caribs, and, due to sampling problems, a combined Creole sample. Due to sexual dimorphism of tooth size, the samples are further subdivided by sex.

As Table 3 indicates, the mean values, as well as the magnitude of observed variation, differ very little among the three populations in the male subsamples.

Table 2. *Differences between Each of the Belizean Samples by Ethnic Group and Geographical Location, Kruskal–Wallis Test*

	Within groups		Between groups		
	Caribs: Punta Gorda Dangriga	Creoles: Punta Gorda Dangriga	Punta Gorda: Carib Creole	Dangriga: Carib Creole	Total: Carib Creole
Shoveling I^1	0.24	0.14	0.03	0.02	0.00
Shoveling I^2	0.31	0.52	0.12	1.49	0.49
Incisor rotation I^1	0.40	2.32	1.00	1.72	0.25
Incisor rotation I^2	7.73**	2.52	0.71	1.90	2.69
Incisor rotation I_1	1.59	0.04	0.01	0.91	2.14
Incisor rotation I_2	18.03***	0.20	1.35	2.98	0.46
Maxillary canine ridges	0.14	2.18	0.83	0.57	0.00
Mandibular canine ridges	0.12	0.03	0.34	0.84	1.20
M^1 Cusp number	0.00	2.01	0.20	2.19	0.77
M^2 Cusp number	1.12	0.23	0.01	0.43	0.22
M_1 Cusp pattern	0.97	1.57	1.20	1.94	0.34
M_2 Cusp pattern	0.03	—	—	—	1.90
Carabelli's Cusp M^1	3.81	3.59	0.94	0.18	0.07
Carabelli's Cusp M^2	1.35	—	—	0.23	2.17
Protostylid M_1	0.14	0.00	0.52	1.03	1.57
Protostylid M_2	0.67	—	—	—	0.05

**$P \leqslant 0.01$. ***$P \leqslant 0.005$.

Table 3. Summary of Means, Standard Errors, and Coefficients of Variation of Belizean Male Odontometrics

Variables	Dangriga (N = 44)			Punta Gorda (N = 21)			Creoles (N = 6)		
	Mean S.E.		CV	Mean S.E.		CV	Mean S.E.		CV
Maxillae									
I1 MD	8.80 ± 0.105		7.94	8.76 ± 0.182		9.53	8.62 ± 0.202		5.73
I1 BL	7.61 ± 0.089		7.79	7.22 ± 0.158		10.01	7.44 ± 0.171		5.63
I2 MD	6.85 ± 0.098		9.52	6.96 ± 0.152		9.99	6.78 ± 0.158		5.71
I2 BL	6.70 ± 0.088		8.70	6.58 ± 0.129		9.00	6.40 ± 0.191		7.30
C MD	8.13 ± 0.088		7.22	8.04 ± 0.116		6.62	8.50 ± 0.253		7.69
C BL	8.87 ± 0.101		7.54	8.51 ± 0.183		9.86	8.81 ± 0.222		6.16
P3 MD	7.28 ± 0.078		7.10	7.36 ± 0.095		5.92	7.24 ± 0.191		6.48
P3 BL	9.87 ± 0.104		6.97	9.88 ± 0.144		6.69	9.67 ± 0.255		6.46
P4 MD	6.88 ± 0.085		8.20	6.89 ± 0.089		5.95	7.05 ± 0.176		6.10
P4 BL	9.81 ± 0.104		7.01	9.89 ± 0.134		6.19	9.67 ± 0.203		5.14
M1 MD	10.56 ± 0.097		6.09	10.40 ± 0.118		5.19	10.23 ± 0.174		4.16
M1 A-BL	11.41 ± 0.094		5.48	11.21 ± 0.108		4.40	10.82 ± 0.215		4.87
M1 P-BL	10.67 ± 0.103		6.42	10.63 ± 0.143		6.15	10.44 ± 0.158		3.72
Mandibles									
I1 MD	5.41 ± 0.098		12.01	5.31 ± 0.129		9.25	5.32 ± 0.130		6.00
I1 BL	6.10 ± 0.116		12.59	5.83 ± 0.116		9.13	5.83 ± 0.224		9.42
I2 MD	5.98 ± 0.069		7.66	5.97 ± 0.098		7.55	5.88 ± 0.151		6.29
I2 ML	6.25 ± 0.082		8.69	6.28 ± 0.099		7.21	6.34 ± 0.236		9.12
C MD	7.14 ± 0.079		7.35	7.17 ± 0.087		5.56	7.27 ± 0.212		7.15
C BL	7.65 ± 0.102		8.82	7.86 ± 0.156		9.11	7.55 ± 0.235		7.62
P3 MD	7.28 ± 0.083		7.58	7.34 ± 0.107		6.70	7.31 ± 0.118		3.94
P3 BL	8.25 ± 0.086		6.88	8.35 ± 0.142		7.78	8.30 ± 0.208		6.14
P4 MD	7.53 ± 0.098		8.38	7.52 ± 0.161		9.83	7.52 ± 0.226		7.37
P4 BL	8.71 ± 0.097		7.42	8.84 ± 0.108		5.61	8.83 ± 0.165		4.56
M1 MD	11.20 ± 0.098		5.80	11.05 ± 0.150		6.23	11.22 ± 0.140		3.05
M1 A-BL	10.51 ± 0.086		5.40	10.43 ± 0.122		5.34	10.25 ± 0.078		1.85
M1 P-BL	10.51 ± 0.093		5.88	10.63 ± 0.137		5.90	10.03 ± 0.129		3.14

Table 4. Summary of Means, Standard Errors, and Coefficients of Variation of Belizean Female Odontometrics

Variables	Dangriga (N = 89)			Punta Gorda (N = 49)			Creoles (N = 20)		
	Mean	S.E.	CV	Mean	S.E.	CV	Mean	S.E.	CV
Maxillae									
I1 MD	8.42	± 0.075	8.36	8.44	± 0.097	8.06	8.35	± 0.154	8.23
I1 BL	7.33	± 0.067	8.57	7.08	± 0.059	5.82	7.22	± 0.124	7.70
I2 MD	6.75	± 0.058	8.16	6.60	± 0.085	9.06	6.56	± 0.125	8.49
I2 BL	6.54	± 0.057	9.07	6.37	± 0.068	7.44	6.36	± 0.123	8.65
C MD	7.55	± 0.054	6.79	7.49	± 0.066	6.18	7.48	± 0.111	6.64
C BL	8.30	± 0.068	7.72	8.13	± 0.072	6.19	8.08	± 0.131	7.25
P3 MD	7.04	± 0.055	7.39	6.94	± 0.065	6.59	6.72	± 0.109	7.26
P3 BL	9.50	± 0.066	6.58	9.46	± 0.082	6.09	9.26	± 0.135	6.51
P4 MD	6.74	± 0.051	7.18	6.78	± 0.074	7.68	6.80	± 0.108	7.09
P4 BL	9.44	± 0.067	6.69	9.46	± 0.096	7.08	9.36	± 0.144	6.87
M1 MD	10.22	± 0.071	6.53	10.27	± 0.087	5.92	10.18	± 0.143	6.27
M1 A-BL	11.02	± 0.062	5.30	10.88	± 0.081	5.22	10.89	± 0.128	5.27
M1 P-BL	10.45	± 0.065	5.87	10.14	± 0.087	6.03	10.20	± 0.136	5.97
Mandibles									
I1 MD	5.18	± 0.054	9.77	5.22	± 0.092	12.36	5.09	± 0.122	10.75
I1 BL	5.95	± 0.201	31.93	5.55	± 0.077	9.68	5.62	± 0.330	26.23
I2 MD	5.80	± 0.052	8.43	5.75	± 0.063	7.67	5.71	± 0.103	8.07
I2 ML	6.01	± 0.063	9.82	5.98	± 0.068	7.93	6.03	± 0.119	8.79
C MD	6.61	± 0.053	7.50	6.53	± 0.055	5.94	6.47	± 0.101	6.97
C BL	7.17	± 0.066	8.68	7.11	± 0.071	7.00	7.03	± 0.102	7.99
P3 MD	7.06	± 0.063	8.39	7.10	± 0.080	7.92	7.02	± 0.127	8.12
P3 BL	7.88	± 0.060	7.17	7.90	± 0.092	8.19	7.71	± 0.234	7.76
P4 MD	7.29	± 0.071	9.16	7.37	± 0.093	8.79	7.26	± 0.144	8.84
P4 BL	8.40	± 0.067	7.48	8.45	± 0.088	7.28	8.37	± 0.135	7.23
M1 MD	10.85	± 0.088	7.63	10.66	± 0.165	10.86	10.70	± 0.204	8.52
M1 A-BL	10.03	± 0.057	5.38	10.01	± 0.079	5.52	9.99	± 0.118	5.30
M1 P-BL	10.18	± 0.070	6.49	10.16	± 0.098	6.73	9.95	± 0.146	6.55

Indeed, discriminant function analysis failed to discern any significant differences among the three groups. This result is somewhat expected, given the very small sample of the Creole males. With this small sample, only comparatively large differences among the samples could be detected with any degree of confidence.

In the female subsample, however, the picture is rather different. Examination of Table 4 illustrates that the Dangriga Carib sample is characterized by the largest dentition, having the largest value for 16 of 26 means, while the Creole sample is clearly the smallest, with only two mean values exceeding those of the other two samples. This pattern is not entirely unexpected. Dahlberg (1963) has characterized Amerindian and African populations as possessors of large dentitions and Europeans as possessors of small dentitions. That the Carib populations, hybrids of Amerindians and Africans, have comparatively larger dentitions than the Creoles, derived from Amerindian and European gene pools, is not surprising.

The values obtained for the Carib samples are in general comparable to published figures for other Amerindian and African dentitions. The Creole sample is, however, interesting in comparison to other figures. Not only is the Creole sample odontometrically smaller than the Carib groups, but they are also generally smaller than a series of Mexican populations characterized by varying degrees of admixture with Europeans.

The four Mexican populations are: San Pablo, an unadmixed Indian community in the state of Tlaxcala; Tlaxcala City, the capital of the state and a trihybrid; and Cuanalan and Saltillo, Tlaxcaltecan transplants of the 16th century, which are also trihybrid groups.

In comparison with the three least admixed Mexican groups, the Creoles exceed the Mexican populations only in the size of the premolars, perhaps reflecting the influence of the large African component in the Creole gene pool (Dahlberg, 1963). Yet, in comparison to the most admixed Mexican population, Saltillo, which is the smallest Mexican group odontometrically, the Creoles have uniformly larger dentitions. The pattern is similar when the Creole sample is compared to a modern English sample (Goose, 1963). Here, the Creoles have larger mean values, both mesiodistally and buccolingually, for all teeth but the first molars. For this single tooth, the English population has somewhat larger values. These general observations are seen in males as well as females.

While these comparisons are consistent with an interpretation of odontometric differentiation in these groups resulting from admixture and hybridization with gene pools characterized by a particular pattern of dental variability, the following discussion indicates that this may be more simplistic than is warranted.

When the Belizean female odontometric data are subjected to discriminant function analysis significant differences among the groups emerge. Examining the population centroids in multidimensional hyperspace by F-tests and the corresponding Mahalanobis distance (Table 5), we find that the Dangriga Caribs

Table 5. *Distance Matrix, Belize*[a]

	Dangriga Caribs	Punta Gorda Caribs	Creoles
Dangriga	–	8.08***	2.89*
Punta Gorda	19.82	–	0.10
Creoles	13.72	0.55	–

[a]F values, top triangle; D^2 values, bottom triangle. ***$P < 0.001$. *$P < 0.05$.

seem rather distinct, whereas the Punta Gorda Caribs are not significantly different from the Creole sample. While this may be viewed as a general geographical differentiation, with the two Carib groups quite distinct from one another, the relationship between the Caribs and Creoles is not clear, since the majority of the Creole sample is from Dangriga. Not too much weight should be given this apparent separation, however, since only a single variable, maxillary molar posterior width, loaded in the discriminant function and hence was able to significantly discriminate among the samples.

With the apparent homogeneity of the Belizean groups, it seemed appropriate to compare them to several Mexican groups in which the relationship between hybridization and dental variability has been fully studied (O'Rourke and Crawford, 1976, 1980; O'Rourke, 1976*a*,*b*; Baume and Crawford, 1978). Such comparisons provide the potential for a more complete assessment of dental variation in relation to hybridization and culture history in Belize.

The Caribs are derived from African and Indian gene pools and the Creoles from African and British. Therefore, it would be expected that the Caribs should show more affinity to San Pablo and Tlaxcala, while the Creoles should be closer to Cuanalan and Saltillo. When discrete dental trait frequencies from the two Belizean groups are compared to corresponding frequencies in the Mexican populations (Table 6), the results show that, as expected, the Creoles are closer to Cuanalan and Saltillo. Here only three and four traits, respectively, are significantly different, while the Creoles differ in five traits with San Pablo and Tlaxcala. The Carib–Mexican comparison indicates that the Caribs are also similar to Tlaxcala and much different than Cuanalan, as is expected. However, the Caribs are also similar to Saltillo and different from San Pablo, which is not expected; although the relatively high African admixture in Saltillo may account for that similarity, the San Pablo likeness is rather surprising.

The total scheme of population interrelationships may be seen in Sanghvi's X^2 distance measures (Table 7). Here, the distances between Caribs and all other groups are about as expected, with small distances between the trihybrid Mexican groups and a large distance from the Indian population of San Pablo. The relatively large magnitude of the distance between Caribs and Creoles is

Table 6. *Differences between Each Mexican and Belizean Sample, Kruskal–Wallis Test*

	Cuanalan		Saltillo		San Pablo		Tlaxcala	
	Carib	Creole	Carib	Creole	Carib	Creole	Carib	Creole
Shoveling I¹	40.18*	9.56*	1.14	0.31	38.07*	9.60*	24.25*	10.47*
Maxillary canine ridges	31.22*	7.60*	11.17*	2.14	6.77*	1.45	1.84	12.75*
Mandibular canine ridges	38.65*	11.55*	34.67*	12.40*	10.76*	5.98*	0.85	2.22
M¹ Cusp number	47.35*	14.16*	100.48*	28.35*	40.16*	15.87*	129.08*	21.21*
M² Cusp number	7.93*	1.17	2.14	0.48	16.65*	0.10	3.26	0.07
M₁ Cusp pattern	1.30	0.0001	0.86	0.01	7.50*	6.50*	14.58*	11.84*
M₂ Cusp pattern	1.21	1.21	0.57	22.80*	51.43*	12.62*	14.58*	5.35*
Carabelli's cusp M¹	6.90*	1.54	0.35	0.36	0.03	0.14	0.03	0.14
Protosyylid M₁	14.45*	1.86	3.40	0.54	4.65*	0.47	3.41	0.48

*$P \le 0.05 = 3.841$.

Table 7. Comparison of Belizean and Mexican Groups

	Carib	Creole	Cuanalan	Saltillo	San Pablo	Tlaxcala
Carib	–	1.76	1.12	1.21	2.27	1.62
Creole	3.09	–	2.10	2.24	1.92	2.59
Cuanalan	1.25	4.41	–	1.12	2.22	1.80
Saltillo	1.45	5.01	1.26	–	1.61	1.16
San Pablo	5.09	3.68	4.93	2.60	–	0.70
Tlaxcala	2.62	6.71	3.24	1.33	4.94	–

[a] Sanghvi's X^2 divergence measure, bottom triangle; distance measure, top triangle.

Table 8. Summary of Discriminant Function Analysis

| | Variable[a] | Standardized coefficients of discriminant function | | | |
		I	II	III	IV
X P3	BL***	−2.08	−0.07	1.31	−1.21
X I2	MD***	1.30	−2.22	1.03	0.48
X P4	MD***	−1.73	−0.89	−2.26	2.55
X M1	A-BL**	1.51	0.15	−1.54	2.40
N P3	MD**	−0.93	−0.22	−0.28	0.12
N M1	A-BL*	0.97	−0.86	−1.08	−2.26
X M1	P-BL*	−0.67	0.81	2.84	−0.85
Eigenvalue		0.65547	0.14801	0.09441	0.05391
Canonical correlation		0.62924	0.35906	0.29371	0.22616
Cumulative proportion of explained dispersion		0.66910	0.82019	0.91656	0.97159

[a] X, Maxilla; N, Mandible. ***$P < 0.001$. **$P < 0.01$. *$P < 0.05$.

unexpected given the previous demonstration of homogeneity, but should be viewed with caution given the small samples of Creoles.

An examination of odontometric variation in females within and between the Belizean and Mexican groupings reveals a similar pattern of variation. Discriminant function analysis of the odontometric data demonstrates that seven variables, five maxillary and two mandibular, significantly discriminate among the eight groups (Table 8). It is clear that variables from the posterior dentition are most important in interpopulation discrimination, since only one of the seven variables contributing to the discrimination is from the anterior dentition (maxillary lateral incisor length). In addition, the particularly high loading of three premolar variables on the first discriminant function may be a reflection of large versus small premolar size in Africans and Amerindians, respectively (Dahlberg, 1963).

Table 9 provides the results of the F-tests and the Mahalanobis D^2 values derived from discriminant function analysis. With the exception of Creole–Carib comparisons, all groups are found to be significantly different from one another. The Mahalanobis generalized distance values for the three Belizean comparisons are by far the smallest, the intra-Mexican comparisons next in magnitude, and the international comparisons the largest. It might be expected that the smallest distances between the Belizean and Mexican groups and hence the greatest affinities would be those populations that have experienced the greatest admixture from African sources, namely Cuanalan and Saltillo. In fact, this is not the case. The smallest distances are between Tlaxcala and all three Belizean groups; yet Tlaxcala has experienced less than half the African admixture than

Table 9. Distance Matrix, Ondontometrics[a]

	Creole	Punta Gorda	Dangriga	San Pablo	Tlaxcala	Cuanalan	Saltillo
Creole	—	0.51	1.39	7.22***	2.81***	5.43***	6.17***
Punta Gorda	0.98	—	2.38*	16.53***	6.80***	10.31***	14.05***
Dangriga	2.32	2.06	—	17.72***	7.96***	11.95***	16.14***
San Pablo	12.41	15.06	11.71	—	3.78***	4.42***	4.66***
Tlaxcala	6.48	10.19	9.93	4.90	—	4.45***	3.10**
Cuanalan	11.21	12.96	12.03	4.66	7.30	—	7.20***
Saltillo	11.13	14.01	12.05	3.70	4.28	8.21	—

[a] F values, upper triangle; D^2 values, lower triangle. ***$P \leq 0.001$. **$P \leq 0.01$. *$P \leq 0.05$.

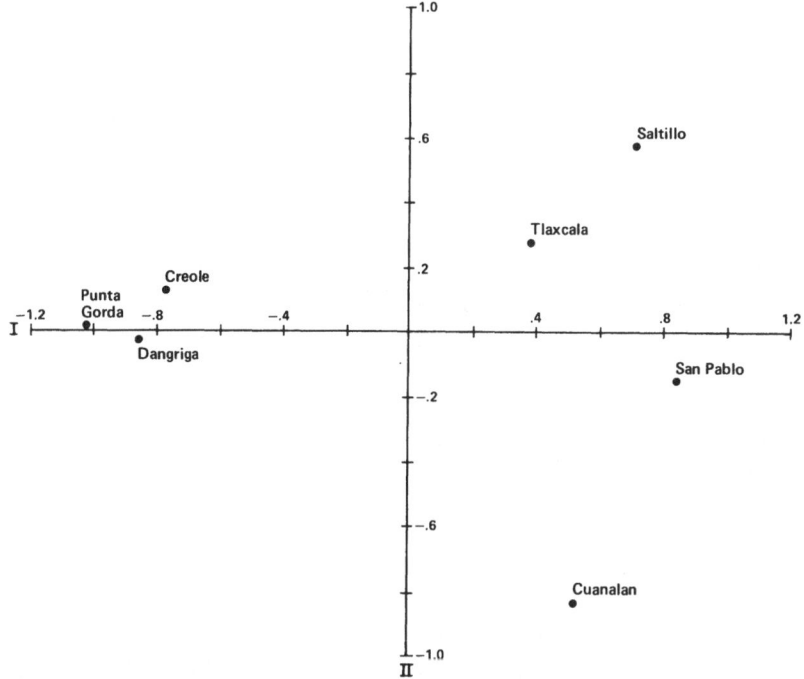

FIGURE 1. Relationship of population mean centroids derived from odontometric data plotted on first two canonical axes.

either Cuanalan or Saltillo. Possible explanations for this unexpected finding will be discussed in the final section.

It is interesting to note that the relative distances between the Belizean groups are altered with the addition of the Mexican populations in the multivariate analysis. For example, while the F-value of the Dangriga–Creole comparison is nonsignificant, the associated D^2 value is actually larger than that between the two Carib groups. This may be merely a function of sample size disparity, since the Creole sample is less than half the size of the two Carib groups. Nevertheless, this analysis reinforces the suggestion of Dangriga's unique position among the Belizean groups, especially since the Punta Gorda–Creole comparison remains nonsignificant. An analogous analysis based on the male subsamples was not attempted, due to small sample sizes.

Plotting the population mean centroids on the first two canonical axes (Fig. 1) emphasizes the relationships just described in the distance matrix. The first canonical axis separates quite distinctly the Belizean from the Mexican groups. The second canonical axis, on the other hand, accentuates the differentiation of the Mexican groups in contrast to the homogeneity of the Belizean groups. It should be noted that although the Belizean groups are rather tightly clustered in the plot, the second canonical axis does separate, to some degree, the Creole sample from the two Carib groups. In its general pattern of population relationships and differentiation, the canonical axis plot based on odontometric variation is quite similar to that found for discrete dental traits using eigenvectorial methods (see Fig. 3).

3.3. Two-Dimensional Representations of Discrete Traits

In an attempt to visualize the variation in discrete dental traits among the Belizean and Mexican populations, two-dimensional eigenvectoral representations were constructed. Each discrete trait was scored as either being present or absent and this score was converted into a frequency. The frequencies of occurrence of these traits were then transformed into a relationship matrix P of scaled trait frequency variances/covariances of dimension $s \times s$, where s is the number of populations (Harpending and Jenkins, 1973; Workman *et al.*, 1973). The relative relationship among populations, represented in two dimensions, was obtained as an eigenvectorial reduction of the variance/covariance matrix. Plots of the populations were obtained by multiplying each eigenvector by the square root of its corresponding eigenvalue. The matrix P describes the variation and covariation of populations over all discrete dental trait data; and another matrix T describes the variations and covariations of the k trait frequencies aggregated over all s populations. The matrix T can be reduced to the same scale as P because they have the same set of nonzero eigenvalues (Harpending and Jenkins, 1973). The reduction of P gives plots of populations along axes corresponding to trait frequencies, and the reduction of T gives plots of traits along axes corresponding to populations (Workman *et al.*, 1976). This procedure facilitates the interpretation of the observed variation among populations by allowing an identification of the dental traits responsible for the populational dispersion. These procedures thus provide clear visual aids for the interpretation of the structural variation among populations. The interpretation of the structural relations within each group is, however, dependent upon independent sources (e.g., historical and enivronmental data) because the distribution of the trait frequencies among populations does not provide inferences as to the processes that produced the observed variation.

The univariate analyses of the relationships among the Belizean populations indicated that the Carib and Creole groups were rather homogeneous. Because of the sample sizes and the fact that no significant differences were found between the Dangriga and Punta Gorda Creoles, these two groups were combined into a single Creole population. Two-dimensional reductions of the P and T matrices for the first two scaled eigenvectors of the two Carib groups and the one Creole group are shown in Fig. 2.

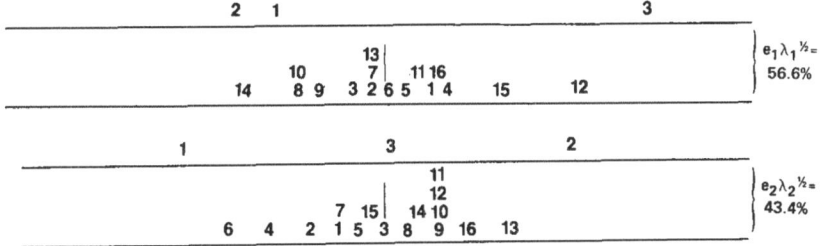

FIGURE 2. Dispersion of three Belizean populations (top) and discrete dental traits (bottom) along eigenvectors associated with the two largest eigenvalues of the P and T matrices. Discrete traits (numbers 1–16) are listed in order in Table 2.

The first axis differentiates the two Carib groups from the Creoles. Traits showing greatest differentiation are (12) M_2 cusp patterns, frequency higher in Caribs, (14) M^1 Carabellis, and (15) M_1 protostylid, with the frequency being highest in the Caribs. Most of the traits cluster near the center, indicating that the differentiation is not great, and the remaining 13 traits do not contribute significantly to the dispersion of the populations. The second axis differentiates between the two Carib groups; however, this differentiation is slight because most of the traits again cluster around the center. The only two traits that could be singled out as contributing to this dispersion are (6) and (4), rotation of I_2 and I^2, respectively. If these three populations are plotted in two dimensions with x and y axes corresponding to the first and second eigenvectors, they form a triangle around the axial center. We can interpret this, along with the lack of extensive differentiation based on the contribution of only a few traits, to indicate a rather homogeneous grouping with only slight differences based on the 16 dental traits.

A comparison among the Belizean populations and Mexican groups seemed appropriate because the analysis might provide some insight into the relationship between hybridization and genetic variability. Groups arrayed on the first two scaled eigenvectors provide a clear picture of the relations among the Mexican and Belizean groups (Fig. 3). The separation between Belizean and Mexican populations was obviously expected. The spatial positions reflect, however, both the history and population composition of these groups.

The populations arrayed along the first eigenvector can be lumped into three groups: (1) San Pablo and Tlaxcala, (2) Cuanalan and Saltillo, and (3) Caribs and Creoles. This dispersion accounts for 54.8% of the variation. San Pablo is an unmixed Indian population in the Valley of Tlaxcala, and Tlaxcala is

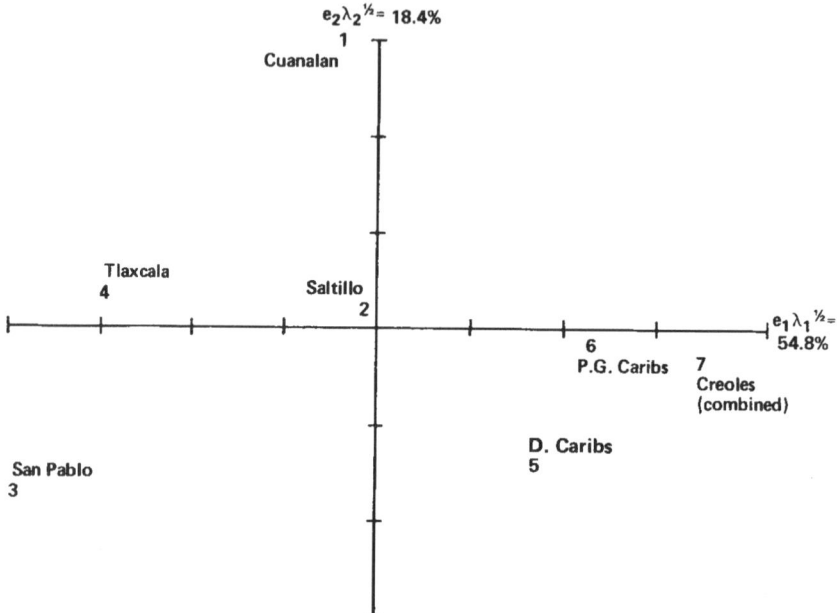

FIGURE 3. Relationship of Belizean and Mexican populations based on discrete dental traits using scaled eigenvectors associated with first and second eigenvalues of the *P* matrix.

a trihybrid consisting primarily of Indian with lesser components of Spanish and African admixture (Crawford *et al.*, 1974, 1976). Cuanalan and Saltillo are intermediate in the plot, reflecting their genetic composition; Cuanalan is a trihybrid (Indian, Spanish, African) and Saltillo is also a trihybrid but with higher African admixture than Cuanalan. As would be expected, Saltillo plotted closest to the Belizean populations (African and Indian admixture). The Creoles occupy the extreme right-hand position, reflecting African and British admixture. The Carib samples are closer to the Mexican groups, and they are composed of both African and Indian components. Traits showing greatest differentiation along the first eigenvector are: (3) M_2 cusp pattern, (7) rotation of I^1, and (12) maxillary canine ridges.

The population dispersion along the second eigenvector, accounting for only 18.4% of the variation, primarily separates San Pablo and Dangriga Caribs from Cuanalan. This separation is difficult to interpret. It may be reflecting the Indian components in San Pablo and the Dangriga Caribs. However, one would expect Tlaxcala and Punta Gorda Caribs to differentiate also. The traits primarily responsible for this configuration are (1) and (2) shoveling of I^1 and I^2, (12) M_2 cusp pattern, and (7) maxillary canine ridges. Traits (7) and (12) also contributed to the dispersion along the first eigenvector.

These analyses suggest that the variation and the resultant differentiation of the Belizean and Mexican populations reflect both the historical connections among these populations and the degree of admixture. The Belizean populations do not, however, show the clear distinctions that the Mexican groups exhibit and form a rather homogeneous cluster with only slight variation.

4. Discussion and Conclusion

Apparently, the clear relationship between hybridization and dental variability that was found in the analysis of the Mexican material is here due to the extremely large and highly significant differences between the Belizean and Mexican groupings. Such precise interrelations are perhaps too specific to be apparent in comparisons of such grossly divergent populations. It is also possible that the sources of the African components in the gene pools of these groups were quite different and the lack of concordance between the highly African Caribs and Creoles of Belize and the Mexican trihybrid groups is a reflection of their diverse origins. In addition, the Indian component among the Mexican groups, primarily Tlaxcaltecan, is different genetically from the Arawak–Carib amalgam of the Black Caribs. The founders of the Tlaxcaltecan populations are known to have migrated south into Central America, while both the Caribs and Arawaks have a South American origin.

The analysis of dental variability in these Belizean groups indicates that not only are they distinct from other Latin American populations to which they are compared, but generally may be considered a rather homogeneous group. For example, Baume and Crawford (1980) have found that on the bases of discrete dental trait asymmetry, both the Belizean and Mexican populations cluster among themselves. That is, the Belizean groups show less average asymmetry, while the Mexican groups show more. This result is unexpected, since, as others discuss in this book, allelic polymorphisms as well as certain other quantitative traits show the Belizeans to exhibit some degree of microdifferentiation. The inability to detect such differentiation in dental variables may be interpreted in several ways. First, the high mobility of the Caribs (Gonzalez, 1969) and, presumably, the Creoles in Belize acts as an homogenizing agent such that continual and uniform gene flow throughout the region operates to impede regional and/or ethnic differentiation. The second factor that may contribute to the uniformity of these groups is time of separation. The groups studied have only been separate entities for less than 200 years. This may simply be not enough time for significant divergence in these complex, convervative polygenic traits.

Work is proceeding on the analysis of dental variability in these groups by replacing the populations as the unit of study with the individual. Such an approach, it is hoped, will allow the assessment of the role of sampling, both statistical and genetic, in the reliability of the population approach to studies of microdifferentiation.

ACKNOWLEDGMENTS

This research was supported in part by a grant from the National Institute of Dental Research, DE0411501, University of Kansas General Research Fund grant #3507-x038, and Biomedical Research Support grants #4349-x706 and 4309-x706. During the data collection and data analyses Dr. M. H. Crawford was supported by a Career Development Award, K04DE028-01.

We would like to thank Drs. Miranda and von Heinkel for their kind help.

References

Bailit, H. L., 1975, Dental variation among populations, *Dent. Clin. N. Am.* **19**(1):125–139.

Bailit, H. L., DeWitt, S. J., and Leigh, R. A., 1968, The size and morphology of the Nasioi dentition, *Am. J. Phys. Anthropol.* **28**:271.

Baume, R. M., and Crawford, M. H., 1978, Discrete dental traits in four Tlaxcaltecan Mexican populations, *Am. J. Phys. Anthropol.* **49**(3):351–360.

Baume, R. M., and Crawford, M. H., 1980, Discrete dental trait asymmetry in Mexican and Belizean groups, *Am. J. Phys. Anthropol.* **52**(3):315–322.

Boyd, R. C., 1972, An odontometric and observational assessment of the dentition, Appendix IV, in *Physical Anthropology of the Eastern Highlands of New Guinea* (R. A. Littwood, ed.), pp. 175–212. University of Washington Press, Seattle, Washington.

Crawford, M. H., 1976, *The Tlaxcaltecans: Prehistory, Demography, Morphology and Genetics,* University of Kansas Anthropology Series, no. 7, Lawrence, Kansas.

Crawford, M. H., Leysbon, W. C., Brown, K., Lees, F., and Johnson, R. S., 1974, Human biology of Tlaxcala, Mexico: II, Blood group, serum, red cell frequencies, and genetic distances of the Indian populations of Mexico, *Am. J. Phys. Anthropol.* **42**:251–268.

Crawford, M. H., O'Rourke, D. H., Lin, P., and Baume, R. M., 1975, Microevaluation in Mexican populations, Paper presented at AAA meetings, San Francisco, California.

Crawford, M. H., Lisker, R., and Briceno, R. P., 1976, Genetic microdifferentiation of two transplanted Tlaxcaltecan populations, in *The Tlaxcaltecans* (M. H. Crawford, ed.), pp. 169–175, University of Kansas Anthropology Series, no. 7, Lawrence, Kansas.

Dahlberg, A. A., 1963, Analysis of the American Indian dentition, in *Dental Anthropology* (D. R. Brothwell, ed.), pp. 149–178, Macmillan, New York.

Friedlaender, J. S., 1975, *Patterns of Human Variation,* Harvard University Press, Cambridge.

Gonzalez, N., 1969, *Black Carib Household Structure,* University of Washington Press, Seattle.

Goose, D. H., 1963, Dental measurement: An assessment of its value in anthropological studies, in *Dental Anthropology* (D. R. Brothwell, ed.), pp. 125–148, Pergamon, Oxford.

Harpending, H., and Jenkins, T., 1973, Genetic distance among South African populations, in *Methods and Theories of Anthropological Genetics* (M. H. Crawford and P. L. Workman, eds.), pp. 177–199, University of New Mexico Press, Albuquerque.

O'Rourke, D. H., 1976a, Odontometric analysis of four Mexican populations of related genetic background, *Am. J. Phys. Anthropol.* **44**(1):197 (abstract).

O'Rourke, D. H., 1976b, Odontometric analysis of four Tlaxcaltecan populations, unpublished Master's thesis, University of Kansas.

O'Rourke, D. H., and Crawford, M. H., 1976, Odontometric analysis of four Tlaxcaltecan communities, in *The Tlaxcaltecans* (M. H. Crawford, ed.), pp. 81–92, University of Kansas Anthropology Series, no. 7, Lawrence, Kansas.

O'Rourke, D. H., and Crawford, M. H., 1980, Odontometric microdifferentiation of transplanted Mexican Indian populations: Cuanalan and Saltillo, *Am. J. Phys. Anthropol.* 52:421–434.

Sofaer, J. A., Niswander, J. D., MacLean, C. J., and Workman, P. L., 1972, Population studies on southwestern Indian tribes, V. Tooth morphology as an indicator of biological distance, *Am. J. Phys. Anthropol.* 37:357–366.

Workman, P. L., Harpending, H., Lalouel, J. M., Lynch, C., Niswander, J. D., and Singleton, R., 1973, Population studies on Southwestern Indian tribes, VI, Papago population structure: A comparison of genetic and migration analyses, in *Genetic Structure of Populations* (N. E. Morton, ed.), pp. 166–194, University Press of Hawaii, Honolulu.

Workman, P. L., Mielke, J. H., and Nevanlinna, H. R., 1976, The genetic structure of Finland, *Am. J. Phys. Anthropol.* 44:341–368.

11

Anthropometry of Black Caribs

PAUL M. LIN

1. Introduction

The primary purpose of this chapter on the anthropometry of the Black Caribs is to assess possible microevolutionary divergence in physique between two populations residing in Livingston, Guatemala, and on St. Vincent Island, West Indies, given 180 years of separation. These populations belonged to the common ancestral group from St. Vincent. References to the historical studies of the Black Caribs in the area are given elsewhere in this volume (see Chapters 1 and 2). Secondarily, variation in the sexual dimorphism of the two populations is discussed.

A division of the samples by sex and age is provided in Table 1. The disproportional sex ratios of the Livingston sample roughly approximate the actual sex ratio of the Black Carib population residing in Livingston. These data evidence the emigration of men under the age of 60 and, to a lesser degree, of the women under the age of 50. Men's migration due to employment opportunities elsewhere has been described by Gonzalez (1969) and in Chapter 3. However, the efflux of women appears to be a relatively recent trend. The sex ratio of the St. Vincent Black Caribs, as reflected by this sample, is lower than that of the Livingston counterpart, again mainly due to the availability of employment. In this study, the samples measured in Sandy Bay, Owia, and Fancy, small villages located on the northern and northeastern coast, are combined to represent a composite St. Vincent Black Carib population.

PAUL M. LIN • Institute of Social and Behavioral Pathology, and Psychiatric Research Unit, Department of Psychiatry, Pritzker School of Medicine, The University of Chicago, Chicago, Illinois 60637.

Table 1. Age Distribution of the Samples

| | Livingston | | St. Vincent | |
Age	Male	Female	Male	Female
17–24	9	13	12	37
25–34	2	9	10	30
35–44	3	16	15	28
45–54	3	24	19	34
55–64	9	29	19	39
65–74	7	21	20	18
75 +	6	13	3	7
Total	39	125	98	193

2. Methods

Thirty-six anthropometric measurements, primarily defined by Martin (1957) and Oliver (1969), were taken by the author in Livingston in 1975 and on St. Vincent in 1979. The 36 variables, which measure the skeletal and soft-tissue dimensions, are analyzed with univariate and multivariate statistical methods in order to describe the total morphological pattern of each group and to delineate intergroup differences.

3. Results

3.1. Sexual Dimorphism

The descriptive statistics on the anthropometry of the Black Caribs given in Tables 2A–2D are concordant with the well-known fact about human physique that the male is larger than the female in skeletal dimensions. However, in a number of soft-tissue dimension variables, the Black Carib females are larger than the males either in the mean values or maximum values, particularly in abdomen circumference, triceps skinfold, and subscapular skinfold. Table 2E summarizes the result of Student's t-test, employing BMDP3D (Dixon and Brown, 1979), to evaluate differences in each variable between the sexes. Those variables, for which degrees of freedom 162 and 289 are assigned to the Livingston and St. Vincent samples, respectively, have variances that are not significantly different according to an F-test. For these variables, t is computed by the formula for pooled variances. For other variables t is computed with separate variances, for which an approximate degree of freedom is given.

The average abdomen circumference of the Livingston females is significantly larger than that of the males, whereas the average abdomen circumference of the St. Vincent females is not larger than that of the males, nor is the sexual difference significant. This interpopulation discordance is due to the

Table 2A. Descriptive Statistics, Livingston Males

Measurement	Mean	S.D.	Kurtosis	Skewness	Minimum	Maximum
Age	55.00	22.34	−1.14	−0.66	17.00	83.00
Weight	63.27	8.24	−0.72	−0.08	47.17	78.02
Sitting height	815.86	30.99	−0.76	−0.16	750.00	864.00
Stature	1703.24	69.40	0.14	−0.21	1532.00	1844.00
Iliospinale height	1025.86	59.01	0.24	0.12	895.00	1151.00
Trochanteric height	952.41	51.71	1.66	0.38	845.00	1111.00
Biacromial width	385.66	19.15	−0.44	0.32	355.00	431.00
Chest width	274.07	20.21	0.91	−0.09	220.00	317.00
Chest depth	202.76	16.19	−0.59	0.00	166.00	230.00
Bicristal width	264.03	12.89	−0.09	−0.13	234.00	288.00
Bitrochanteric width	309.21	13.43	3.80	1.38	285.00	355.00
Upper limb length	802.31	34.84	0.19	0.02	730.00	885.00
Upper arm length	338.69	21.48	−0.48	−0.04	290.00	380.00
Forearm length	271.52	18.71	2.13	−0.94	213.00	304.00
Hand length	192.10	11.91	−0.07	−0.21	163.00	214.00
Hand width	87.79	4.44	0.02	−0.51	77.00	96.00
Thigh length	454.55	39.96	1.06	0.82	375.00	563.00
Leg length	451.97	28.00	0.37	−0.33	378.00	501.00
Foot length	269.90	13.87	−0.19	0.63	249.00	303.00
Foot width	109.72	8.61	0.56	0.12	94.00	132.00
Head circumference	569.45	16.36	0.54	−0.68	529.00	600.00
Upper arm circumference	272.66	28.78	−0.89	−0.09	222.00	320.00
Chest circumference	871.35	63.72	−0.71	−0.25	735.00	980.00
Abdomen circumference	794.72	74.00	0.02	0.18	652.00	972.00
Calf circumference	334.69	27.26	−0.51	0.28	287.00	394.00
Triceps skinfold	7.79	4.03	0.86	1.12	3.00	19.00
Subscapular skinfold	9.31	2.77	−1.04	0.33	5.00	14.00
Head length	190.72	6.60	−0.35	−0.55	177.00	202.00
Head width	153.41	6.22	−0.62	−0.41	140.00	163.00
Minimum frontal width	107.31	6.78	1.13	0.24	93.00	126.00
Bizygomatic width	141.21	6.94	−0.34	0.08	127.00	156.00
Bigonial width	106.00	6.00	−0.05	−0.38	93.00	118.00
Nasal height	59.76	5.12	−0.54	0.00	50.00	70.00
Nasal width	45.03	3.25	0.35	0.78	40.00	53.00
Nasal index	75.85	7.94	−0.79	0.09	62.69	92.16
Upper face height	88.10	7.10	−0.84	−0.24	75.00	101.00
Morphological face height	130.66	8.25	−0.56	−0.50	113.00	144.00
Head height	135.59	5.19	−0.43	−0.35	123.00	145.00

difference in abdomen dimension between the Livingston and St. Vincent male groups. While the average abdomen circumference is practically identical between the Livingston and St. Vincent female groups (844.1 versus 844.7 mm), the Livingston male group is much leaner than the St. Vincent male group in this variable (794.7 versus 852.1 mm). Correspondingly, the average subscapular skinfold of the Livingston males is thinner than that of the St. Vincent males (9.3 versus 12.6 mm). In short, the St. Vincent males are bulkier than the Livingston males. The difference in body bulk can be best observed in the weight variable,

Table 2B. Descriptive Statistics, Livingston Females

Measurement	Mean	S.D.	Kurtosis	Skewness	Minimum	Maximum
Age	52.58	17.64	−0.68	−0.30	17.00	88.00
Weight	60.15	11.74	1.23	0.87	39.92	104.78
Sitting height	772.88	30.10	−0.40	0.07	704.00	842.00
Stature	1566.12	53.59	−0.22	0.06	1437.00	1718.00
Iliospinale height	945.88	44.03	−0.07	−0.15	822.00	1045.00
Trochanteric height	886.64	39.74	−0.26	0.11	796.00	987.00
Biacromial width	349.14	17.43	−0.61	−0.02	309.00	391.00
Chest width	268.80	27.08	1.19	0.81	208.00	362.00
Chest depth	191.68	20.97	0.13	0.75	159.00	253.00
Bicristal width	260.26	20.38	7.22	1.59	221.00	375.00
Bitrochanteric width	307.41	19.21	3.70	0.56	240.00	395.00
Upper limb length	725.68	30.00	−0.24	0.05	644.00	803.00
Upper arm length	311.61	15.83	−0.41	−0.31	269.00	345.00
Forearm length	239.81	17.36	−0.21	0.03	197.00	282.00
Hand length	174.30	8.79	−0.24	−0.33	149.00	191.00
Hand width	77.37	3.54	0.87	−0.31	64.00	85.00
Thigh length	425.05	28.88	−0.13	0.11	352.00	502.00
Leg length	401.41	28.55	0.28	−0.46	315.00	460.00
Foot length	244.47	11.62	−0.44	−0.10	216.00	270.00
Foot width	98.94	6.87	−0.18	0.13	84.00	120.00
Head circumference	562.82	22.48	1.02	0.06	496.00	624.00
Upper arm circumference	285.52	37.88	0.69	0.60	215.00	430.00
Chest circumference	849.80	98.95	0.26	0.72	650.00	1125.00
Abdomen circumference	844.14	118.99	0.09	0.58	617.00	1182.00
Calf circumference	329.73	31.30	−0.02	0.33	262.00	429.00
Triceps skinfold	15.22	5.70	0.50	0.59	4.00	36.00
Subscapular skinfold	18.87	8.00	−0.30	0.53	6.00	40.00
Head length	182.60	7.10	−0.09	−0.21	160.00	197.00
Head width	146.69	6.04	2.12	−0.69	120.00	159.00
Minimum frontal width	104.06	5.68	1.08	0.28	88.00	125.00
Bizygomatic width	133.26	5.70	1.57	−0.11	111.00	150.00
Bigonial width	102.32	5.71	0.68	0.49	89.00	120.00
Nasal height	55.92	4.48	−0.10	−0.22	45.00	67.00
Nasal width	42.09	2.98	−0.42	0.13	34.00	49.00
Nasal index	75.67	7.33	−0.06	0.38	59.70	97.78
Upper face height	81.68	7.06	0.45	0.03	63.00	104.00
Morphological face height	121.78	7.84	0.08	0.17	101.00	143.00
Head height	129.54	4.92	0.30	0.24	118.00	143.00

the average weight being 63.27 and 68.10 kg for the Livingston and St. Vincent males, respectively ($t = -2.38$, siginificant at the 0.02 level for d.f. = 135).

Seven variables in the Livingston physique and four in the St. Vincent physique are not significant in Student's t-test. In terms of these univariate statistics, the sexual dimorphism of the Livingston population is less pronounced than that of the St. Vincent population. Both populations show no significant sex differences in bicristal width, bitrochanteric width, or upper arm circumference,

Table 2C. Descriptive Statistics, St. Vincent Males

Measurement	Mean	S.D.	Kurtosis	Skewness	Minimum	Maximum
Age	49.18	17.04	−0.97	−0.25	17.00	80.00
Weight	68.10	9.92	1.23	0.92	48.99	101.61
Sitting height	848.36	36.00	−0.18	0.29	775.00	938.00
Stature	1685.54	68.00	0.19	0.15	1511.00	1873.00
Iliospinale height	1032.65	51.36	0.72	0.55	919.00	1205.00
Trochanteric height	933.24	48.70	1.33	0.80	839.00	1111.00
Biacromial width	390.53	16.95	−0.15	−0.27	339.00	429.00
Chest width	284.45	19.09	1.48	−0.43	211.00	333.00
Chest depth	195.51	12.92	3.57	1.33	172.00	253.00
Bicristal width	258.92	15.76	−0.73	0.20	230.00	292.00
Bitrochanteric width	305.64	18.93	2.40	−0.50	228.00	356.00
Upper limb length	771.85	35.00	1.56	0.12	650.00	893.00
Upper arm length	323.94	15.89	0.76	−0.21	270.00	367.00
Forearm length	253.83	18.03	1.83	0.41	205.00	324.00
Hand length	195.10	16.13	14.17	2.60	156.00	292.00
Hand width	87.71	5.94	8.33	−2.02	56.00	99.00
Thigh length	520.00	32.93	0.89	0.51	454.00	620.00
Leg length	412.56	24.48	0.34	0.57	365.00	491.00
Foot length	256.89	13.91	0.57	0.47	223.00	303.00
Foot width	102.00	7.02	−0.34	0.26	87.00	120.00
Head circumference	551.01	18.26	−0.88	0.15	517.00	592.00
Upper arm circumference	279.48	31.02	5.31	−0.94	131.00	372.00
Chest circumference	926.62	60.99	−0.01	0.31	800.00	1100.00
Abdomen circumference	852.14	78.98	2.16	1.34	740.00	1148.00
Calf circumference	361.16	23.88	0.02	0.12	306.00	425.00
Triceps skinfold	7.00	2.59	3.95	1.84	3.80	17.00
Subscapular skinfold	12.55	4.38	8.04	2.45	7.00	37.00
Head length	187.36	7.65	−0.29	−0.46	168.00	202.00
Head width	147.24	4.93	−0.53	−0.29	136.00	158.00
Minimum frontal width	109.33	5.01	0.65	0.69	101.00	126.00
Bizygomatic width	138.95	5.75	−0.10	−0.09	123.00	152.00
Bigonial width	106.77	6.29	−0.19	−0.46	90.00	118.00
Nasal height	51.54	3.43	1.05	−0.07	40.00	62.00
Nasal width	43.98	3.86	−0.41	−0.11	34.00	51.00
Nasal index	83.69	8.95	2.71	0.83	64.29	122.50
Upper face height	77.85	6.07	0.17	0.53	68.00	94.00
Morphological face height	123.10	7.85	0.45	0.45	106.00	149.00
Head height	144.90	10.22	1.00	−0.64	112.00	167.00

while the St. Vincent population shows no significant sex difference in abdomen circumference. In sum, the Black Caribs show the least sexual dimorphism in the width and circumference of the torso and the circumference of limbs.

3.2. Factor Analysis

Human physique in a population context can be conceived as an aggregate of corporal subcomponents. Some components appear to be common to all

Table 2D. Descriptive Statistics, St. Vincent Females

Measurement	Mean	S.D.	Kurtosis	Skewness	Minimum	Maximum
Age	43.88	17.60	−1.07	0.12	16.00	86.00
Weight	62.90	12.59	3.25	1.33	42.18	117.03
Sitting height	791.96	35.46	0.06	0.16	706.00	900.00
Stature	1571.26	71.61	6.06	−0.69	1150.00	1847.00
Iliospinale height	962.58	49.92	−0.43	0.24	845.00	1086.00
Trochanteric height	877.09	48.37	−0.22	0.18	748.00	1008.00
Biacromial width	353.92	16.88	0.24	0.26	307.00	405.00
Chest width	269.05	25.13	2.64	1.29	225.00	375.00
Chest depth	186.55	22.52	3.68	1.18	121.00	301.00
Bicristal width	262.24	20.55	1.74	0.98	223.00	350.00
Bitrochanteric width	306.90	19.12	0.23	0.28	264.00	366.00
Upper limb length	706.18	32.14	−0.42	0.13	632.00	785.00
Upper arm length	293.63	18.35	0.06	−0.15	242.00	340.00
Forearm length	234.76	18.36	3.83	0.66	182.00	334.00
Hand length	177.85	8.76	−0.44	0.13	160.00	202.00
Hand width	78.33	4.22	0.50	0.27	68.00	94.00
Thigh length	497.56	30.46	−0.18	0.05	413.00	573.00
Leg length	379.03	23.09	−0.21	0.08	310.00	435.00
Foot length	234.79	14.90	11.29	1.82	207.00	339.00
Foot width	91.26	6.79	0.46	0.06	70.00	115.00
Head circumference	546.37	18.94	−0.13	0.29	503.00	600.00
Upper arm circumference	278.37	39.88	2.19	1.23	211.00	440.00
Chest circumference	888.03	84.73	1.41	0.98	719.00	1215.00
Abdomen circumference	844.67	115.80	0.88	0.85	614.00	1237.00
Calf circumference	354.02	31.95	1.66	0.89	289.00	483.00
Triceps skinfold	16.40	6.74	1.58	1.04	3.20	45.20
Subscapular skinfold	21.22	9.34	0.48	0.96	6.40	50.00
Head length	180.02	10.88	20.38	−3.50	112.00	205.00
Head width	141.28	6.05	4.77	−0.92	107.00	156.00
Minimum frontal width	106.75	5.28	−0.18	0.14	92.00	122.00
Bizygomatic width	130.97	6.27	0.41	0.20	112.00	152.00
Bigonial width	100.47	6.46	2.61	−0.71	72.00	115.00
Nasal height	49.26	3.86	−0.22	−0.05	39.00	59.00
Nasal width	39.63	3.36	−0.29	0.24	32.00	49.00
Nasal index	80.79	7.87	−0.37	0.01	62.71	102.50
Upper face height	74.06	5.45	−0.10	0.00	56.00	88.00
Morphological face height	115.37	6.73	−0.15	0.32	100.00	136.00
Head height	138.40	9.91	0.22	−0.55	106.00	159.00

populations, while others are apparently unique to a specific population. The NT-SYS computer program analysis (Rohlf *et al.*, 1969) was performed in order to delineate the common and unique components of factor structures of human physique. With the eigenvalue $\geqslant 1$ criterion, the varimax solution yielded nine factors for the Livingston and St. Vincent male groups and eight factors for the female groups. Only those loadings greater than an arbitrary cutoff point of 0.5 are summarized in Tables 3A–3D. The decimal point is omitted for clarity of presentation.

Table 2E. Student's t-Test, Males versus Females

Measurement	Livingston males versus females			St. Vincent males versus females		
	t	D.F.	*P*	*t*	D.F.	*P*
Age						
Weight	2.01	93	0.047	3.85	240	0.000
Sitting height	7.66	162	0.000	12.76	289	0.000
Stature	13.28	162	0.000	13.08	289	0.000
Iliospinale height	8.33	53	0.000	11.21	289	0.000
Trochanteric height	10.09	162	0.000	9.34	289	0.000
Biacromial width	11.26	162	0.000	17.47	289	0.000
Chest width	1.26	162	0.210 NS	5.34	289	0.000
Chest depth	3.22	162	0.002	4.30	285	0.000
Bicristal width	0.76	162	0.450 NS	−1.40	289	0.162 NS
Bitrochanteric width	0.33	162	0.742 NS	−0.53	289	0.597 NS
Upper limb length	13.90	162	0.000	15.97	289	0.000
Upper arm length	7.36	51	0.000	13.91	289	0.000
Forearm length	10.10	162	0.000	8.42	289	0.000
Hand length	8.53	50	0.000	9.88	127	0.000
Hand width	12.91	52	0.000	13.96	148	0.000
Thigh length	4.35	51	0.000	5.96	289	0.000
Leg length	9.72	162	0.000	11.48	289	0.000
Foot length	11.61	162	0.000	12.22	289	0.000
Foot width	8.09	162	0.000	12.61	289	0.000
Head circumference	1.75	162	0.000	2.00	289	0.046
Upper arm circumference	−1.87	162	0.064 NS	0.26	242	0.794 NS
Chest circumference	1.72	103	0.089 NS	4.45	256	0.000
Abdomen circumference	−3.06	103	0.003	0.69	265	0.493 NS
Calf circumference	1.03	162	0.306 NS	2.14	249	0.033
Triceps skinfold	−9.58	98	0.000	−17.05	274	0.000
Subscapular skinfold	11.72	162	0.000	−10.41	289	0.000
Head length	6.61	162	0.000	5.97	289	0.000
Head width	6.38	162	0.000	8.42	289	0.000
Minimum frontal width	2.75	162	0.007	4.00	289	0.000
Bizygomatic width	6.93	55	0.000	10.55	289	0.000
Bigonial width	3.72	162	0.000	7.93	289	0.000
Nasal height	5.22	162	0.000	4.94	289	0.000
Nasal width	5.18	162	0.000	7.63	289	0.000
Nasal index	−0.37	162	0.708 NS	2.84	289	0.005
Upper face height	4.92	162	0.000	5.39	289	0.000
Morphological face height	6.37	162	0.000	8.76	289	0.000
Head height	6.34	162	0.000	5.23	289	0.000

The salient feature of the sex difference of the Black Carib physique in factor analysis is that the anthropometric variables are relatively more highly intercorrelated in the male groups than in the female samples. None of the communalities for the Livingston male group falls below 0.5. In the St. Vincent male group four variables yield communalities smaller than 0.5. The female

Table 3A. Varimax Solution, Livingston Males

Measurement	Factor									h^2
	1	2	3	4	5	6	7	8	9	
Age							−555			692
Weight	897									975
Sitting height						503				933
Stature		936								968
Iliospinale height		934								943
Trochanteric height		943								958
Biacromial width										652
Chest width	888									881
Chest depth								688		721
Bicristal width						732				639
Bitrochanteric width						727				804
Upper limb length		759							518	982
Upper arm length		864								878
Forearm length									808	723
Hand length					676					884
Hand width					803					774
Thigh length		676								662
Leg length		653								695
Foot length		696								787

	I	II	III	IV	V	VI	VII	VIII	IX	h²
Foot width										610
Head circumference		678								787
Upper arm circumference	915									929
Chest circumference	846									841
Abdomen circumference	737									885
Calf circumference	778						548			641
Triceps skinfold	558				633					740
Subscapular skinfold	749									681
Head length										710
Head width		883								872
Minimum frontal width		730								735
Bizygomatic width		744								709
Bigonial width	503		802							623
Nasal height										877
Nasal width			−714							710
Nasal index			786							853
Upper face height			815							814
Morphological face height							−523			813
Head height							552			545
Eigenvalue	10.08	6.12	3.58	2.57	2.30	1.67	1.37	1.17	1.07	
Percent of trace	33.67	20.47	11.95	8.60	7.68	5.58	4.57	3.91	3.57	

Trace = 29.93
Percent of the total variance accounted for = 78.76

Table 3B. Varimax Solution, Livingston Females

Measurement	\multicolumn{8}{c}{Factor}								h^2
	1	2	3	4	5	6	7	8	
Age						630			690
Weight	902								939
Sitting height		827							561
Stature		859							901
Iliospinale height		863							770
Trochanteric height									772
Biacromial width					501				616
Chest width	742								669
Chest depth	784								757
Bicristal width									636
Bitrochanteric width	611						538		738
Upper limb length		878							914
Upper arm length		678							896
Forearm length		607						548	848
Hand length		563							744
Hand width					555				465
Thigh length									230
Leg length		744							610
Foot length		522							678
Foot width					577				497

Head circumference									333
Upper arm circumference	877								843
Chest circumference	876								904
Abdomen circumference	848								828
Calf circumference	705								698
Triceps skinfold	825								775
Subscapular skinfold	866								815
Head length									522
Head width			654						411
Minimum frontal width									463
Bizygomatic width			593						503
Bigonial width			598						409
Nasal height									782
Nasal width				841					732
Nasal index						697			982
Upper face height				−823					600
Morphological face height				714					569
Head height				658					159
Eigenvalue	10.82	5.52	2.94	1.85	1.54	1.05	0.86	0.68	
Percent of trace	42.83	21.85	11.65	7.31	6.09	4.16	3.41	2.70	

Trace = 25.26
Percent of the total variance accounted for = 66.47

Table 3C. Varimax Solution, St. Vincent Males

Measurement	1	2	3	4	5	6	7	8	9	h^2
Age	514							590		584
Weight	867	649								947
Sitting height	935									570
Stature	943									919
Iliospinale height										936
Trochanteric height		652								977
Biacromial width		749								615
Chest width										732
Chest depth		519								620
Bicristal width		512								690
Bitrochanteric width	687									677
Upper limb length	641									926
Upper arm length										679
Forearm length									679	718
Hand length	814									537
Hand width	699									469
Thigh length	633									734
Leg length										772
Foot length			820							773
Foot width							555			425

	I	II	III	IV	V	VI	VII	VIII	IX	h²
Head circumference										876
Upper arm circumference	744									683
Chest circumference	786				541					866
Abdomen circumference	646									866
Calf circumference	579				777					635
Triceps skinfold					788					702
Subscapular skinfold		682								827
Head length										577
Head width										629
Minimum frontal width										455
Bizygomatic width			778							615
Bigonial width										310
Nasal height						850				708
Nasal width						850				844
Nasal index				812						996
Upper face height				734						730
Morphological face height										697
Head height										478
Eigenvalue	13.41	3.88	2.15	1.82	1.68	1.13	1.07	0.92	0.73	
Percent of trace	50.05	14.48	8.05	6.82	6.26	4.20	3.99	3.43	2.72	

Trace = 26.79
Percent of the total variance accounted for = 70.50

Table 3D. Varimax Solution, St. Vincent Females

Measurement	\multicolumn{8}{c}{Factor}								h^2
	1	2	3	4	5	6	7	8	
Age						722			632
Weight	886								938
Sitting height		805							412
Stature		940							729
Iliospinale height		913							901
Trochanteric height									898
Biacromial width		509							565
Chest width	871								845
Chest depth	757								709
Bicristal width	751								750
Bitrochanteric width	722								671
Upper limb length		899							888
Upper arm length		765							685
Forearm length								700	742
Hand length		704							736
Hand width									562
Thigh length		764							659
Leg length		856							765
Foot length		558							529
Foot width							483		435

Head circumference								404
Upper arm circumference	896							863
Chest circumference	920							897
Abdomen circumference	770							700
Calf circumference	725							785
Triceps skinfold	793							701
Subscapular skinfold	875							844
Head length								178
Head width			678					497
Minimum frontal width			631					633
Bizygomatic width			659					643
Bigonial width			519					435
Nasal height		836						817
Nasal width				758				810
Nasal index				904				997
Upper face height		713						579
Morphological face height		638						553
Head height								240
Eigenvalue	10.94	2.22	1.84	1.28	1.03	0.73	0.65	
Percent of trace	42.68	8.66	7.17	4.99	4.01	2.86	2.53	

Trace = 25.63
Percent of the total variance accounted for = 66.47

samples yield eight and seven communalities smaller than 0.5 for the Livingston and St. Vincent groups, respectively. Despite low communalities, the small values of residual correlations (not presented in this chapter) indicate that factor analysis is appropriate for the present data sets.

Together the communalities and residual correlations indicate that, with the exception of the Livingston male group, the Black Carib physique is characterized by the marginality of a number of variables in their correlation with other variables, notably hand width, foot width, head circumference, head width, minimum frontal width, bigonial width, and head height. This information may be interpreted in terms of the hand and foot widths being the most distal part of the physique and the head dimensions forming a component independent of the rest of the physique.

The physical components as delineated by factors are presented in Table 4. The first two factors, each representing body bulk, or general size, and body linearity, are well-known factors common to all populations. Head laterality, consisting of head, minimum frontal, bizygomatic, and bigonial widths, and facial linearity, consisting of nasal upper facial, and morphological heights, together account for from 21% (Livingston males) to 15% (St. Vincent males) of the total variance. In the male groups the head laterality component includes head circumference. Extremity component, in the form of hand and foot length and width, and hip laterality component rank next in the proportion of variance they contribute. The upper limb component accounts for the smallest proportion of variance in all four groups.

It will be seen in Table 4 that there is notable concordance between sexes and groups. Intersex concordance is observed in nasal index (factor 4), hand length (factor 5), nasal width (factors 7 and 6) in the Livingston population, and foot width (factor 7) and nasal index (factors 6 and 5) in the St. Vincent population. While not an anthropometric measurement, age is included in factor analysis. In both sexes of the Livingston population, age is correlated with nasal width. In the St. Vincent population age turns out to be a unique factor not significantly correlated with any other variables. In the Livingston population nasal index is negatively correlated with the facial linearity component (factor 4), whereas it is positively correlated with nasal width in the St. Vincent population (factors 6 and 5). The nose form is scrutinized more closely in the following.

The male groups are concordant in the upper arm and forearm lengths (factor 9) and the female groups in forearm length (factor 8). Overall, intersex similarities within a population are greater than interpopulation like-sex similarities. This interpretation is consistent with Mahalanobis D^2 distances presented in Table 5. and Fig. 1.

The factor analysis presented here indicates sex and population differences in configurations of variables. A BMDP7M stepwise discriminant analysis (Dixon and Brown, 1979) was performed on the 37 variables, including nasal index, to

Table 4. Components of Black Carib Physique[a]

| Component | Livingston | | | | St. Vincent | | | |
| | Males | | Females | | Males | | Females | |
	Factor	Composition	Factor	Composition	Factor	Composition	Factor	Composition
Body bulk	1		1		2		1	
Body linearity	2		2		1		2	
Head laterality	3		3		3		4	
Facial inearity	4	−Nasal index	4	−Nasal index	4		3	
Extremity	5	Hand length, Hand width, Foot width	5	Hand length, Foot length	7	Foot width	7	Foot width
Nose width	6	Nose width, −Head height, −Triceps skinfold	6	Nose width	6	Nasal index	5	Nasal index
Hip laterality	7		7					
Age					8		6	
Upper limb	9	Upper arm forearm	8	Forearm	9	Upper arm forearm	8	Forearm

[a] The negative sign indicates negative correlation of a part in composition with the component.

Table 5. *Mahalanobis D^2 Distance and Corresponding F Statistic between Paired Groups[a]*

	Livingston males	Livingston females	St. Vincent males	St. Vincent females
Livingston males	–	15.99	44.57	54.84
Livingston females	20.60	–	52.95	35.29
St. Vincent males	53.89	126.06	–	16.45
St. Vincent females	77.11	116.03	46.33	–

[a] The F matrix is in the lower triangle, the D^2 matrix in the upper triangle. $P < 0.01$ for all F values (d.f. = 22, 430).

determine which variables most effectively discriminate groups on the basis of one-way analysis of variance F statistic for testing H_0: $\mu_{1v} = \mu_{2v} = \cdots = \mu_{gv}$ between groups on variables = 1, . . . , 37. Table 5 presents 10 variables, in decreasing order of F values, for which the mean values in the groups are most different. The D^2 biological distances are also graphically represented in Fig. 1. All F values are significant at the 0.01 level.

As may be expected, the D^2 distances are the greatest in cross-sex-population pairings, i.e., between the Livingston males and St. Vincent females and between Livingston females and St. Vincent males. The distances between the sexes within the same populations are the smallest. The interpopulation differences between like sexes are intermediate in magnitude. These D^2 distances indicate, therefore, that the sexual dimorphism in the Black Carib physique, when the 37 anthropometric variables are considered simultaneously, is of a lesser magnitude than the interpopulation differences between like sexes.

The variables that show most sex differences in both populations are hand width, biacromial width, bitrochanteric width, chest width, sitting height, and minimum frontal width. Subscapular skinfold and triceps skinfold are highly intercorrelated, and either variable can be considered as the second most discriminating variable. It is to be noted that the males and females differ mostly

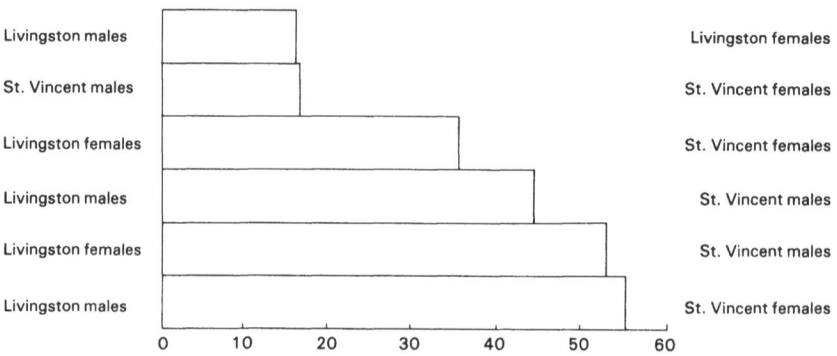

FIGURE 1. Mahalanobis D^2 distance between paired groups.

in the lateral dimensions or widths in various parts of the body. The hand width alone can discriminate the sexes effectively.

3.3. Discriminant Analysis

Discriminant analysis is also performed to delineate the like-sex interpopulational difference between the Livingston and St. Vincent samples. As Table 5 indicates, there is a remarkable concordance between the two populations in the configuration of variables that most effectively discriminate sex. Five variables rank among the top eight most discriminating variables in both sex groups: nasal height, thigh length, trochanteric height, hand length, and iliospinale height. Furthermore, there is a perfect concordance between the two matched sex groups in the directions of difference in average values of the five variables. The average nasal height, trochanteric height, and iliospinale height of the Livingston males and females are larger than those of their St. Vincent counterparts. The reverse is true of thigh length and hand length. The Livingston males and females have significantly longer legs than the St. St. Vincent males and females ($t = 7.36$ for d.f. $= 135$; $t = 7.35$ for d.f. $= 225$). Conversely, the Livingston males and females have significantly shorter thighs than the St. Vincent males and females ($t = -9.04$ for d.f. $= 135$; $t = -21.16$ for d.f. $= 316$). The Livingston and St. Vincent male groups differ significantly in all variables except 12: stature, iliospinale height, biacromial width, bicristal width, bitrochanteric width, hand length, hand width, upper arm circumference, triceps skinfold, minimum frontal width, bizygomatic width, and bigonial width. The Livingston and St. Vincent female groups do not differ significantly in eight variables: stature, trochanteric height, chest width, bicristal width, bitrochanteric width, upper arm circumference, abdomen circumference, and triceps skinfold.

The causes for these interpopulation differences are apparently due mostly to different sets of complex interplay between the genetic component and environment, including such factors as diet and motor habit. One feature is more amenable to a genetic interpretation: the nasal morphology. The Livingston males and females have significantly longer and wider noses than their St. Vincent counterparts ($t = 8.13$ for d.f. $= 36$, and $t = 14.10$ for d.f. $= 316$, respectively). A more apt description of interpopulation difference in nose form can be made with nasal index. The average nasal index of the Livingston male group is 75.85 (S.D. $= 7.94$), and that of the St. Vincent male group is 83.69 (S.D. $= 8.95$). The average nasal index is 75.67 (S.D. $= 7.33$) for the Livingston female group and 80.79 (S.D. $= 7.87$) for the St. Vincent female group. Although they all fall in the mesorhine class (70.00–84.99), there is a considerable variation in nasal index, which reflects substantial variations in nasal length and width across the populations and between the sexes.

Table 6. *Ten Most Discriminating Variables in Stepwise Discrimination Analysis*

Step	Among four groups	Males versus females		Livingston versus St. Vincent	
		Livingston	St. Vincent	Males	Females
1	Thigh length	Hand width	Biacromial width	Nasal height	Thigh length
2	Upper arm length	Subscapular skinfold	Triceps skinfold	Thigh length	Trochanteric height
3	Trochanteric height	Stature	Hand width	Trochanteric height	Nasal height
4	Triceps skinfold	Bitrochanteric width	Foot width	Iliospinale height	Hand length
5	Biacromial width	Chest circumference	Bitrochanteric width	Hand length	Foot length
6	Nasal height	Biacromial width	Chest width	Head width	Head height
7	Hand length	Chest width	Sitting height	Morphological face height	Upper arm length
8	Iliospinale height	Iliospinale height	Minimum frontal width	Bicristal width	Iliospinale height
9	Upper arm circumference	Sitting height	Bizygomatic sidth	Weight	Nasal width
10	Chest circumference	Minimum frontal width	Bicristal width	Triceps skinfold	Calf circumference

3.4. Analysis of Variance

Stepwise discriminant analysis (Table 6) indicates that nasal height is one of the three variables that most discriminate the like-sex groups. Being clearly a sensitive indicator of sex difference, nasal height merits a close examination. As a generalization of the t-test already discussed (Table 2), analysis of variance, or ANOVA for short, was performed to test the differences among the means of the four groups simultaneously. In applying ANOVA (Lin, n.d.) to the present data, two questions are to be asked: (1) Are the differences among the four sample means on nasal length or nasal width greater than what would be expected if the samples were drawn from the same population, or, stated as a null hypothesis, are the means of the populations from which the samples are drawn equal (H_0: $m_A = m_B = m_C = m_D$)?; and (2) What can be said about the variation in nasal length or nasal width from one group to another?

The analysis performed is a two-factor design, inevitably limited by non-experimental work, unlike the common applications of ANOVA, in which experimental treatments are imposed by random allocation. The data are classified by two factors – sex and population (i.e., Livingston and St. Vincent) – to fit a two-way classification. Nevertheless, sex and population represent potential sources of variation whose main effects and interaction deserve a close scrutiny. The variance is decomposed into constituent parts of components by partitioning the total sums of squares in a two-way orthogonal analysis of variance (Tables 7 and 8). The effects of the sex and population factors on the sample ($N = 455$) are sorted out, leaving aside the question of the environmental component, by

$$E(Y_{ij}) = \mu + \alpha_i + \beta_j + (\alpha\beta)_{ij} + \xi_{ijk}$$

where μ equals the parametric mean of the population (i.e., the Livingston and St. Vincent populations combined); α_i denotes the row constants, i.e., the ith differential or main effect of factor sex (or *due sex*) measuring the deviation of the sex means from the overall population mean; β_j denotes the column constants, the jth differential effect of factor population (or *due population*) measuring the deviation of the population means from the overall mean; and ξ_{ijk} is an error or residual term, which is required to be independent, normal, with zero means and variance σ^2, this variance being the same in all parts of the ANOVA table.

One may assume a possible effect of both sex and population classifications on the mean value of each observation of Y_{ij} at the ith row and jth column with an *additive* model. If the effects of sex and population are additive, that is, if interpopulation differences in nasal length produce the same effect whether the subjects belong to either sex, and likewise, intersex differences in this variable produce the same effect whether the subjects belong to either population, then there will be no significant quantity due to interaction, $(\alpha\beta)_{ij}$. On the contrary, Table 7 shows that there is a sizeable quantity of sum of squares, $88.711(F =$

Table 7. Two-Way Analysis of Variance, Nasal Length

Source of variation	Degrees of freedom	Sum of squares	Mean square	F	Significance of F
Main effects	2	5845.734	2922.867	179.096	0.000
Sex	1	813.753	813.753	49.862	0.000
Population	1	5403.672	5403.672	333.105	0.000
Sex−population interaction	1	88.711	88.711	5.436	0.020
Explained	3	5934.445	1978.148	121.209	0.000
Error	451	7360.367	16.320		
Total	454	13294.813	29.284		

Table 8. Two-Way Analysis of Variance, Nasal Width

Source of variation	Degrees of freedom	Sum of squares	Mean square	F	Significance of F
Main effects	2	1419.943	709.971	61.714	0.000
Sex	1	986.333	986.333	85.737	0.000
Population	1	574.289	574.289	49.920	0.000
Sex−population interaction	1	3.011	3.011	0.262	0.609
Explained	3	1422.957	474.319	41.230	0.000
Error	451	5188.402	11.504		
Total	454	6611.359	14.562		

5.436, d.f. $= 1$, $P < 0.02$), which represents the differential effect of the combination of the ith level of sex and jth level of population not accounted for by the sum of $\mu + \delta_i + \beta_j$.

The data in Table 7 show (1) that each of the main effects, sex and population, is significant ($P < 0.001$), and (2) that the effect of sex varies between the two populations, and similarly, the effect of population is not uniform between the sexes. The interaction component indicates certain dependence of the effect of sex upon population, and *vice versa*. It can be concluded that the sex and population factors are not simply additive. The combination of sex and population factors contributes to the observed level of phenotypic expression of nasal length. ANOVA of nasal width (Table 8) shows that while both main effects of sex and population factors are significant ($P < 0.001$), the effect due to the sex−population interaction is not. One-way analysis of variance (tables not presented) on nasal length and nasal width among the four group means yield signficant F values of 121.199 and 41.227 (d.f. $= 3$, 451), respectively. Because rejection of the overall H_0 only indicates that something other than chance is generating the differences among the four group means, it is necessary to conduct a specific comparison to specify in more detail the source of the

Table 9. Multiple Comparisons among Four Group Means of Nasal Index

	SNK	Scheffe	k
$\bar{Y}_4 - \bar{Y}_1 = 83.6910 - 75.1561 = 8.5349$	3.8967	4.2383	4
$\bar{Y}_3 - \bar{Y}_1 = 80.7917 - 75.1561 = 5.6356$	3.3066	3.9303	3
$\bar{Y}_4 - \bar{Y}_2 = 83.6910 - 75.6682 = 8.0228$	2.5412	3.0206	3
$\bar{Y}_2 - \bar{Y}_1 = 75.6682 - 75.1561 = 0.5121$	2.9063	4.1060	2 N.S.
$\bar{Y}_3 - \bar{Y}_2 = 80.7917 - 75.6682 = 5.1235$	1.8195	2.5707	2
$\bar{Y}_4 - \bar{Y}_3 = 83.6910 - 80.7917 = 2.8993$	1.9655	2.7768	2

Livingston males	Livingston females	St. Vincent females	St. Vincent males
$\bar{Y}_1$	$\bar{Y}_2$	$\bar{Y}_3$	$\bar{Y}_4$
75.1561	75.6682	80.7917	83.6910

Conclusions:

$\mu_1 = \mu_2 < \mu_3 < \mu_4$

Table 10. Multiple Comparisons among Four Group Means of Nasal Length

	SNK	Scheffe	k
$\bar{Y}_4 - \bar{Y}_1 = 60.2820 - 49.2642 = 11.0178$	1.8308	1.9913	4
$\bar{Y}_3 - \bar{Y}_1 = 55.9200 - 49.2642 = 6.6558$	1.0958	1.3024	3
$\bar{Y}_4 - \bar{Y}_2 = 60.2820 - 51.5408 = 8.7412$	1.8066	2.1472	3
$\bar{Y}_2 - \bar{Y}_1 = 51.5408 - 49.2642 = 2.2766$	0.9958	1.4069	2
$\bar{Y}_3 - \bar{Y}_2 = 55.9200 - 51.5408 = 4.3792$	1.0832	1.5304	2
$\bar{Y}_4 - \bar{Y}_3 = 60.2820 - 55.9200 = 4.3620$	1.4725	2.0803	2

St Vincent males	St. Vincent females	Livingston females	Livingston males
$\bar{Y}_1$	$\bar{Y}_2$	$\bar{Y}_3$	$\bar{Y}_4$
49.2642	51.5408	55.9200	60.2820

Conclusions:

$\mu_1 < \mu_2 < \mu_3 < \mu_4$

Table 11. Multiple Comparisons among Four Group Means of Nasal Width

	SNK	Scheffe	k
$\bar{Y}_4 - \bar{Y}_1 = 45.0513 - 39.6321 = 5.4192$	1.5371	1.6719	4
$\bar{Y}_3 - \bar{Y}_1 = 42.9796 - 39.6321 = 3.3475$	0.9938	1.1812	3
$\bar{Y}_4 - \bar{Y}_2 = 45.0513 - 42.0880 = 2.9633$	1.4694	1.7466	3
$\bar{Y}_2 - \bar{Y}_1 = 42.0880 - 39.6321 = 2.4559$	0.7740	1.0940	2
$\bar{Y}_3 - \bar{Y}_2 = 42.9796 - 42.0880 = 0.8916$	0.9094	1.2849	2 N.S.
$\bar{Y}_4 - \bar{Y}_3 = 45.0513 - 42.9796 = 2.0727$	1.2761	1.8029	2

St. Vincent females	Livingston females	St. Vincent males	Livingston males
$\bar{Y}_1$	$\bar{Y}_2$	$\bar{Y}_3$	$\bar{Y}_4$
39.6321	42.0880	42.9796	45.0513

Conclusions:

$\mu_1 < \mu_2 = \mu_3 < \mu_4$

significant overall F. For performing such specific comparisons, the stepwise Student–Newman–Keuls (SNK) (Sokal and Rohlf, 1969) and simultaneous Scheffe (Scheffe, 1959) multiple contrast methods were employed. For $\alpha = 0.05$ and 455 degrees of freedom in the independent standard deviation s for the range w of k groups, the percentiles of the distribution $Q = w/s$ [interpolated from Pearson and Hartley (1954)] are as follows:

k	2	3	4
Q	2.81	3.23	3.65

From the Q the least significant ranges (LSR) are computed for nasal index, nasal length, and nasal width. Scheffe's ranges are computed from a single range value, 3.55. All pertinent information for and from the *a posteriori* tests is presented in Tables 9–11.

The Scheffe *post hoc* criterion yields more stringent critical values than the SNK approach. The Scheffe ranges are therefore more conservative. At any rate, the two tests yield the same results of multiple comparisons; all but the Livingston males–Livingston females comparison on nasal index ($0.5121 <$ 1.8195 or 2.5707) and the Livingston females–St. Vincent males comparison on nasal width ($0.8916 < 0.90943$ or 1.2849) are significant.

4. Discussion

The ranking of group means of nasal length shows that the Livingston population possesses larger noses than the St. Vincent population. However, there is no discernible pattern with regard to sex. That is, the males have longer noses than the females in the Livingston population, but the reverse is true in the St. Vincent population. In nasal width the males have greater mean values than the females, and in both sexes the Livingston population has wider noses than the St. Vincent population. As mentioned earlier, the Livingston population has significantly longer noses in terms of nasal index with t-tests, the rank order of nasal index being Livingston males first, Livingston females second, St. Vincent females third, and St. Vincent males last. Again, there is no consistent pattern with regard to sex in nasal length. As will be seen from Tables 9 and 10, the rank orders of group means of nasal index and nasal length are reverses of each other, indicating that nasal length is a more important variable than nasal width in nasal morphology. The information on nasal index is therefore redundant.

Factor analysis, presented earlier, suggests that phenotypic expressions of nasal length and nasal width are possibly controlled either by two separate sets of genetic components or by only one set differentially. It is also possible, and most likely, that there exist two sets of partially overlapping genetic components, thus producing differential phenotypic effects relating to nasal length and nasal width. In addition, a sex genetic component interacts with the former components as a third factor. Whatever the nature of the genetic architecture, the data from factor analysis and ANOVA suggest that the genetic component relating to the phenotypic expression of nasal width exerts a systematic effect that does not achieve significant difference for either sex factor or population factor separately. However, there are significant sex differences in regard to nasal length. This interpretation is consistent with the data from stepwise discriminant analysis and factor analysis. That is (1) nasal length is one of the three variables that discriminate sexes most effectively (Table 6), and (2) the facial linearity component, which includes nasal length, is more important in factor rank order than the factor delineating nasal width (Tables 3 and 4). These factor rank orders are as follows:

Livingston males	factors 4 and 6
Livingston females	factors 4 and 6
St. Vincent males	factors 4 and 6
St. Vincent females	factors 3 and 5

For lack of sufficient familial data, it is not feasible to partition the variability in Black Carib physique into genetic and environmental components or to estimate heritability for each trait. Nevertheless, the present data allow appropriate univariate and multivariate statistical analyses to describe the Black Carib physique in body components or regions and to delineate intergroup morphological differences and variations in terms of 37 anthropometric variables and the patterns of their aggregates.

The data indicate that the net effects of genetic—environment interaction produce differential phenotypic manifestations in single traits or body components. Nasal length appears to be one of the variables, the phenotypic manifestations of which are more sensitive to the effects of genetic action than that of environmental influence. Within the genetic component the sex factor manifests itself differentially from one trait to another and from one body component to another. A seemingly inordinate amount of discussion is devoted to nose morphology, with a suggestion that sets of genetic components interact differentially, leading to various phenotypic expressions, and that the phenotypic variations must be analyzed with appropriate statistical methods.

The partitioning of the variation in Black Carib nose morphology, assumed to be under the effects of genetic component more than the environmental influence, as the climate is highly similar between Livingston and St. Vincent, provides some insight into population architecture of the Black Caribs. ANOVA of a number of variables, while not presented, suggests that the phenotypic variance in some body components is not due to additive genetic variation, while in others the variance appears to conform to an additive model.

5. Conclusion

Two conclusions can be drawn from the present study: (1) The interaction of sex-influenced variability and population-specific variability creates a synergistic effect. That is, the effects of two or more factors in their interdependence contribute a significant amount of positive increment to the expression of some variables. (2) The interpopulation sex differences or variances are smaller than interpopulation like-sex differences or variances. These biological expressions are no doubt due to the history of certain degrees of isolation, interbreeding, and mating systems of the Black Carib populations of Livingston and St. Vincent. The interpretation of the anthropometric data presented is to be corroborated by ethnohistorical and serological investigations reported elsewhere in the volume.

ACKNOWLEDGMENTS

Collection of the data on the St. Vincent Black Caribs was made possible by Wichita State University General Research Fund 3615-22.

The author acknowledge the UCLA Health Sciences Computing Facility for providing programs BMDP3D and BMDP7M with the support of the National Institutes of Health Special Research Resource Grant RR-3.

References

Dixon, W. J., and Brown, M. B., 1979, *BMD Biomedical Computer Programs*, University of California Press, Berkeley.

Gonzalez, N. L. S., 1969, *Black Carib Household Structure*, University of Washington Press, Seattle.

Lin. P. M., n.d., MSGP, Multivariate Statistical and Graphic Computer Programs, unreleased.

Martin, R., 1957, *Lehrbuch der Anthropologie*, Band I, Gustav Fischer Verlag, Stuttgart.

Oliver, G., 1969, *Practical Anthropometry*, Charles C. Thomas, Springfield, Illinois.

Pearson, E. S., and Hartley, H. O., 1954, *Biometrika Tables for Statisticians*, Vol. 1, Cambridge University Press, New York.

Rholf, F. G., Kishpaugh, J., and Bartcher, R., 1969, *NT-SYS, Numerical Taxonomy System of Multivariate Statistical Programs*, University of Kansas, Lawrence.

Scheffe, H. A., 1959, *The Analysis of Variance*, Wiley, New York.

Sokal, R. R., and Rohlf, F. J., 1969, *Biometry*, W. H. Freeman, San Francisco.

12

Factors Influencing Blood Pressure Level among the Black Caribs of St. Vincent Island

JANIS HUTCHINSON, PAUL M. LIN, and MICHAEL H. CRAWFORD

1. Introduction

Variation in blood pressure level, like many other physical and behavioral traits, is the product of both environmental and genetic factors. Both components have been extensively examined by a number of researchers (Lowe, 1964; Miall, 1967; Langford *et al.*, 1968; Pickering, 1968; Joossens, 1973; Biron *et al.*, 1976; Lee, 1978; Feinleib *et al.*, 1979; Havlik *et al.*, 1979b; Voors *et al.*, 1979; Canessa *et al.*, 1980). A major problem in understanding the etiology and epidemiology of blood pressure is determining the quantitative contribution of genetic versus environmental influences. Such quantification can be used to illuminate factors that affect blood pressure distributions and variation. The genetic contribution to blood pressure is customarily estimated by means of heritability (h^2) (Harburg *et al.*, 1977; Rose *et al.*, 1979; Havlik *et al.*, 1979b; Weinberg *et al.*, 1979). Although the standard error of these estimates may be

JANIS HUTCHINSON AND MICHAEL H. CRAWFORD ● Laboratory of Biological Anthropology, University of Kansas, Lawrence, Kansas 66045. PAUL M. LIN ● Institute of Social and Behavioral Pathology, and Psychiatric Research Unit, Department of Psychiatry, Pritzker School of Medicine, The University of Chicago, Chicago, Illinois 60637.

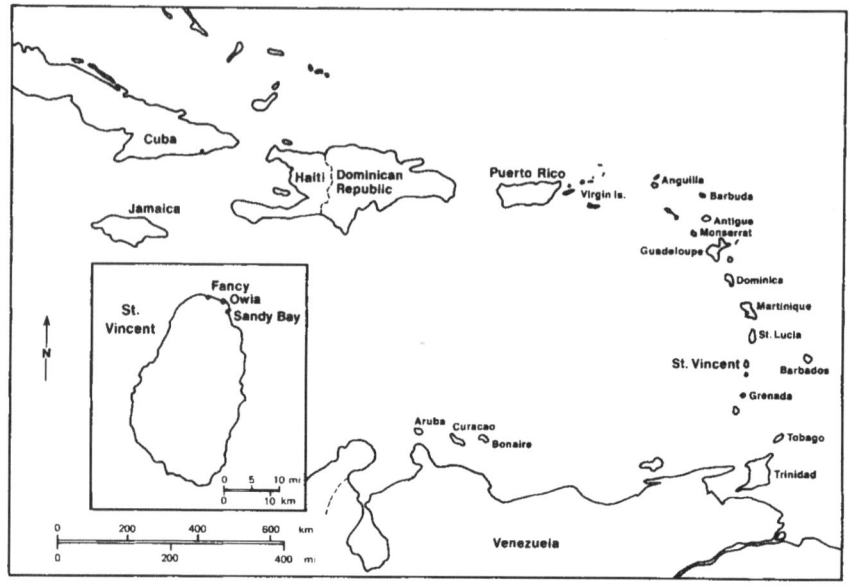

FIGURE 1. Geographical location of St. Vincent in the Lesser Antilles.

high (thereby increasing the possible range of the true value), such measures do demonstrate maximum and minimum levels of heritable variation.

The environmental effects of this phenotype are difficult to assess since a large number of external factors may be involved. Since these environmental and cultural factors vary from population to population, comparison between groups is complex and in some cases inappropriate. Also, the interactive influence of both genes and environment on blood pressure must be considered. A holistic approach may produce results that differ from those achieved by analyzing each component separately. An interactive model is difficult to construct since all factors cannot be examined simultaneously. However, path-analytic models have been constructed that employ an assortment of environmental and biological components simultaneously. The present study aims to investigate these relationships in terms of hybridization, familial, and anthropometric variability.

2. Methods

2.1. Populations Studied

If a genetic component for blood pressure exists, the relatives of propositii should possess similar pressures. This association has been demonstrated by McIlhany et al. (1975), Schull et al. (1977), Havlik et al. (1979a), Rose et al. (1979), Morton et al. (1980), and Kreiger et al. (1980). Such familial relationships

Table 1. Numerical and Sex Distribution of the Population Sample from St. Vincent Island, Collected during the Summer of 1979

Village	Males	Females	Total
Sandy Bay	71	122	193
Owia	46	86	132
Fancy	36	60	96
Total	153	268	421

were examined in three communities, Sandy Bay, Owia, and Fancy, on the island of St. Vincent (Fig. 1) in the Caribbean. Table 1 provides a subdivision of the sample into the numbers of males and females studied in each community. The age of the individuals who participated in the study varies from 10 to 90 years. All blood pressure readings were taken by a single researcher while each subject was in a seated position with the left arm resting on a table. A baumanometer with a 14-cm-wide compression cuff positioned at heart level was used to record systolic and diastolic, phase V, pressures.

2.2. Familial Analysis

Familial similarity is examined on the basis of correlation and regression analyses among genetically related individuals. In the St. Vincent study, correlation coefficients are computed utilizing the BMDP1R computer program on 68 mother—offspring pairs, 32 father—offspring pairs, and 70 sib pairs. Age and sex are standardized with the formula $Y_i - b(s_i - \bar{x})$, where Y_i is the individual's blood pressure reading, b is the regression coefficient (for the subject's unadjusted blood pressure regressed on father, or mother, or sib unadjusted blood pressure), s_i is the subject's age, and $\bar{x}$ is the mean age for the sample.

Heritability estimates for each familial cohort are computed using regression analysis (BMDP1R). These estimates are calculated for mother—offspring and father—offspring cohorts. Sibship heritability estimates are not computed since a common environment is shared in terms of economic responsibility and social interaction, thus inflating apparent genetic variability.

2.3. Hybrid Analysis

Blood pressure level has also been associated with skin reflectance measurement. Such a relationship was reported by Boyle (1970) based on blacks residing in Charleston County, South Carolina. This study indicates that darker skinned individuals have a greater propensity for high blood pressure than lighter skinned individuals. The exact nature of this relationship is not fully understood; however, a phenotypic description of it is possible.

A serological analysis of 373 Black Caribs was carried out by the Minneapolis Blood Bank for the following systems: ABO, MNSs, and Rhesus. Gene frequencies for C, c and E, e of the Rhesus system, along with the ABO and MNSs systems, are utilized in the estimates of admixture. Gene frequencies for black Americans from New York and Miami, Florida were averaged (Mourant *et al.*, 1976). The West African population includes an averaged gene frequency for populations from Sierre Leone, Nigeria, Senegal, Liberia, and the Ivory Coast (Mourant *et al.*, 1976). Gene frequencies for Arawak and Caribs (Carawak) are also averaged (Geerdink *et al.*, 1974). Both populations, Carawak and West African, make up the ancestral populations of the Black Caribs on St. Vincent Island.

Roberts and Hiorns' and "true least squares" methods (Roberts and Hiorns, 1962, 1965; Elston and Stewart, 1971) were utilized to estimate the percentages of Indian and African genes in the Black Carib gene pool. Both methods assume that the gene frequencies of the ancestral populations are represented by the composite groups used, Carawak and West African, and that drift and selection are absent (Crawford, 1976). Estimation of amount of admixture is computed from the known gene frequencies of the West African, Carawak, and St. Vincent populations. Individual estimates of admixture are calculated by considering each individual on St. Vincent as a separate hybrid population. Thus, individual admixture estimates can range from 0 to 100% West African or Carawak contribution to the gene pool.

The possible relationship between degree of African ancestry and elevation of arterial blood pressure level was examined. The sample was subdivided into normotensive and hypertensive cohorts, and a test of association between the degree of African admixture and blood pressure level was tested. A diastolic reading above 95 mm Hg was considered hypertensive; any reading below this level was considered normotensive. This standard is in accordance with the Conference on Methodology in Epidemiological Studies in Cardiovascular Disease, which met in Princeton, New Jersey in 1959 (Lee, 1978). An R × C (row by column) test of independence is used to examine associations between African admixture and age for hypertensives (Sokal and Rohlf, 1969). This method alleviates computations of the χ^2 test when the matrix exceeds two rows or columns or corrects for small cell size, and it is usually the more exact test. The R × C test of independence utilizes the G-test, which corresponds to a χ^2 analysis. This formula is

$$G = 2[(\Sigma f \ln f \text{ for the cell frequencies})$$

$$- (\Sigma f \ln f \text{ for the row and column totals}) + N \ln N \text{ for the grand total}]$$

2.4. Anthropometric Analysis

Both environmental and genetic factors are involved in blood pressure and anthropometric variability. The genetic component to blood pressure is composed

*Table 2. Anthropometric Traits Collected during the Summer
of 1979*

1. Weight	20. Foot width
2. Sitting height	21. Head circumference
3. Stature	22. Upper arm circumference
4. Suprasternal height	23. Chest circumference
5. Iliospinale height	24. Abdomen circumference
6. Trochanteric height	25. Calf circumference
7. Biacromial width	26. Triceps skinfold
8. Chest width	27. Subscapular skinfold
9. Chest depth	28. Head length
10. Bicristal width	29. Head width
11. Bitrochanteric width	30. Minimum frontal width
12. Upper limb length	31. Bizygomatic width
13. Upper arm length	32. Bigonial width
14. Forearm length	33. Nasal height
15. Hand length	34. Nasal width
16. Hand width	35. Upper facial height
17. Thigh length	36. Morphological facial height
18. Leg length	37. Head height
19. Foot length	

of polygenes, while the environmental contribution includes the ingestion of
sodium chloride, other biochemical elements, stress, and acculturation (Hamilton
et al., 1954; Dahl, 1963; Scotch, 1963; Harburg *et al.,* 1973; Guyton *et al.,*
1974; McGarvey and Baker, 1979). Although anthropometrics are the interactive
products of both polygenetic and environmental elements, they also contribute
to variability in blood pressure level. Certain traits have been repeatedly associated with blood pressure variability, for example, body weight (Tibblin *et al.,*
1967; Boyle, 1970; Hsu *et al.,* 1977), torso dimensions, stature (Hanna and
Baker, 1979), and body composition (Siervogel *et al.,* 1982). Concomitant traits,
such as upper arm circumference and triceps skinfold, also influence blood
pressure variability (Khosla and Lowe, 1965; Taylor, 1967; Langford *et al.,*
1968). Estimation of the quantitative contribution of anthropometric measurements to arterial pressure may vary, depending upon the biological makeup of
the population. The Black Caribs of St. Vincent Island present an opportunity to
examine the numerical contribution of anthropometrics to blood pressure
variability in a hybrid population.

Thirty-seven anthropometric variables were examined in order to determine possible associations with systolic and diastolic pressures among 287 Black
Caribs (Table 2). The selected measurements have previously been associated
with blood pressure variability and most are linked to the physiology of blood
pressure. This subsample includes (1) weight, (2) sitting height, (3) stature, (4)
anterior trunk height, (5) biacromial width, (6) chest width, (7) chest depth,
(8) abdominal height, (9) upper arm circumference, (10) chest circumference,

(11) abdomen circumference, (12) triceps skinfold, (13) subscapular skinfold, and (14) body mass index = weight (in grams)/stature^2 (in cm).

Stepwise multiple regression (BMDP2R) was used to identify body dimensions that contribute to variability in both systolic and diastolic pressures. The multiple R^2 analysis yields the proportion of variation in the dependent variable (blood pressure) that can be explained by the independent variables (anthropometrics). The F-to-enter values measure the proportion of variation in the independent variable that contributes to variability in the dependent trait and reveal the importance of specific variables in predicting blood pressure. The F-to-enter was set at 1.0 for the selected variables and 2.0 for the total sample of measurements. Anthropometrics were standardized for age and sex using regression analysis. The residuals were then utilized as the independent variables, while blood pressure was designated as the dependent variable.

The direction of anthropometric variability between hypertensives and normotensives was also examined for selected variables. t-Tests were used to identify significant differences between mean anthropometric characters for hypertensive versus normotensive males and females. For this analysis a systolic reading above 160 mm Hg was considered hypertensive; any reading below this level was considered normotensive (Boyle, 1970). For diastolic pressure, subjects with readings in excess of 95 mm Hg were considered hypertensive, while any reading below this level was placed in the normotensive category.

Discriminant analyses were utilized to distinguish between hypertensives and normotensives based upon selected anthropometric variables. A χ^2 analysis was used to determine if the classifications are due to nonrandom processes.

3. Results

3.1. Familial Correlations

Table 3 summarizes the observed familial correlations, heritability estimates, and their standard errors for systolic and diastolic pressures. Only sibship correlations are significant for both systolic and diastolic pressure. Mother–offspring correlations are significant for diastolic pressure, but not for systolic pressure. Father–offspring correlations are not significant; this could be due to a number of factors, such as small sample size, with only 32 father–offspring pairs. These correlations, along with the heritability estimates, indicate considerable homogeneity in blood pressure level among relatives.

3.2. Hybridization

Table 4 summarizes the observed gene frequencies for Carawaks (Carib–Arawak hybrid), Black Caribs on St. Vincent, West Africans, and black Americans, using the ABO, MNSs, and Rhesus systems. Except for the *MS* and *NS* genotypes,

Table 3. Familial Aggregation of Black Carib Blood Pressure

Relationship	Correlation	h^2	S.E.
Systolic blood pressure			
Mother–offspring	0.22	0.296	0.162
Father–offspring	0.13	0.134	0.184
Sibship	0.24*		
Diastolic blood pressure			
Mother–offspring	0.30*	0.434	0.168
Father–offspring	0.14	0.138	0.180
Sibship	0.27*		

*$P < 0.05$.

Table 4. Gene Frequency Distribution for Carawaks, the Black Caribs of St. Vincent, West Africans, and Black Americans

	Carawaks	St. Vincent Black Caribs	West Africans	Black Americans
ABO				
A	0.0075	0.1574	0.2724	0.2620
B	0.0000	0.0978	0.2408	0.2520
O	0.9925	0.7448	0.4868	0.4860
Rhesus				
Ce	0.5685	0.0736	0.0683	0.0881
cE	0.2970	0.2548	0.0787	0.1441
ce	0.0437	0.4441	0.5733	0.3383
CE	0.0235	0.0041	0.0000	0.0000
Ce	0.5685	0.0396	0.0086	0.0449
ce	0.0438	0.1838	0.2525	0.3846
MNSs				
MS	0.1590	0.0533	0.0948	0.0885
Ms	0.4235	0.4003	0.3494	0.4015
NS	0.0820	0.0951	0.0429	0.0718
Ns	0.3355	0.4513	0.5129	0.4382

Black Carib gene frequencies are indistinguishable from Carawak and West African patterns. This table also indicates a tendency for greater similarity in gene frequencies between Black Caribs and West Africans. Such a relationship can also be demonstrated using admixture estimates, which show that 73% of the sample received one-half or more of these genes from an African ancestor.

If blood pressure level is examined by age cohort for Black Caribs, the Carajas of Brazil (Lowenstein, 1961), Black Americans (Comstock, 1957), and the Ilora of Western Nigeria (Abraham *et al.*, 1960), the uniqueness of the St. Vincent sample is demonstrated (see Fig. 2). Among the Carajas and West

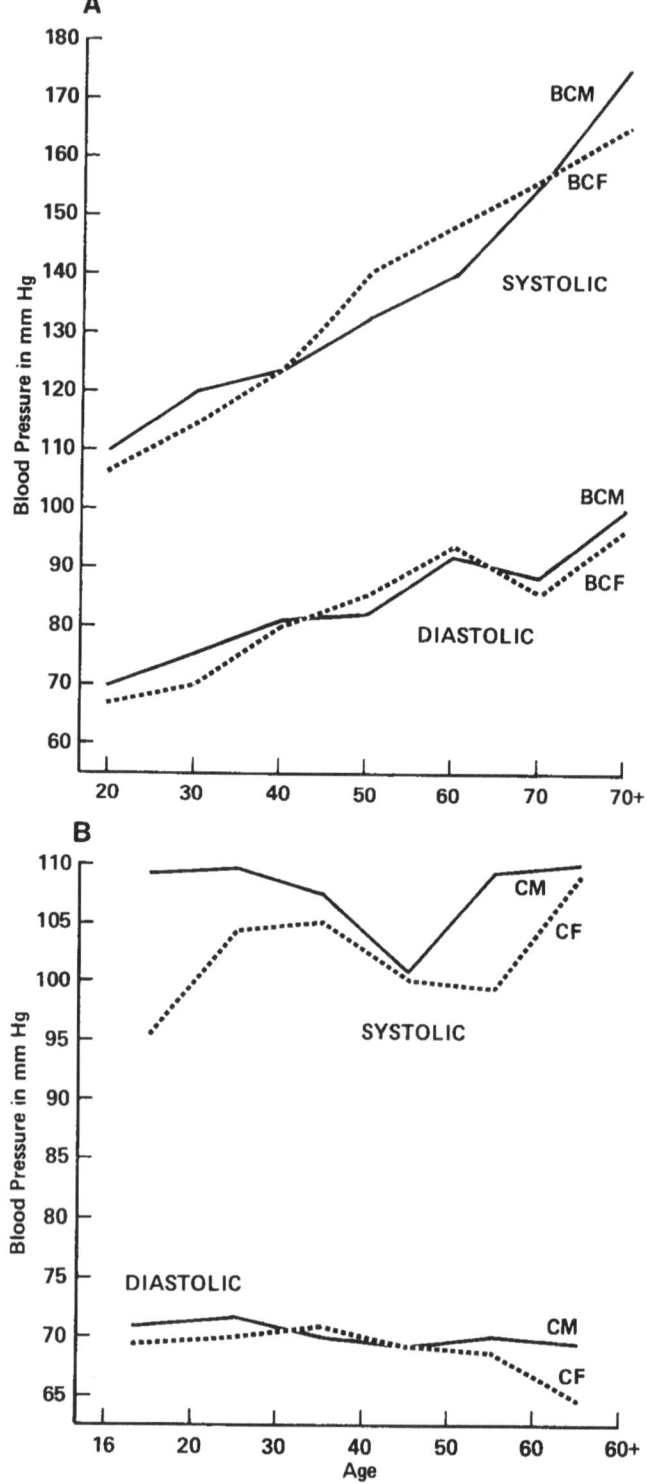

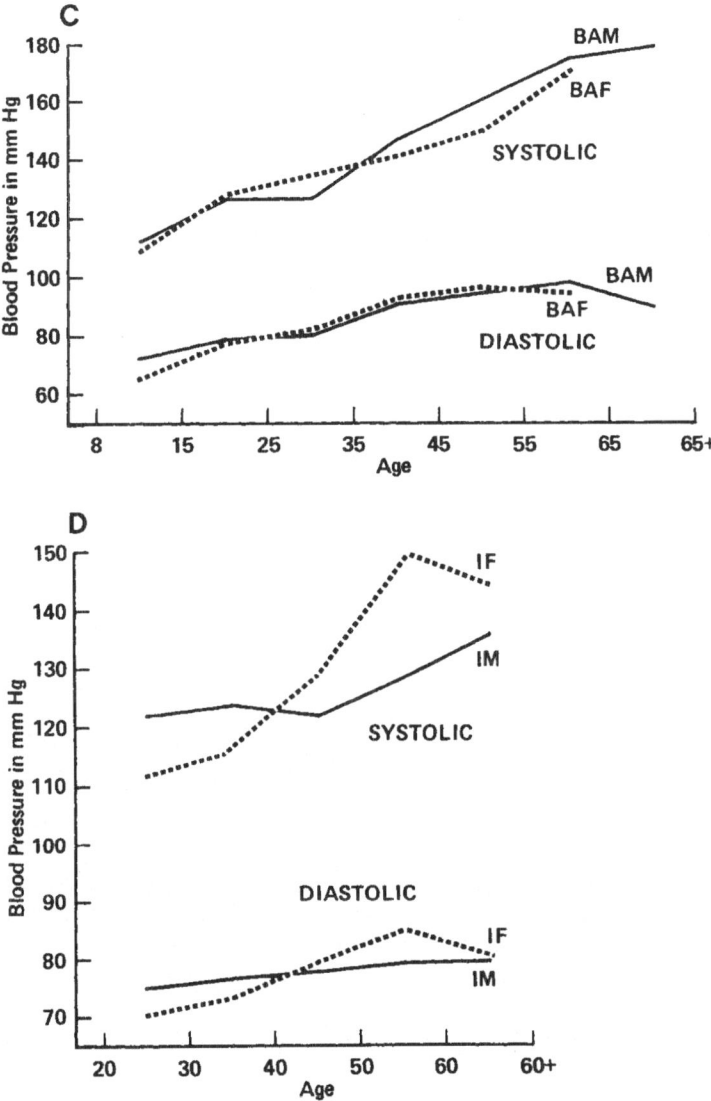

FIGURE 2. Blood pressure distribution by age and sex for (A) the Black Caribs (BC) of St. Vincent, (B) the Carajas (C) of Brazil, (C) black Americans (BA) from Muscogee County, Georgia, and (D) the Ilora (I) of Western Nigeria. M, males; F, females.

Africans, diastolic blood pressure increases gradually with age. On the other hand, in black American and in St. Vincent samples, both males and females show an increase in pressure with age, with the latter group exhibiting pronounced increments in arterial pressure. The fact that both hybrid groups

Table 5. The Distribution of African Admixture among Normotensive and Hypertensive Cohorts[a]

Percent African admixture	Normotensive	Hypertensive
0.00–0.24	34	7
0.25–0.49	44	16
0.50–0.74	85	18
0.75–1.00	146	23

[a] $\chi^2 = 5.32$ with three degrees of freedom.

Table 6. Numerical Distribution of Hypertensives by Age Group within African Admixture Cohorts[a]

Age	0.0–0.49	0.50–0.74	0.75–1.0
20–49	5	5	4
50–59	10	5	10
60–69	5	5	4
70–89	3	3	5

[a] $G = 1.189$, $\chi^2 = 5.991$ with two degrees of freedom at the 0.05 level.

demonstrate increases in pressure with age may suggest strong genic influence on arterial pressure. However, sharp increments among the admixed groups may also be explained by a number of corresponding contributory environmental factors.

The relationship between African admixture and blood pressure on St. Vincent was chosen for additional analysis because of similarities in gene frequencies with West African and black American populations. Also, both hybrid populations, which exhibit increments in pressure with age, are the descendants of West African groups. Table 5 provides the numbers of normotensive and hypertensive individuals by quartile degree of African admixture. A slight increase in the number of hypertensives with increments in the percent of African admixture was observed, but this increase is not significant.

Table 6 tests the hypothesis that the slight increase noted among hypertensives is due to an increase in the number of older individuals in the higher ($\geqslant 50\%$) African admixture cohorts. The R x C test of independence reveals that each admixture cohort possesses essentially the same age distribution of hypertensives. Also, a one-way analysis of variance using both hypertensive and normotensive individuals suggests that each admixture group is comparable in age composition.

Table 7. Mean Distribution x̄ of Selected Anthropometric Traits by Age Cohort among Males, N = 99

Age / N	10–20 / 28	21–30 / 18	31–40 / 24	41–50 / 22	51–60 / 27	61–70 / 26	71–90 / 9
Stature, mm	1670.8	1660.9	1678.3	1696.6	1680.9	1674.6	1716.9
Sitting height, mm	838.9	844.4	848.6	847.6	843.9	846.9	853.5
Weight, kg	67.3	67.0	67.8	70.2	66.0	68.5	67.1
Anterior trunk height, cm	1363.3	1356.2	1377.6	1395.5	1381.5	1384.9	1410.6
Biacromial width, cm	383.0	389.8	385.5	394.7	390.0	390.0	386.7
Chest width, cm	274.4	281.0	283.0	287.6	281.6	290.4	275.2
Chest depth, cm	185.0	192.9	184.0	196.8	193.0	204.6	197.1
Abdominal height, cm	771.7	774.0	758.4	767.8	767.9	773.0	781.7
Upper arm circumference, cm	470.3	391.2	528.2	296.5	468.6	313.4	538.9
Chest circumference, cm	3661.9	4456.8	2662.3	5219.4	4318.5	2592.9	3215.1
Abdomen circumference, cm	1793.4	3172.3	2939.7	2773.8	1811.0	2588.7	2085.7
Triceps skinfold, mm	8.0	5.6	6.6	7.1	6.0	7.4	6.5
Subscapular skinfold, mm	53.6	38.2	23.6	41.5	41.2	39.1	18.5
Systolic pressure, mm Hg	115.4	126.3	124.4	128.4	138.7	156.2	168.5
Diastolic pressure, mm Hg	69.1	83.1	84.0	81.0	91.0	89.5	108.2

Table 8. Mean Distribution $\bar{x}$ of Selected Anthropometric Traits by Age Cohort among Females, N = 188

Age N	10–20 46	21–30 57	31–40 43	41–50 33	51–60 50	61–70 24	71–90 15
Stature, mm	1587.2	1572.7	1580.1	1580.2	1580.4	1539.4	1519.5
Sitting height, mm	788.9	786.1	799.8	796.9	797.4	788.6	747.2
Weight, kg	59.2	58.7	66.2	68.7	65.9	59.3	58.5
Anterior trunk height, cm	1296.9	1278.9	1288.3	1294.3	1294.8	1262.4	1235.7
Biacromial width, cm	357.5	353.0	355.0	357.1	355.5	349.8	349.2
Chest width, cm	259.1	258.8	273.2	278.2	275.4	266.9	275.7
Chest depth, cm	174.3	173.7	185.8	194.4	191.5	192.4	212.1
Abdominal height, cm	721.0	702.0	706.2	707.6	708.8	695.6	702.4
Upper arm circumference, cm	356.4	378.7	408.7	418.8	311.4	338.7	294.5
Chest circumference, cm	3461.2	3918.7	4508.9	4378.8	3939.9	3317.4	3281.1
Abdomen circumference, cm	2821.1	3190.5	2729.2	2696.2	2737.1	3623.8	3093.1
Triceps skinfold, mm	15.1	14.4	16.3	20.2	17.3	14.3	14.9
Subscapular skinfold, mm	42.0	34.5	29.7	20.5	21.5	23.1	7.9
Systolic pressure, mm Hg	102.5	108.4	120.9	143.9	152.8	165.2	187.7
Diastolic pressure, mm Hg	66.2	68.6	76.7	87.2	96.5	90.9	107.0

Table 9. Stepwise Regression of Anthropometric Variables on Systolic Pressure

Variable entered	R^2	F-to-enter
Males		
1. Chest depth	9.96	10.5140
2. Minimum frontal width	16.06	6.8216
3. Bizygomatic width	22.44	7.6483
4. Abdomen circumference	25.48	3.7527
5. Chest circumference	31.80	8.4461
6. Biacromial width	35.63	5.3421
7. Calf circumference	39.06	5.0143
8. Bicristal width	41.09	3.0316
9. Subscapular skinfold	44.28	4.9854
10. Upper limb height	45.99	2.7208
Females		
1. Chest depth	9.04	18.3893
2. Calf circumference	18.96	22.5280
3. Head circumference	23.82	11.6782
4. Bitrochanteric width	26.79	7.3854
5. Minimum frontal width	29.14	6.0008
6. Hand width	32.07	7.7564
7. Iliospinale height	33.65	4.2580
8. Morphological facial height	35.34	4.6476
9. Abdomen circumference	36.38	2.9039
10. Chest width	37.20	2.2823

3.3. Anthropometric Relationship to Hypertension

Table 7 provides the mean distribution of anthropometric traits and blood pressure by age group for males. Weight and subscapular skinfold measurements are highest in the 41–50 age cohort, followed by a gradual decrease. Individuals in the 41–90 age groups also exhibit enlarged chest depth. Measures of adipose tissue deposition, such as subscapular skinfold and triceps skinfold, reveal a gradual increase with age, and this process is most notable in the 41–50 age cohort, when males are at increased risk of high blood pressure. Also, as expected, both systolic and diastolic pressures increase with age.

Table 8 summarizes the mean distribution of anthropometric traits for females by age group. Subscapular skinfold decreases with age among females. However, the 41–50 age cohort shows an acceleration of blood pressure level along with increments in the means for weight, triceps skinfold, upper arm circumference, chest width, and chest depth. Again, as expected, females exhibit an elevation in blood pressure level with age.

The total sample of anthropometric variables is included in a multiple regression analysis (Tables 9 and 10). The R^2 analysis indicates that the

Table 10. Stepwise Regression of Anthropometrics on
Diastolic Pressure

Variable entered	R^2	F-to-enter
Males		
1. Biacromial width	9.83	10.3524
2. Calf circumference	14.71	5.3871
3. Abdomen circumference	20.28	6.4937
4. Head height	25.05	5.8552
5. Thigh length	31.10	7.9836
6. Foot length	33.34	3.0358
7. Forearm length	36.15	3.9156
8. Chest circumference	37.81	2.3504
9. Upper limb length	39.38	2.2434
10. Head length	40.88	2.1925
Females		
1. Chest depth	11.17	23.2565
2. Calf circumference	16.70	12.2267
3. Bitrochanteric width	22.44	13.5345
4. Head circumference	26.35	9.6740
5. Minimum frontal width	28.64	5.8012
6. Hand width	30.43	4.6320
7. Upper arm length	32.24	4.7747
8. Morphological facial height	33.28	2.7689
9. Forearm length	34.09	2.1723

anthropometric variables included in this study account for 45.99% and 37.20% of the variation in systolic pressure for males and females, respectively. The F-to-enters reveal that the chest region is an important contributor to variation in male systolic pressure. For females, the pattern is more variable, with calf circumference, head circumference, bitrochanteric width, chest depth, and hand width contributing to systolic pressure variability.

Analysis of diastolic pressure based upon the total sample of traits (Table 10) indicates that 34.09% of female diastolic pressure and 40.88% of male diastolic pressure are related to these body dimensions. Similarly, for males, chest measurements, such as biacromial width, and abdomen circumference are important contributors to diastolic pressure variability. For females, chest depth, calf circumference, and bitrochanteric width are significant in determining diastolic pressure. Therefore, upper torso laterality and lower limb linearity appear to be important variables for determining male diastolic pressure, while the body dimensions for females are more variable.

A subsample of anthropometric variables is regressed on systolic pressure for males and females separately (Table 11). The F-to-enters show that only triceps skinfold and biacromial width for males and chest depth for females significantly contribute to systolic pressure variability. The R^2 analysis provides

Table 11. Stepwise Regression of Selected Anthropometrics on
Systolic Pressure

Variable entered	R^2	F-to-enter
Males		
1. Triceps skinfold	3.06	3.0666
2. Biacromial width	4.94	1.8961
Females		
1. Chest depth	2.35	4.4799

Table 12. Stepwise Regression of Selected Anthropometrics on
Diastolic Pressure

Variable entered	R^2	F-to-enter
Males		
1. Biacromial width	5.48	5.62338
2. Chest depth	7.43	2.0271
3. Upper arm circumference	9.39	2.0542
Females		
1. Weight	2.61	4.9829
2. Chest circumference	3.53	1.7579
3. Subscapular skinfold	4.33	1.5422
4. Triceps skinfold	4.88	1.0578

the proportion of variation in systolic pressure explained by variation in these body dimensions. The variables presented here contribute 4.94% and 2.35% to variability of systolic pressure for males and females, respectively.

Table 12 gives the results of the selected sample of traits regressed on diastolic pressure for males and females. The F-to-enters show that biacromial width, chest depth, and upper arm circumference contribute significantly to diastolic pressure variability among males, while weight, chest circumference, subscapular skinfold, and triceps skinfold are related to diastolic pressure among females. For males it appears that torso dimensions are important measures of diastolic pressure variability, while among females fat measurements are more important. For males 9.39% and for females 4.88% of diastolic pressure variability are explained by variation in the subsample of these variables.

The next step in the analysis of blood pressure attempts to demonstrate the direction of anthropometric variability between hypertensives and normotensives. Table 13 gives the mean distribution of body dimensions for systolic hypertensives and systolic normotensives by sex. The means for weight, sitting height, stature, anterior trunk height, biacromial width, chest width, chest depth, abdominal height, and triceps skinfold are greater in the male hypertensive

Table 13. Mean Distribution of Selected Anthropometric Variables for Systolic Hypertensives and Systolic Normotensives

	Males		Females	
	Hypertensives	Normotensives	Hypertensives	Normotensives
Weight, kg	70.34	67.28	62.78	63.11
Sitting height, mm	857.40	844.34	783.80	793.50
Stature, mm	1710.13	1676.19	1556.61	1575.06
Anterior trunk height, cm	1412.47	1376.58	1273.25	1286.64
Biacromial width, cm	394.20	388.74	353.06	354.51
Chest width, cm	284.00	283.77	274.53	268.41
Chest depth, cm	203.33[a]	193.47[a]	198.14[a]	184.27[a]
Abdominal height, cm	787.27[a]	766.43[a]	703.47	707.01
Upper arm circumference, cm	400.47	419.25	327.05	370.33
Chest circumference, cm	2558.33	3985.13	3117.75	4088.35
Abdominal circumference, cm	1486.93	2667.74	3339.39	2951.05
Triceps skinfold, mm	7.60	6.50	14.44	16.59
Subscapular skinfold, mm	33.07	37.59	17.67[a]	28.96[a]

[a] Significant at $\alpha = 0.05$.

Table 14. Mean Distribution of Selected Anthropometric Variables for Diastolic Hypertensives and Diastolic Normotensives

	Males		Females	
	Hypertensives	Normotensives	Hypertensives	Normotensives
Weight, kg	69.69	67.08	63.43	62.95
Sitting height, mm	846.28	846.34	789.10	792.29
Stature, mm	1695.69	1676.48	1564.21	1573.39
Anterior trunk height, cm	1395.20	1377.57	1280.03	1285.11
Biacromial width, cm	396.20[a]	387.32[a]	354.42	354.18
Chest width, cm	289.00	282.05	271.66	269.05
Chest depth, cm	200.32	193.16	194.60[a]	184.98[a]
Abdominal height, cm	781.60[a]	765.53[a]	703.10	707.15
Upper arm circumference, cm	456.08	403.00	353.89	364.11
Chest circumference, cm	3693.68	3794.38	3226.68	4048.36
Abdominal circumference, cm	1807.84	2718.89	3061.97	3016.15
Triceps skinfold, mm	6.76	6.63	15.10	16.45
Subscapular skinfold, mm	34.48	37.05	16.71[a]	29.35[a]

[a] Significant at $\alpha = 0.05$.

Table 15. Discriminant Analysis of Systolic Hypertensives versus Systolic Normotensives[a]

	Percent correctly classified	Hypertensives	Normotensives	Total	χ^2
Males					
Hypertensives	47.1	8	9	17	0.058
Normotensives	70.7	24	58	82	14.098
Females					
Hypertensives	38.5	15	24	39	2.076
Normotensives	69.1	46	103	149	21.806

[a] $\chi^2 = 3.841$ with one degree of freedom.

cohort. However, using a t-test to examine significant differences between means, we find that only the means for chest depth and abdominal height are significantly different at the 0.05 level between hypertensive and normotensive males.

When considering systolic pressure among females, only the means for chest width, chest depth, and abdominal circumference are greater in the hypertensive cohort. The means for chest depth and subscapular skinfold are significantly different between hypertensive and normotensive females. Although subscapular skinfold is greater in the female normotensive cohort, one would expect the opposite; this may be related to sample size, since there are only 36 systolic hypertensive females versus 152 systolic normotensive females. Only the means for chest depth are significant for both males and females.

Table 14 gives the mean distribution of anthropometric traits for diastolic hypertensives and normotensives by sex. For males, all anthropometric characters except chest circumference, abdominal circumference, and subscapular skinfold are greater in the hypertensive cohort. However, only the means for biacromial width and abdominal height are significantly different between diastolic hypertensive and normotensive males.

For females only the means for weight, chest width, chest depth, and abdominal height are greater in the female hypertensive cohort. Again, the means for chest depth and subscapular skinfold are significantly different between hypertensive and normotensive females. Although the mean for chest depth is not significantly different for males, it is almost significant, and it appears that, given the measurements and population presented here, this variable is important in influencing blood pressure variability in both sexes.

The last phase of this study uses discriminant analysis to distinguish between systolic hypertensives and systolic normotensives (Table 15). Only systolic normotensives could be classified into the correct group more often than

Table 16. Discriminant Analysis of Diastolic Hypertensives versus Diastolic Normotensives[a]

	Percent correctly classified	Hypertensives	Normotensives	Total	χ^2
Males					
Hypertensives	48.0	12	13	25	0.040
Normotensives	58.1	31	43	74	1.946
Females					
Hypertensives	31.6	12	26	38	5.158
Normotensives	64.7	53	97	150	12.906

[a] $\chi^2 = 3.841$ with one degree of freedom.

expected by chance. The χ^2 values for these cohorts are significant at the 0.05 level. The small sample sizes for the hypertensive groups may be responsible for their insignificant χ^2 values. Categorization of males was based primarily on chest circumference and abdominal circumference, while females were distinguished by weight and chest depth.

When considering diastolic pressure (Table 16), only females are classified with greater accuracy than expected by chance. For females only subscapular skinfold contributes significantly to the discrimination, while biacromial width was the only important variable for males.

4. Discussion

4.1. Familial Correlations

Examination of other types of familial cohorts also demonstrates the important relationship between genes and blood pressure level. For instance, Havlik et al. (1979b) examined blood pressure similarities between father–son/father–daughter pairs and corresponding relationships for mothers. They found that correlations ranged between 0.10 and 0.17 for systolic pressure, while correlations for diastolic pressure ranged between 0.13 and 0.16. (These correlations are lower than the coefficients presented here, probably due to the partitioning of sons' and daughters' pressures.) Overall, it appears that genes may contribute as much as 20% to blood pressure variability.

Miall et al. (1962) in Jamaica and Johnson et al. (1965) in Tecumseh, Michigan, found higher sib–sib correlations than parent–offspring correlations, suggesting the involvement of a strong genetic component for blood pressure. However, studies in Montreal and New Zealand demonstrate the opposite (Tyroler, 1977). When considering mother–offspring diastolic pressure versus sibship diastolic pressure among the Black Caribs, higher correlations are found among the former group. This suggests considerable environmental effect upon blood pressure on this island. Such conflicting results illustrate the difficulty in estimating the genetic contribution involved in blood pressure. The Montreal, New Zealand, and Black Carib studies are also "not consistent with a simplistic hypothesis of commonly shared environments, that is, one which would predict a strong similarity among age contemporaneous sib pairs and lower correlations in parent–offspring pairs" (Tyroler, 1977, p. 617).

Familial similarity has also been examined using adoptive children. Although the environment is the same, Biron *et al.* (1976) found that adopted children show no significant aggregation of blood pressure level with their adoptive parents or adoptive siblings. Comparison of blood pressure correlation coefficients among consanguine families versus families with adopted members support the conclusion that genes contribute significantly to blood pressure level.

The importance of the genic contribution to blood pressure level also appears to differ between diastolic and systolic pressures. Since diastolic pressure is a measure of arterial pressure during relaxation of the ventricles (Anthony and Kolthoff, 1975), internal environmental factors are of lesser importance. Consequently, factors such as cardiac minute output and peripheral resistance do not play a major role in influencing diastole. On the other hand, systole is a measure of arterial pressure during contraction of the ventricles, when many physiological elements are at work (Anthony and Kolthoff, 1975). The lower heritability estimates for systolic pressure may be an indication of the predominant role of these internal environmental factors in influencing systole. On the other hand, since the environment is constant, diastolic pressure is primarily a measure of the genetic influence on arterial pressure.

4.2. Hybridization and Blood Pressure

A significant relationship between African admixture and blood pressure has been demonstrated by other researchers (Boyle, 1970; MacLean *et al.*, 1974). MacLean *et al.* (1974) found that arterial pressure increased with increments in percent of African admixture, but noted that the results may be confounded by environmental factors. Since neither unacculturated West Africans nor Amerindians show increases in blood pressure with age (although hypertension does exist among these groups) and since Black Caribs are more similar to black Americans in blood pressure level, such increases in blood pressure may be indicative of a strong environmental component. For instance, in both cultures, black American and Black Carib, skin color plays an important role in creating stress. In the U. S., occupation, housing, and living conditions contribute to stress among black Americans. This is also true of Black Caribs, who are low on the social and economic ladder on St. Vincent, since very dark individuals (considered Negroes, although many also have Carib ancestors) are put on a lower social level than "Black Caribs." Stress produced by this type of categorization may contribute to increased blood pressure level among dark-skinned individuals. Therefore, dark skin may be an easily quantified characteristic that can be associated with blood pressure level; however, this association may mask the true relationship between high stress (exemplified by dark skin) and increased arterial pressure.

4.3. Body Build and Blood Pressure

The overall contribution of anthropometrics to blood pressure variability is low. Barnicot et al. (1972) attributed 13.8% of the variation in systolic pressure and 11.8% of the variation in diastolic pressure to variability in anthropometric characters. The present study attributes between 2% and 45% of the variation in blood pressure to body measurements. It should be noted that the proportion of variation in blood pressure explained by anthropometrics will vary depending upon the traits utilized in the analysis.

Variability in blood pressure level appears to be related to different anthropometric traits for males versus females. For females, overall fatness, as measured by skinfold, and chest depth appear to be related to blood pressure variability, while for males, torso dimensions such as biacromial width and chest depth influence blood pressure. Biacromial width and chest depth are related to overall torso size, and since other concomitant torso dimensions are also important among males, this area of the body appears to be more important than overall fatness, as among females. Following this line of reasoning, two components appear to influence blood pressure variability: overall weight and torso dimensions for females and torso size for males. Large torso size may be important because it is indicative of a large heart, which would increase the flow of blood through the arteries. Such increments coupled with a viscous blood flow would increase blood pressure. Therefore torso size is linked indirectly to the physiology of blood pressure in that a large torso will increase the flow of blood through the arteries and thereby increase blood pressure.

The importance of torso size and weight to blood pressure variability has been reported in other studies. Hanna and Baker (1979) discriminated between hypertensives and normotensives on the basis of anthropometrics. They found that hypertensives exhibited increased overall fatness and enlarged torso size. Goldring et al. (1977) found that both weight and height were significantly correlated with systolic and diastolic pressures. However, when the effect of weight was removed, height became unimportant. The association between obesity and hypertension has long been noted; however, the addition of torso dimensions introduces a complicating variable to the relationship between obesity and blood pressure. Although the degree of obesity, as measured by skinfold measurements, may be small, if such individuals have a large torso, their risk of becoming hypertensive is elevated. In conclusion, a closer examination of anthropometrics is needed to determine the genetic versus environmental factors influencing these traits, since the relationship between blood pressure and anthropometrics is more complex than previously believed.

5. Conclusion

This chapter has examined the genetic component of blood pressure by investigating familial inheritance of arterial pressure and by identifying the relationship between African admixture and blood pressure level. When considering familial inheritance of blood pressure, heritability estimates are the primary means of revealing the importance of genes in determining blood pressure level. The heritability estimates computed in the preceding analysis revealed that between 13% and 30% of the variation in blood pressure level is due to the action of genes. These estimates are always higher for diastolic than systolic pressure, indicating that the former is under greater genetic control. This is not to say that more or different genes control diastolic versus systolic pressure, but, more likely, that systolic pressure is influenced by more internal environmental mechanisms. Therefore, although heritability estimates are usually higher for diastolic pressure, we should not assume that a different number of genes or different genes are acting on systolic pressure. Instead, we should examine systolic pressure in order to identify environmental factors that may modify systole.

Unlike the family method, hybrid analysis attempts to reveal variation in blood pressure level due to the inheritance of genes from African ancestors. This model hypothesized that increments in African admixture are associated with increases in blood pressure level. Although there was a slight increase in blood pressure level as African admixture increased, this hypothesis was not borne out.

A number of studies on skin color and African admixture stimulated interest in this analysis, although these studies were clouded by confounding environmental factors. This appears to be true in the case of the preceding analysis as well. It seems likely that other factors, such as stress, are more strongly related to African admixture level than previously considered. It is these factors, and not African admixture, that are the true modifiers of blood pressure.

Variation in blood pressure level based on the anthropometric analysis reflects variation in both genes and environmental factors controlling body dimensions. Although the proportion of variation in blood pressure level associated with anthropometrics is high, 45%, this is probably an overestimate. The large number of variables included in the analysis may have produced spurious associations, since F values are forced into the regression equation. However, even though a large number of measurements were included, the analysis revealed that variables related to the physiology of blood pressure are the best predictors of arterial pressure level. While determination of the proportion of variation in blood pressure level controlled by anthropometrics is important, of comparable import are specific body dimensions associated with blood pressure variation. This chapter has identified dimensions of the torso as the most important region of the body influencing blood pressure level. While overall fatness is still an influential component, torso dimensions appear to be of comparable importance.

These analyses have demonstrated the importance of various factors related to blood pressure variation. The next step in the study of blood pressure among the Black Caribs of St. Vincent is to determine the interactive effect of genes, culture, and other external environmental factors on arterial pressure. Path analysis will be used to carry out this endeavor. The goal of such an analysis is to eliminate the overlap among the various factors related to blood pressure variation and to determine the true relationship among these factors. The use of this method can demonstrate which factors can easily alter blood pressure level.

References

Abrahams, D. G., Alele, C. A., and Barnard, B. G., 1960, The systemic blood pressure in a rural West African community, *West Afr. Med. J.* 9:45–58.

Anthony, C. P., and Kolthoff, N. J., 1975, *Textbook of Anatomy and Physiology*, C. V. Mosby, St. Louis.

Barnicot, N., Bennett, F., Woodburn, J., Pilkington, T., and Antonis, A., 1972, Blood pressure and serum cholesterol in the Hadza of Tanzania, *Hum. Biol.* 44:87–116.

Biron, P., Mongeau, J., and Bertrand, D., 1976, Familial aggregation of blood pressure in 558 adopted children, *Can. Med. Assoc. J.* 115:773–774.

Boyle, E., 1970, Biological patterns in hypertension by race, sex, body weight and skin color, *J. Am. Med. Assoc.* 213:1637–1643.

Canessa, M., Adragna, N., Solomon, H., Connolly, T., and Tosteson, D., 1980, Increased sodium–lithium countertransport in red cells of patients with essential hypertension, *N. Engl. J. Med.* 302:772–805.

Comstock, G. W., 1957, An epidemiological study of blood pressure levels in a biracial community in the southern United States, *Am. J. Hyg.* 65:271–315.

Crawford, M. H., 1976, *The Tlaxcaltecans: Prehistory, Demography, Morphology and Genetics*, University of Kansas Publications in Anthropology, no. 7, Lawrence, Kansas.

Dahl, L. K., 1963, Metabolic aspects of hypertension, *Annu. Rev. Med.* 14:69–98.

Elston, R. C., and Stewart, J., 1971, A general model for the genetic analysis of pedigree data, *Hum. Hered.* 21:523–543.

Feinleib, M., Garrison, R. J., Stallones, L., Kannel, W. B., Castelli, W. P., and McNamara, P. M., 1979, A comparison of blood pressure, total cholesterol and cigarette smoking in parents in 1950 and their children in 1970, *Am. J. Epidemiol.* 110:291–303.

Geerdink, R. A., Nijenhuis, L. E., van Loghem, E., and Sjoe, E. L. F., 1974, Blood groups and immunoglobulin groups in Trio and Wajana Indians from Surinam, *Am. J. Hum. Genet.* 26:45–53.

Goldring, D., Londe, S., Sivakoff, M., Hernandez, A., Britton, C., and Choi, S., 1977, Blood pressure in a high school population, *J. Pediatr.* 9:884–889.

Guyton, A. C., Coleman, T. G., Cauley, A. W., Manning, R. D., Norman, R. A., and Fenigson, J. D., 1974, A systems analysis approach to understanding long-range arterial blood pressure control and hypertension, *Clin. Res.* 35:150–174.

Hamilton, M., Pickering, G. W., Fraser-Roberts, J. A., and Sowry, G. S. C., 1954, The etiology of essential hypertension. 4. The role of inheritance, *Clin. Sci.* **13**:273–304.

Hanna, J. M., and Baker, P. T., 1979, Biocultural correlates to the blood pressure of Samoan migrants in Hawaii, *Hum. Biol.* **51**:481–497.

Harburg, E., Erfurt, J. C., Chape, C., Hauenstein, L. S., Schull, W. J., and Schork, M. A., 1973, Socioecological stressor areas and black–white blood pressure: Detroit, *J. Chronic Dis.* **26**:595–611.

Harburg, E., Schork, M. A., Erfutt, J. C., Schull, W. J., and Chape, C., 1977, Heredity, stress and blood pressure, a family set method – II, *J. Chronic Dis.* **30**:649–658.

Havlik, R. J., Garrison, R. J., Katz, S., Ellsion, R. C., Feibleib, M., and Myrianthopoulos, N. C., 1979a, Detection of genetic variance in blood pressure of 7 year old twins, *Am. J. Epidemiol.* **109**(5):512–516.

Havlik, R. F., Garrison, R. J., Feibleib, M., Kannel, W. B., Castelli, W. P., and McNamara, P. M., 1979b, Blood pressure aggregation in families, *Am. J. Epidemiol.* **10**:304–312.

Hsu, P., Mathewson, F., and Rabkin, S., 1977, Blood pressure and body mass index patterns – A longitudinal study, *J. Chronic Dis.* **30**:93–113.

Johnson, D., Epstein, F. H., and Kjelsberg, M. O., 1965, Distribution and familial studies of blood pressure and serum cholesterol levels in a total community – Tecumseh, Michigan, *J. Chronic Dis.* **18**:147–160.

Joossens, J. V., 1973, Salt and hypertension, water hardness and cardiovascular death rate, *Triangle* **12**:9–16.

Khosla, T., and Lowe, C. R., 1965, Arterial pressure and arm circumference, *Br. J. Prev. Soc. Med.* **19**:159–163.

Krieger, H., Morton, N. E., Rao, D. C., and Azevedo, E., 1980, Familial determinants of blood pressure in northeastern Brazil, *Hum. Genet.* **53**:415–418.

Langford, H. G., Watson, R. L., and Douglas, B. H., 1968, Factors affecting blood pressure in population groups, *Trans. Assoc. Am. Phys.* **81**:135–146.

Lee, K., 1978, A genetic analysis of serum cholesterol and blood pressure levels in a large pedigree, Institute of Statistics Mimeo Series, no. 1174, University of North Carolina at Chapel Hill.

Lowe, C. R., 1964, Arterial pressure, physique, and occupation, *Br. J. Prev. Soc. Med.* **18**:115–124.

Lowenstein, F. W., 1961, Blood pressure in relation to age and sex in the tropics and sub-tropics, *Lancet* **1**:389–392.

MacLean, C. J., Adams, M. S., Leyshon, W. C., Workman, P. L., Reed, T. E., Gershowitz, H., and Weitkamp, L. R., 1974, Genetic studies on hybrid populations. III. Blood pressure in an American Black community, *Am. J. Hum. Genet.* **26**:614–626.

McGarvey, S. T., and Baker, P. T., 1979, The effects of modernization and migration on Samoan blood pressures, *Hum. Biol.* **51**:461–479.

McIlhany, M. L., Shaffer, J. W., Hines, E. A., and Zlotowitz, H. I., 1975, The heritability of blood pressure: An investigation of 200 pairs of twins using the cold pressor test, *Johns Hopkins Med. J.* **136**:57–64.

Miall, W. E., 1967, Age, sex, body habitus, family, in *Epidemiology of Hypertension* (J. Stamler, R. Stamler, and T. N. Pullman, eds.), pp. 60–69, Grune and Stratton, New York.

Miall, W. E., Kass, E. H., Ling, J., and Stuart, K. L., 1962, Factors influencing arterial pressure in the general population in Jamaica, *Br. Med. J.* **2**:497–506.

Morton, N. E., Gulbrandsen, C. I., Rao, D. C., Rhoads, G. G., and Kagan, A., 1980, Determinants of blood pressure in Japanese–American families, *Hum. Genet.* **53**:261–506.

Mourant, A. E., Kopeć, A. C., and Domaniewska-Sobczak, K., 1976, *The ABO Blood Groups,* Oxford University Press, London.

Pickering, G., 1968, *High Blood Pressure,* Grune and Stratton, New York.

Roberts, D. F., and Hiorns, R. W., 1962, The dynamics of racial intermixture, *Am. J. Hum. Genet.* **14**:261–277.

Roberts, D. F., and Hiorns, R. W., 1965, Methods of analysis of genetic composition of a hybrid population, *Hum. Biol.* **37**:38–43.

Rose, R. J., Miller, J. Z., Grim, C. E., and Christian, J. C., 1979, Aggregation of blood pressure in the families of identical twins, *Am. J. Epidemiol.* **109**(5):503–511.

Schull, W. J., Harburg, E., Schork, M. A., Weener, J., and Chape, C., 1977, Heredity, stress and blood pressure, a family set method – III, *J. Chronic Dis.* **30**:659–669.

Scotch, N. A., 1963, Sociocultural factors in the epidemiology of Zulu hypertension, *Am. J. Public Health* **53**:1205–1213.

Siervogel, R. M., Roche, A. F., Chumlea, W. C., Morris, J. G., Webb, P., and Knittle, J. L., 1982, Blood pressure, body composition, and fat tissue cellularity in adults, *Hypertension* **4**(3):382–385.

Sokal, R. R., and Rohlf, F. J., 1969, *Biometry: The Principles and Practice of Statistics in Biological Research,* Freeman, San Francisco.

Taylor, H. L., 1967, Body composition and elevated blood pressure: A comment, in *Epidemiology of Hypertension* (J. Stamler, R. Stamler, and T. N. Pullman, eds.), pp. 101–109, Grune and Stratton, New York.

Tibblin, G., Hjortzbert-Norlund, H., and Aurell, E., 1967, Body build, blood pressure and hypertensive eye-ground changes, in *Epidemiology of Hypertension* (J. Stamler, R. Stamler, and T. N. Pullman, eds.), pp. 110–121, Grune and Stratton, New York.

Tyroler, H. A., 1977, The Detroit project studies of blood pressure, *J. Chronic Dis.* **30**:613–624.

Voors, A. W., Berenson, G. S., Dalferes, E. R., Webber, L. S., and Shuler, S. E., 1979, Racial differences in blood pressure control, *Science* **204**:1091–1094.

Weinberg, R., Shear, C. L., Avet, L. M., Frerichs, R. R., and Fox, M., 1979, Path analysis of environmental and genetic influences on blood pressure, *Am. J. Epidemiol.* **109**(5):588–596.

13

Quantitative Analyses of the Dermatoglyphic Patterns of the Black Carib Populations of Central America

PAUL M. LIN, V. BACH-ENCISO, MICHAEL H. CRAWFORD, JANIS HUTCHINSON, DIANE SANK, and BRIAN SANK FIRSCHEIN

1. Introduction

While blood group and protein systems have been widely utilized for the study of hybridization and population structure, there is a paucity of such estimates based upon quantitative traits. In part, this apparent neglect is due to the environmental sensitivity of quantitative traits such as anthropometrics, skin color, odontology, and dermatoglyphics. However, Friedlaender (1975), Sokal and Friedlaender (1982), and Froehlich and Giles (1981) have examined an assortment of ethnohistorical and evolutionary problems on the basis of dermatoglyphics.

PAUL M. LIN • Institute of Social and Behavioral Pathology, and Psychiatric Research Unit, Department of Psychiatry, Pritzker School of Medicine, The University of Chicago, Chicago, Illinois 60637. V. BACH-ENCISO, MICHAEL H. CRAWFORD, and JANIS HUTCHINSON • Laboratory of Biological Anthropology, University of Kansas, Lawrence, Kansas 66045. DIANE SANK • Department of Anthropology, The City College, City University of New York, New York, New York 10031, and Human Genetics and Biological Variations Laboratory, N. S. Kline Psychiatric Research Institute, Orangeburg, New York 10962. BRIAN SANK FIRSCHEIN • Human Genetics and Biological Variations Laboratory, N. S. Kline Psychiatric Research Institute, Orangeburg, New York 10962.

In this volume, several chapters examine the relationship between quantitative trains and population genetic structure. For example, Byard *et al.* (Chapter 9) focus upon skin color and admixture. Similarly, O'Rourke *et al.* (Chapter 10) employ odontological characteristics to measure the genetic structure of Black Carib groups.

On the basis of dermatoglyphics, this chapter focuses upon three related problems: (1) Does an underlying universal factor structure, as observed in other human groupings, exist among the Black Caribs and Creoles? (2) Is the R-matrix method of Harpending and Jenkins (1973) applicable to dermatoglyphic data? (3) What is the relationship between genetics, as defined by dermatoglyphics, and geography among the Black Carib and Creole populations?

2. Populations Sampled

Black Carib populations are a mixture of West Africans and Amerindians who were transplanted to the coastal areas of the Gulf of Honduras from St. Vincent Island in the Lesser Antilles. In 1797, the British deported the majority of these Black Caribs from St. Vincent to the island of Roatan in the Gulf of Honduras. However, the people did not remain there long and emigrated to the coast of Honduras. The population expanded rapidly and subsequently spread east and west along coastal Honduras and into Guatemala, Belize, and Nicaragua.

Dermal prints of Black Carib and Creole populations are represented by five samples: Livingston from the coast of Guatemala, Belize City in Belize,

Table 1. Population Sample Sizes Used in Analyses of Dermatoglyphics

Location number	Males	Females	Total	Reference
Black Caribs				
1 Livingston, Guatemala	70	146	216	This analysis
2 Belize City, Belize	25	44	69	This analysis
3 Corozal, Honduras	55	65	120	This analysis
5 Sambo Creek, Honduras	55	61	116	This analysis
4 Punta Gorda (Roatan), Honduras	24	52	76	This analysis
Others				
7 Tlaxcala, Tlaxcala, Mexico	55	70	125	Crawford *et al.* (1976a), Lin *et al.* (1979), and this analysis
8 San Pablo, Tlaxcala, Mexico	85	131	216	Crawford *et al.* (1976a), Lin *et al.* (1979), and this analysis
6 Barcelona, Spain	169	186	355	Lin *et al.* (1979) and this analysis

Corozal and Sambo Creek from Honduras, and Punta Gorda from the island of Roatan, located proximal to the coast of Honduras (Table 1).

The Livingston data were collected by Paul M. Lin and Michael H. Crawford during a field study in Guatemala in 1975. Analyses of the genetic data from this group indicate that the Black Carib gene pool consists of approximately 70% African, 29% Indian, and about 1% European admixture (Crawford et al., 1981).

The Belize City dermatoglyphic sample was obtained in 1976 by Paul M. Lin from students at a local school. The majority of the people of Belize City view themselves ethnically as Creoles, which is interpreted here to consist primarily of African and European ancestry (British or Spanish) with some Amerindian gene flow coming either from the Central American Maya or from the Black Caribs (Crawford et al., Chapter 16 in this volume).

The three Black Carib samples from Honduras — Corozal, Sambo Creek, and Punta Gorda — were collected in 1970 by Diane Sank, and the dermatoglyphic patterns and ridge counts were scored by Diane Sank and Brian Sank Firschein. These prints were obtained from school children between the ages of 7 and 16 years. Additional demographic and genetic data are not available for these towns, but they are identified ethnically as Black Carib.

Due to the complexity of triracial admixture among Black Carib and Creole peoples, several other populations are used for comparison of dermatoglyphic data in various aspects of the analysis. (See Table 1 for sample sizes.) The two Mexican populations, San Pablo and Tlaxcala, were collected by the University of Pittsburgh research team in 1969 from the state of Tlaxcala in central Mexico. These two populations have been treated extensively elsewhere regarding demography, genetics, and dermatoglyphics (Crawford, 1976). Demographic history and genetic analyses confirm that San Pablo is a Tlaxcaltecan Indian community with minimal, if any, European admixture. The city of Tlaxcala is representative of the highly admixed Mestizo population and is a trihybrid amalgam of about 24% European, 67% Indian, and some African, about 9% (Crawford et al., 1976b).

The Spanish dermatoglyphics were collected in 1974 by Dr. Jose Egozcue and his colleagues at an elementary and secondary school in Barcelona, Spain. These finger and palm prints were analyzed in the Laboratory of Biological Anthropology at the University of Kansas. The individuals in this sample are taken as representative of the population of Spain since they are from families who came from all parts of the nation. This sample represents a cross section of Barcelona's economic hierarchy, with the working class as well as the middle and upper middle classes being represented.

3. Methods of Dermatoglyphic Analysis

Dermatoglyphic techniques follow the methods established by Cummins and Midlo (1943) and Holt (1968) for pattern identification and ridge counting.

Table 2. Frequencies of Pattern Types (in Percent)

	Whorls		Ulnar loops		Radial loops		Arches	
	Right	Left	Right	Left	Right	Left	Right	Left
Livingston males ($N = 70$)								
1	54.3	36.2	38.6	53.6	0.0	0.0	7.1	10.1
2	41.4	37.7	41.4	43.5	4.3	2.9	12.9	15.9
3	27.5	36.2	65.2	56.5	1.4	1.4	5.8	5.8
4	69.6	53.6	30.4	43.5	0.0	0.0	0.0	2.9
5	20.0	15.9	78.6	82.6	0.0	0.0	1.4	1.4
Total	39.2		53.5		1.0		6.3	
Livingston females ($N = 146$)								
1	46.6	39.7	40.4	40.4	1.4	2.7	11.6	17.2
2	30.3	29.5	53.1	53.4	6.9	6.2	9.7	11.0
3	22.1	26.7	71.7	66.4	0.0	0.0	6.2	6.8
4	46.6	42.5	50.7	54.1	0.7	0.7	2.0	2.7
5	9.6	9.0	87.0	86.9	0.0	0.0	3.4	4.1
Total	30.2		60.4		1.9		7.5	
Belize City males ($N = 25$)								
1	48.0	28.0	36.0	52.0	0.0	0.0	16.0	20.0
2	32.0	32.0	52.0	56.0	8.0	4.0	8.0	8.0
3	12.0	12.0	80.0	76.0	0.0	0.0	8.0	12.0
4	36.0	28.0	60.0	68.0	0.0	0.0	4.0	4.0
5	24.0	8.0	72.0	88.0	0.0	0.0	4.0	4.0
Total	26.0		64.0		1.2		8.8	
Belize City females ($N = 44$)								
1	43.2	40.9	47.7	47.7	0.0	4.6	9.1	6.8
2	34.1	45.5	50.0	38.6	9.1	6.8	6.8	9.1
3	18.6	11.4	76.7	79.5	0.0	0.0	4.7	9.1
4	43.2	36.4	56.8	63.6	0.0	0.0	0.0	0.0
5	4.5	6.8	95.5	93.2	0.0	0.0	0.0	0.0
Total	28.5		64.9		2.0		4.6	
Corozal males ($N = 55$)								
1	41.8	38.2	45.5	50.9	0.0	0.0	12.7	10.9
2	34.5	25.5	47.3	50.9	5.5	9.1	12.7	14.5
3	25.5	21.8	65.5	70.9	0.0	0.0	9.1	7.3
4	40.0	40.0	54.5	52.7	1.8	1.8	3.6	5.5
5	5.5	5.5	92.7	90.9	0.0	0.0	1.8	3.6
Total	27.7		62.3		1.8		8.2	
Corozal females ($N = 65$)								
1	44.6	26.2	38.5	58.5	1.5	3.1	15.4	12.3
2	32.3	30.8	47.7	35.4	6.2	13.8	13.8	20.0

Table 2. (Continued)

	Whorls		Ulnar loops		Radial loops		Arches	
	Right	Left	Right	Left	Right	Left	Right	Left
3	20.0	20.0	73.8	69.2	1.5	3.1	4.6	7.7
4	43.1	41.5	47.7	55.4	3.1	0.0	6.2	3.1
5	6.2	12.3	92.3	86.2	0.0	0.0	1.5	1.5
Total	27.7		60.5		3.2		8.6	
Sambo Creek males ($N = 55$)								
1	52.7	49.1	43.6	45.5	0.0	0.0	3.6	5.5
2	40.0	36.4	40.0	47.3	14.5	10.9	5.5	5.5
3	27.3	20.0	70.9	76.4	1.8	1.8	0.0	1.8
4	47.3	38.2	50.9	60.0	0.0	0.0	1.8	1.8
5	14.5	9.1	85.4	90.9	0.0	0.0	0.0	0.0
Total	33.5		61.1		2.9		2.5	
Sambo Creek females ($N = 61$)								
1	49.2	37.7	37.7	44.3	0.0	3.3	13.1	14.8
2	26.2	24.6	54.1	44.3	3.3	14.8	16.4	16.4
3	9.8	18.0	83.6	62.3	0.0	1.6	6.6	18.0
4	36.1	36.1	62.3	60.7	0.0	1.6	1.6	1.6
5	13.1	10.0	85.2	88.3	0.0	0.0	1.6	1.7
Total	26.1		62.2		2.4		9.2	
Punta Gorda males ($N = 24$)								
1	66.7	45.8	33.3	54.2	0.0	0.0	0.0	0.0
2	50.0	37.5	33.3	45.8	16.7	16.7	0.0	0.0
3	33.3	47.8	62.5	47.8	4.2	0.0	0.0	4.3
4	54.2	45.8	45.8	50.0	0.0	4.2	0.0	0.0
5	4.2	4.2	95.8	91.7	0.0	4.2	0.0	0.0
Total	39.0		56.0		4.6		0.4	
Punta Gorda females ($N = 52$)								
1	51.9	42.3	34.6	44.2	0.0	0.0	13.5	13.5
2	28.8	28.8	53.8	48.1	3.8	11.5	13.5	11.5
3	25.0	28.8	69.2	61.5	1.9	1.9	3.8	7.7
4	44.2	44.2	53.8	51.9	0.0	1.9	1.9	1.9
5	11.5	7.7	86.5	88.5	0.0	1.9	1.3	1.9
Total	31.3		59.2		2.3		7.2	

The methods of scoring were carefully standardized among the various researchers.

Table 2 lists the percentage frequencies for pattern types in the five Black Carib populations subdivided by individual digit and hand as well as a total frequency of pattern type. It should be noted that there is considerable digital variability in all of these populations and that a simple pattern frequency total masks this variation and results in further information loss. We suggest that

Table 3. Ridge Counts

| | Right hand | | | | | | Left hand | | | | | |
| | Ulnar loop | | Radial loop | | Whorl | | Ulnar loop | | Radial loop | | Whorl | |
Digit	Mean	S.D.	Mean	S.D.	Mean	S.D.	Mean	S.D.	Mean	S.D.	Mean	S.D.
Livingston males												
I	14.28	4.92	0	0	18.26	4.38	12.13	4.61	0	0	17.64	3.92
II	10.30	3.80	12.40	2.97	15.50	3.04	10.52	3.60	5.50	2.12	15.23	3.99
III	10.89	4.03	12.50	2.12	18.00	3.29	12.54	3.29	0	0	17.38	3.65
IV	12.59	4.52	0	0	17.21	3.64	13.57	4.51	0	0	18.78	3.31
V	12.66	3.48	0	0	16.42	3.18	12.60	3.55	0	0	18.09	2.26
Livingston females												
I	12.10	5.09	17.00	7.07	17.44	4.01	11.40	4.02	12.00	5.39	16.40	3.63
II	9.95	4.14	12.36	4.84	14.36	4.69	9.09	3.72	8.17	6.46	15.37	4.20
III	11.63	4.10	20.00	0	16.84	4.71	12.19	4.31	8.00	0	17.79	4.04
IV	13.82	5.83	10.00	0	18.91	4.32	14.32	5.13	15.00	0	18.86	4.04
V	12.82	4.13	0	0	15.77	3.79	12.38	4.06	0	0	15.67	2.74
Belize City males												
I	16.67	5.12	0	0	19.42	4.60	14.77	5.57	0	0	18.14	4.95
II	9.85	4.14	12.00	0	16.63	4.90	10.54	3.46	3.00	0	14.25	3.58
III	11.10	4.13	0	0	17.67	4.04	11.90	3.99	0	0	16.00	7.81
IV	14.56	4.80	0	0	15.67	6.02	13.71	4.44	0	0	17.43	5.00
V	12.00	3.87	0	0	15.00	6.39	12.36	4.10	0	0	17.50	3.54
Belize City Females												
I	13.71	5.47	0	0	16.95	3.76	12.19	3.98	18.50	4.95	17.61	3.50
II	9.50	4.06	13.50	8.35	14.87	4.22	10.80	2.27	13.25	9.29	13.84	4.59
III	10.61	3.38	0	0	14.50	2.56	12.10	3.57	0	0	23.00	18.14
IV	14.04	4.93	0	0	17.32	4.08	12.93	5.41	0	0	18.25	4.93
V	11.71	3.95	0	0	12.00	1.41	11.88	4.62	0	0	12.67	2.52

Corozal males												
I	13.35	4.91	0	0	20.70	5.00	12.76	4.79	0	0	18.76	4.81
II	9.46	3.99	15.33	2.08	17.26	4.98	9.70	4.07	11.67	4.50	16.07	3.27
III	11.92	4.23	10.00	0	17.57	3.80	12.51	4.11	0	0	18.92	2.43
IV	13.64	5.49	14.00	0	20.05	5.00	13.28	4.59	6.00	0	20.78	4.17
V	13.02	5.44	0	0	16.67	3.51	13.29	5.49	0	0	17.00	2.65
Corozal females												
I	12.56	5.97	18.00	0	18.35	3.91	11.16	4.50	11.50	6.36	16.56	3.72
II	9.90	4.21	7.25	5.18	15.76	4.27	10.24	4.42	10.00	5.57	15.60	2.66
III	11.25	5.01	8.00	0	15.75	5.14	11.11	4.69	16.00	6.08	16.23	4.49
IV	13.85	5.52	11.00	5.66	19.32	3.78	15.03	5.12	0	0	19.00	9.44
V	12.15	4.41	0	0	16.75	2.75	12.67	4.27	0	0	16.00	6.73
Punta Gorda males												
I	16.33	4.21	0	0	19.00	5.15	14.62	3.04	0	0	18.36	3.01
II	8.38	4.21	14.00	6.96	15.92	3.48	11.64	3.50	12.75	10.21	17.44	2.35
III	13.07	4.46	7.00	0	15.88	3.40	13.09	3.33	0	0	17.91	4.59
IV	16.77	3.70	0	0	20.23	3.35	16.43	3.20	0	0	20.09	2.43
V	15.13	3.95	0	0	20.00	0	14.44	2.87	0	0	16.00	5.00
Punta Gorda females												
I	13.06	4.44	9.00	0	18.56	4.61	11.57	3.69	14.00	0	19.77	3.96
II	11.29	4.07	8.00	5.66	16.33	3.87	12.59	3.88	10.00	4.82	16.67	3.16
III	12.06	3.73	0	0	17.62	2.84	12.71	4.56	0	0	17.53	3.60
IV	14.32	5.19	0	0	19.30	3.82	15.70	5.66	0	0	19.14	4.03
V	14.11	4.47	0	0	17.83	2.14	14.02	4.48	17.00	0	18.00	5.10

(continued)

Table 3 (Continued)

	Right hand						Left hand					
	Ulnar loop		Radial loop		Whorl		Ulnar loop		Radial loop		Whorl	
Digit	Mean	S.D.	Mean	S.D.	Mean	S.D.	Mean	S.D.	Mean	S.D.	Mean	S.D.
Sambo Creek males												
I	15.46	8.26	0	0	20.69	5.03	14.54	6.32	0	0	19.41	3.97
II	10.14	5.27	11.75	4.13	15.87	3.84	11.26	3.90	8.83	5.47	15.45	4.90
III	11.55	4.32	5.00	0	16.87	3.85	13.95	4.38	10.00	0	19.82	4.29
IV	15.10	4.98	0	0	20.12	4.13	15.13	4.46	0	0	19.91	5.12
V	14.00	5.02	0	0	17.38	5.37	13.96	4.37	0	0	17.80	5.50
Sambo Creek females												
I	13.52	6.27	0	0	18.47	4.11	13.32	4.90	8.00	0	18.13	4.65
II	9.86	4.58	13.00	2.83	14.94	4.48	9.89	3.87	6.14	2.34	17.60	4.85
III	11.75	4.02	0	0	18.33	5.35	11.58	4.86	0	0	17.46	5.07
IV	13.32	5.04	0	0	18.91	4.72	13.97	4.88	10.00	0	18.64	5.55
V	12.16	4.87	0	0	18.25	2.92	11.69	5.10	0	0	16.33	3.72

Table 4. Pattern Intensity Index (PII) and Total Ridge Count (TRC)

	Males				Females			
	PII		TRC		PII		TRC	
	Mean	S.D.	Mean	S.D.	Mean	S.D.	Mean	S.D.
Livingston	13.19	4.2	130.3	42.6	12.29	3.8	124.8	46.6
Belize City	11.72	4.2	123.0	54.6	12.42	3.2	124.4	42.5
Corozal	11.96	4.0	131.1	53.7	11.91	3.6	121.2	47.7
Sambo Creek	13.09	3.2	146.1	45.9	11.67	3.9	120.1	54.7
Punta Gorda	13.96	2.8	156.0	30.0	12.42	3.6	134.2	49.7
Tlaxcala, Mexico	12.93	3.3	141.3	52.5	13.14	3.6	137.9	51.0
San Pablo, Mexico	14.45	3.5	152.2	54.4	13.64	3.3	140.1	48.4
Spanish	12.52	3.7	139.5	55.4	12.19	3.5	116.6	50.3

dermatoglyphic analyses by finger should be published as part of the descriptive statistics of future publications.

Table 3 presents a summary of mean digital ridge counts by pattern type. The mean ridge count for whorls is computed by the conventional practice of taking the larger of the two ridge counts.

Total ridge count (TRC) is the sum of the ridge counts of each digit using the larger count from whorl patterns. Pattern intensity index (PII) represents the sum of the triradii: two for whorls, one for loops, and zero for arches (Table 4).

3.1. Analytic Methods

The R-matrix technique for analysis has the advantage of utilizing all traits simultaneously for obtaining a composite picture of relationships among the populations. It has been demonstrated in the analysis of pattern type frequencies that interdigital variability is important for understanding the dermatoglyphic character of a population. Pattern type identification has several advantages in speed and consistency of identification when compared with ridge counting in data analysis. In addition, pattern frequencies per digit and hand are frequently found in the published literature for comparative purposes, whereas ridge counts per digit are infrequently published.

The R-matrix analysis of Harpending and Jenkins (1973, 1974) was adapted for use with frequencies of pattern types per digit and hand in a manner similar to allelic frequencies. This method permits the calculation of a variance—covariance matrix that utilizes all available traits simultaneously so that

$$r_{ii} = \sum_{i=1}^{k} \frac{(p_{ik} - \bar{p}_k)(p_{jk} - \bar{p}_k)}{\bar{p}_k(1 - \bar{p}_k)}$$

where $\bar{p}$ is the mean frequency per k traits. Principal coordinates analysis presents the relationship among populations as revealed by digital pattern types. Eigenvectors, scaled by the square root of their eigenvalues, are computed from this in order to represent the relationships among samples on a multidimensional scale. Another matrix is constructed to represent the variation and covariation of K trait frequencies over all L populations, providing a plot of dermatoglyphic traits along axes corresponding to the population axes.

A matrix of Euclidean distances between pairs of populations can also be calculated from the R-matrix so that

$$d^2 \; = \; r_{ii} + r_{jj} - 2r_{ij}$$

Paired distances between samples can be compared by a matrix fitting method developed by Lalouel (1973), which permits rotation of matrices to maximum congruence from which a correlation is estimated. This MATFIT method estimates the degree to which dermatoglyphic data resemble geographical distance, or distance based on any other measure, such as blood genetics or migration. Since genetic and migration matrices are unavailable for all the Black Carib populations, dermatoglyphic traits are compared only to a matrix of geographical distances measured in kilometers using great circle routes.

4. Results

4.1. Descriptive Statistics

This section describes the observed dermatoglyphic variations of five Black Carib populations: Livingston, Belize City, Corozal, Punta Gorda, and Sambo Creek. Forty variables pertaining to pattern types and ridge counts on both radial and ulnar sides of fingertips of both hands are analyzed.

The salient features of pattern types of the combined Black Caribs are summarized as follows (Fig. 1):

1. A generally W-shaped plot characterizes the distribution of ulnar loops over the five digits.
2. Its reverse counterpart is observed in the frequency distribution of whorls.
3. Low frequencies of arches taper downward from the thumb to the little finger.
4. Even lower incidences characterize radial loops; their curve roughly parallels that of arches.
5. Of all pattern types, ulnar loops have the highest frequency on the little finger, followed by the middle and the ring finger.
6. Correspondingly, the frequency of arches is lowest on the little finger and slightly higher on the middle finger.

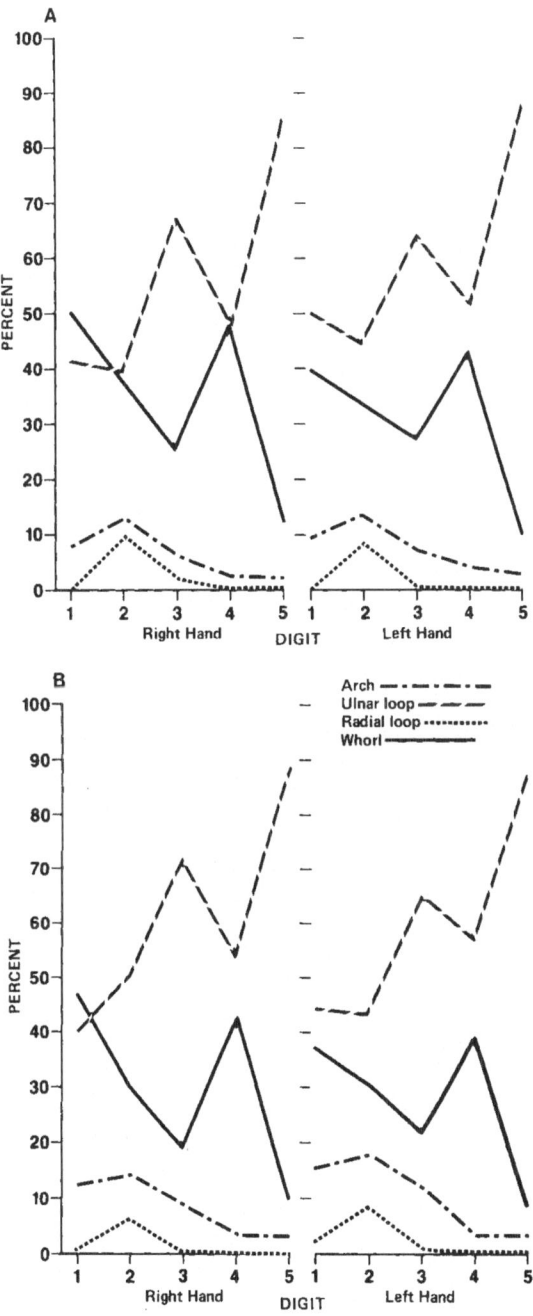

FIGURE 1. Frequency distribution of pattern types for combined Black Carib groups. (A) Males, (B) females.

7. As found for most populations, the index finger has a higher frequency of radial loops than any other finger.

8. Both sexes show some bilateral asymmetry in the thumb, which has a higher incidence of ulnar loops on the right hand than on the left. This asymmetry is not observed in Livingston females, Corozal males, and Sambo Creek males. Whether or not bilateral asymmetry of this sort is a universal phenomenon can be determined only from additional data.

A bivariate plot of PII and TRC for the five Black Carib groups, the two Mexican groups, and the Spanish samples indicates a positive correlation between these two variables (Fig. 2). However, the regression line is calculated utilizing only eight of these groups. Since both variables are not always reported, only three populations are added for comparison: U.S. whites from Boston (Plato *et al.*, 1975) and two U.S. black samples from Boston (Steinberg *et al.*, 1975) and New York City (Quazi *et al.*, 1977). For females, San Pablo and Tlaxcala are at one extreme, and Punta Gorda is distinct from the other Black Carib groups. This agrees with the ridge count analysis and MATFIT results. In the female samples there is a very close relationship between the PII–TRC correlation and the geographical proximities between Livingston and Belize City and between Corozal and Sambo Creek. However, in the male samples these relationships are less obvious. This sex-specific phenomenon may be explained by the vastly different migration patterns of the males when compared to the females.

The ridge counts, excepting those on the ulnar side of the radial loop, are plotted in Fig. 3. The following phenomena should be noted:

1. With the exception of the ridge counts of whorls on the ulnar sides of the ring and little fingers, the ridge counts of whorls are greater than that of ulnar loops.

2. The distributions of ulnar loops and the radial sides of whorls are parallel.

3. The ulnar side of whorls is not in an overall parallel relationship with that of the others.

The data thus suggest one of the defects inherent in the conventional methods of ridge counts. By only considering the larger of ridge counts of whorls on either radial or ulnar side, important information is missed. Our data, which indicate that the ridge counts on the ulnar side of whorls behave differently from that of the radial side of both whorls and ulnar loops, suggest that effectively differentiated, if not separate, sets of genes operate to bring about the observed phenomena. The rare occurrence of radial loops hinders exploration of the possibility that the ridge counts on the ulnar side are controlled by similar, if not the same, sets of genes for both whorls and radial loops. The differences in the levels and shapes of paired frequency distributions in Fig. 3 will be discussed using Hotelling's T^2 and profile analysis to test parallelism, levels, and flatness hypotheses in a forthcoming paper by Lin and Crawford.

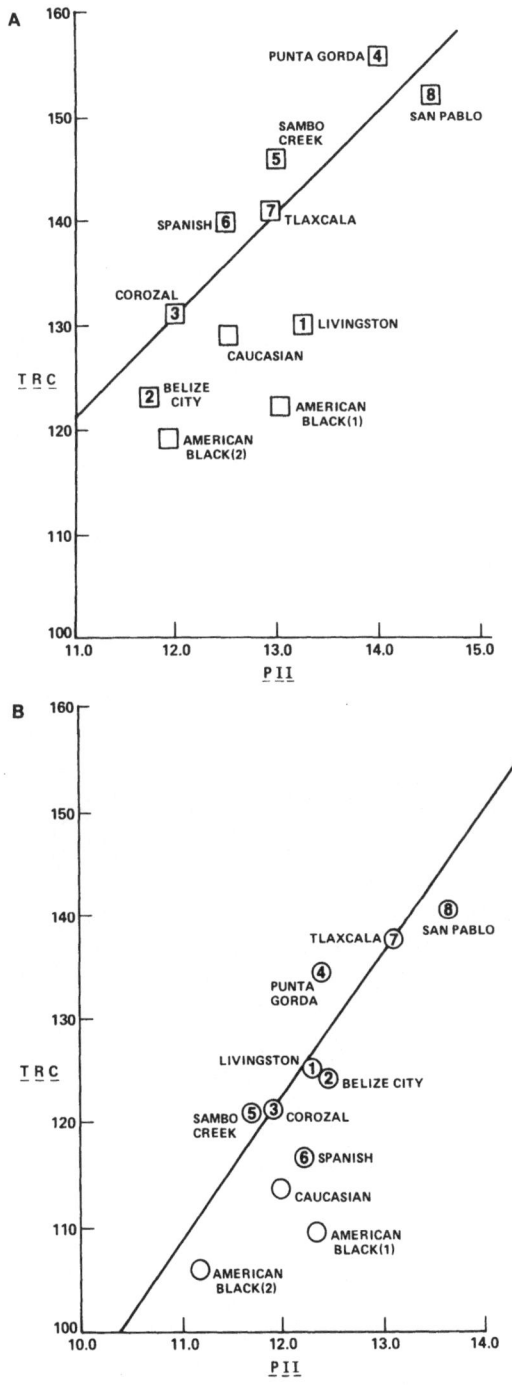

FIGURE 2. A bivariate plot and correlation of (A) pattern intensity index (PII) and (B) total ridge count (TRC) of various human populations.

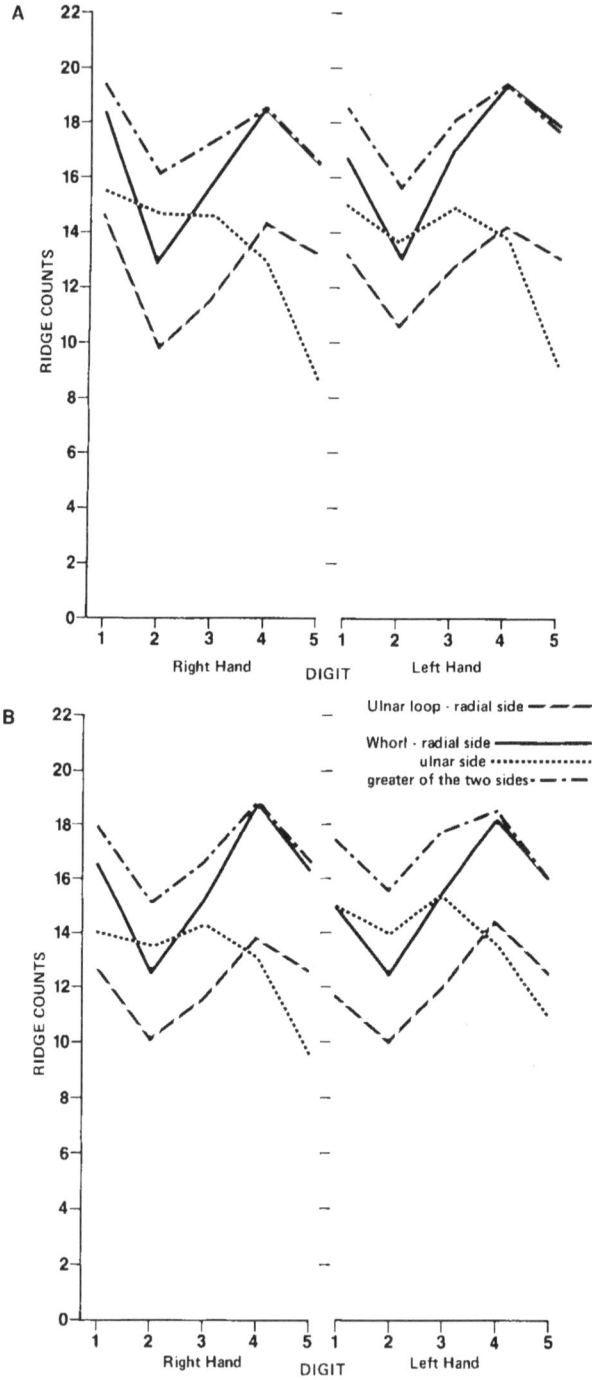

FIGURE 3. A comparison of (A) male and (B) female Black Carib ridge count frequencies per pattern and side of hand.

4.2. Intrapopulation Analysis

At any rate, our observations lead to a question of the genetic architecture of components that underlie the phenotypic expressions of pattern types and fingertip ridges. In order to deal with this question, factor analysis with Kaiser's varimax rotation (Lin, n.d.) was performed on combined groups of males and females separately. The eigenvalue $\geqslant 1$ criterion was applied to determine the number of factors to be extracted after principal components analysis, yielding nine factors for both male and female groups. The varimax solution is summarized in Table 5. For simplicity the decimal point is omitted. The large communalities, h^2, and small coefficients in the residual correlation matrices (not presented) indicate that factor analysis is appropriate for the data. The nine factors account for 76.27% and 74.0% of the total variance for the male and female groups, respectively. In Table 5 only those loadings greater than the arbitrary cutoff value of 0.500 are presented.

The outstanding features of factor structure are as follows:

1. In both sexes, factor 1 defines both pattern types and ridge counts on the ulna side of the index and middle fingers of both hands. More specifically, factor 1 relates primarily to the index finger, as this finger consistently and distinctly yields higher loadings than the middle finger.
2. The ring and little fingers together constitute one factor of ridge counts on the radia side (males: factor 3, females: factor 2). This factor has no counterpart in the index and middle fingers.
3. The remaining factors relate to single fingers.
4. The separate factors of pattern types and ridge counts on the ulnar side of the ring and little fingers (males: factors 3 and 4; females: factors 4 and 6), together are complementary to factor 1.
5. With the exception of factor 3 of the males and factor 2 of the females, the pattern types and ridge counts on the radial side form the lowest ranking factors (factors 7, 8, and 9 of both sexes) on the index, middle, ring, and little fingers.
6. The thumb is an exception to point 5 in that the pattern types and ridge counts on the radial side form a factor that ranks third in the female group. The thumb always represents unique factors, thus indicating the independence of the thumb from all other fingers (males: factors 5 and 6; females: factors 3 and 5). The factors relating to the thumb are in the middle range of factor ranking.

In the semigraphical representation given below, the factors of the male group are left in their "natural"ranking order, and the factors of the female group are rearranged so as to be paired with the male counterparts. Factor 8 has no counterparts between the sexes and is therefore omitted.

Table 5A. Varimax Solution, Females[a]

Variable	Factor									h^2
	1	2	3	4	5	6	7	8	9	
Radial side										
Right hand										
1			690							6777
2							650			6080
3										4307
4									779	6923
5								837		8674
I			747							7589
II							648			7569
III		(450)								7081
IV		649								7275
V		650								6822
Left hand										
1			827							7237
2							798			7417
3		545								5303
4									676	6203
5								870		8852
I			792							7940
II							700			7991
III		656								7697
IV		692								7514
V		684								7343
Ulnar side										
Right hand										
1				770						7701
2	687									6595
3	796									7454
4						768				7583
5					841					7877
I						798				8389
II	733									7704
III	788									7481
IV						699				7950
V					886					8492
Left hand										
1					839					8244
2	604									6853
3	742									6967
4						788				7492
5					827					7579
I					862					8698
II	704									7445
III	752									6842
IV						765				8140
V					877					8335
V_p	5.083	4.183	3.650	3.385	3.301	3.242	2.949	2.041	1.807	

[a] The Arabic numerals identify the digits for triradial counts (0 or 1), and the Roman numerals for ridge counts. V_p is the variance explained by each of the factors.

Table 5B. Varimax Solution, Males[a]

Variable	Factor									10^3h^2
	1	2	3	4	5	6	7	8	9	
Radial side										
Right hand										
1						799				7743
2							685			6486
3								777		7563
4									600	6226
5									877	8691
I						743				7523
II							738			7289
III								(496)		6858
IV			703							8095
V			767							8370
Left hand										
1						781				7476
2							686			6050
3								694		6681
4								708		6879
5									867	8321
I						695				7724
II							665			7385
III								(435)		7580
IV			660							8410
V			780							8476
Ulnar side										
Right hand										
1					663					7794
2	775									7212
3	590									7248
4		765								6876
5				826						7876
I					751					8165
II	803									7973
III	598									7519
IV		796								8258
V				877						8538
Left hand										
1					859					8390
2	780									7605
3	566									7135
4		689								6870
5				778						7672
I					887					8870
II	814									7902
III	601									7758
IV		710								7590
V				831						7986
V_p	4.830	4.164	3.443	3.241	3.216	3.189	3.080	2.991	2.351	

[a] See footnote to Table 5A.

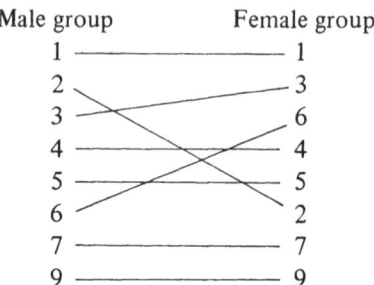

Six of the eight lines are in level parallels or near parallels, suggesting some relationship between the two series of factors in rank order. We approach the problem of measuring the degree of correspondence between these two rankings by computing a rank correlation coefficient τ obtained from Kendall's S statistic (Kendall, 1970). The τ coefficient is defined by

$$\tau = \frac{S}{\frac{1}{2}n(n-1)}, \qquad S = P - Q$$

where P is the number of pairs that are ranked in the *same* order by the male and female groups, Q is the number of pairs in which the rankings are in opposite order, and $\frac{1}{2}n(n-1)$ is the total number of pairs of factors.

A significance test of the null hypothesis that the male ranking is independent of the female ranking can be conveniently done on S. The null expectation of S (as of τ) is zero.

By the formula cited above, the rank correlation coeficient τ of the present data is 0.57. The correlation is positive and substantial, though far from perfect. The sum of the scores from factors 1–9 is $S = 16$. To determine whether or not a relationship exists, the table of probability that S (for τ) attains or exceeds a specified value (Kendall, 1970, p. 173). (Appendix Table 1) is entered for $n = 8$. The probability value for $S = 16$ is 0.031 (one tail) or 0.062 (two tail). Therefore, a significant direct relationship exists between the sexes in factor ranking.

In summary, the data from factor analysis strongly support the "universals" hypothesis proposed by the authors (Crawford *et al.*, 1976a; Lin *et al.*, 1979). The hypothesis holds that (1) the observable and observed qualitative and quantitative features of dermatoglyphics are underlaid by highly structured genetic components, and (2) the underlying structure is such that it phenotypically expresses itself specifically or differentially in a I–III-II–IV-V tripartite configuration. It should be added that the universals hypothesis has been foreshadowed by a number of earlier workers (e.g., Roberts and Coope, 1975).

In factor structure the thumb is independent of all other fingers. The index and middle fingers form one unit, and the ring and little fingers form the third unit. Thus, a cleavage exists between the thumb and the index—middle fingers and between the index–middle fingers and the ring–little fingers. We propose to call these invariant factor units "eigen–structures." The reasons for the tripartite structure are unclear, but explanations may be sought in the anatomy of innervation, functional requisites for tactility and mechanical contact (gripping), or embryological development, or, most likely, their various combinations.

A corollary of the universals hypothesis is that in the absence of fundamental differences in the configurations of dermatoglyphic features, statistical discriminations among populations and between sexes would yield ambiguous results. As a matter of fact, computer analyses based upon the BMD7M programs (Dixon and Brown, 1979) provide indeterminate classifications. With stringent jackknifing, only 31.4% of the males (14 variables) and 30.4% of the females (24 variables) are classified correctly. These poor classifications provide a dramatic contrast with a 95.8% correct classification among the same five populations and between sexes yielded by 22 of the 38 anthropometric variables. Clearly, few generalizations can be made from discriminant analysis.

1. In both sexes the five populations are most different in the ridge counts on the radial side of the left index finger.
2. With the exceptions of the radial-side ridge counts of the left index finger, the radial-side pattern types of the right middle finger, and the ulnar-side pattern types of the left ring fingers, different sets of variables emerge as the 10 most discriminating variables between the sexes, indicating a lack of concordance of effectively discriminating variables between the sexes (Table 6).
3. There is no significant agreement between the sexes in the rankings of Mahalanobis D^2 distances ($\tau = 0.33$, $P > 0.11$) or in the rankings of F values ($\tau = 0.38$, $P > 0.11$) (Table 7).

Table 6. Ten Most Discriminating Variables among the Five Populations in Discriminant Analysis

| | Male groups | | | Female groups | | |
Step	Digit	Hand	Side	Digit	Hand	Side
1	II	Left	Radial	II	Left	Radial
2	5	Right	Ulnar	IV	Left	Radial
3	I	Right	Ulnar	5	Right	Radial
4	4	Left	Ulnar	3	Left	Ulnar
5	I	Right	Radial	II	Right	Ulnar
6	V	Left	Ulnar	2	Right	Ulnar
7	V	Right	Radial	4	Left	Ulnar
8	5	Right	Radial	II	Left	Ulnar
9	2	Left	Radial	I	Left	Radial
10	3	Left	Radial	III	Right	Ulnar

Table 7. A Comparison of Mahalanobis D^2 Distances and F Statistics between Paired Groups of Males and Females[a]

	Livingston	Belize City	Corozal	Punta Gorda	Sambo Creek
Males					
Livingston	–	2.051	1.080	1.506	1.448
Belize City	2.52**	–	1.472	3.613	1.341
Corozal	2.23**	1.71*	–	1.524	0.898
Punta Gorda	1.74*	2.91**	1.67*	–	1.217
Sambo Creek	2.93**	1.54	1.66	1.32	–
Females					
Livingston	–	1.443	1.514	1.015	1.008
Belize City	1.85**	–	2.445	2.377	1.711
Corozal	2.59**	2.45**	–	1.593	1.160
Punta Gorda	1.50	2.18**	1.78*	–	1.023
Sambo Creek	1.65*	1.67*	1.40	1.11	–

[a] The F matrix is in the lower triangle, the D^2 matrix in the upper triangle. *: Significance at the 5% level. **: Significance at the 1% level. Males, d.f. = 14, 208. Females, d.f. = 24, 331.

4. The biological distances, summarized in Table 6, suggest that the Belize City and Punta Gorda male populations are the furthest apart and the females are nearly as far apart. This finding may be a correlate of geographical distance.

5. In both sexes, overall, partings with the Sambo Creek population yield small D^2 distances and correspondingly small F values.

6. No population is consistently far apart in biological distance from other populations. Nevertheless, point 5 suggests that the Sambo Creek population appears to have been a centroid, as it were, of migratory networks of the Black Caribs in the region.

4.3. Interpopulation Comparison

4.3.1. R-Matrix Analysis

Traditionally males and females have been treated separately in dermatoglyphic analyses. Demographic data on the Black Caribs also suggest that there may be differences in migration patterns for males and females. The R-matrix analyses are therefore performed on males and females separately.

Figure 4 provides a two-dimensional plot of the five Black Carib samples of males, in which the first scaled eigenvector explains 57% of the variation and the second explains 22%. As has been observed in most other principal component treatments of dermatoglyphic pattern frequencies, the first axis usually reflects the triradius number, which can be expressed by the PII. In this case, Belize City has the lowest PII, 11.72, while the other populations increase in

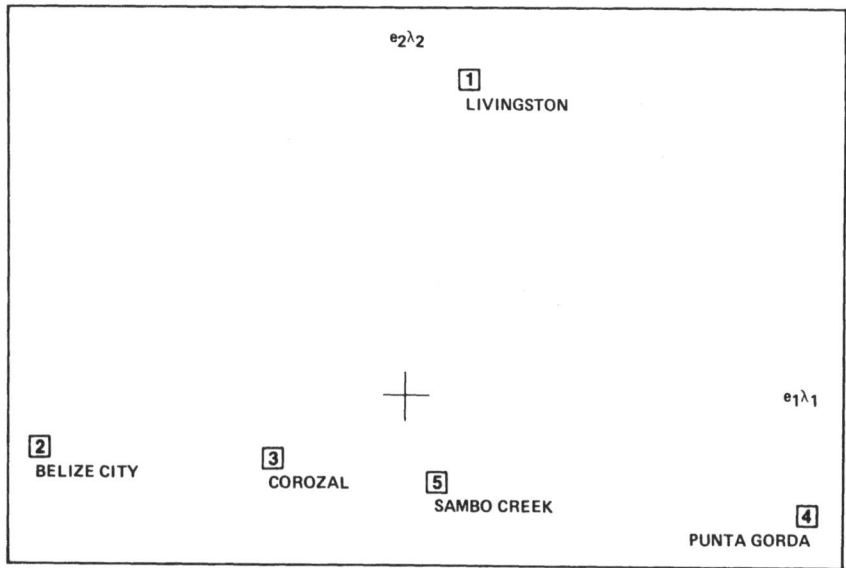

FIGURE 4. Two-dimensional least-squares "genetic map" of five male Black Carib populations.

value along the first axis, with Punta Gorda exhibiting the highest value, 13.96 (see Table 4). On the second axis, Livingston is separated from the other four Carib populations partly as a result of the high frequency of whorls, especially on digits IV and V.

The two-dimensional eigenvectorial plot of female dermatoglyphics differs considerably from the male sample (Fig. 5). Here Punta Gorda, Sambo Creek, Livingston, and Corozal are clustered along the first axis, which contributes only 39% of the variation, while Belize City is separated from the cluster. Corozal is separated from the other four populations along the second axis, which accounts for 28% of variation. Neither axis conforms to a gradient based upon PII. A mean of the r_{ii} values from the R-matrix, which expresses the average variance within the data matrix, is lower for the female matrix (0.011) than for the male (0.028). Thus, these populations exhibit less variability among the female elements than among the males and probably reflect random differences.

The matrix of Euclidean distances based on digital pattern frequencies (Table 8) provides a composite measure between pairs of populations in which the total variability can be compared to other matrices of paired distances using the MATFIT method of Lalouel (1973). Figure 6 compares the interpopulational distances from dermatoglyphics to geographical distances (in kilometers) for both males and females. Punta Gorda appears to be divergent dermatoglyphically from the other four populations. Correlations between dermatoglyphics and geography are higher (0.638) for females than for males (0.352). Since distance

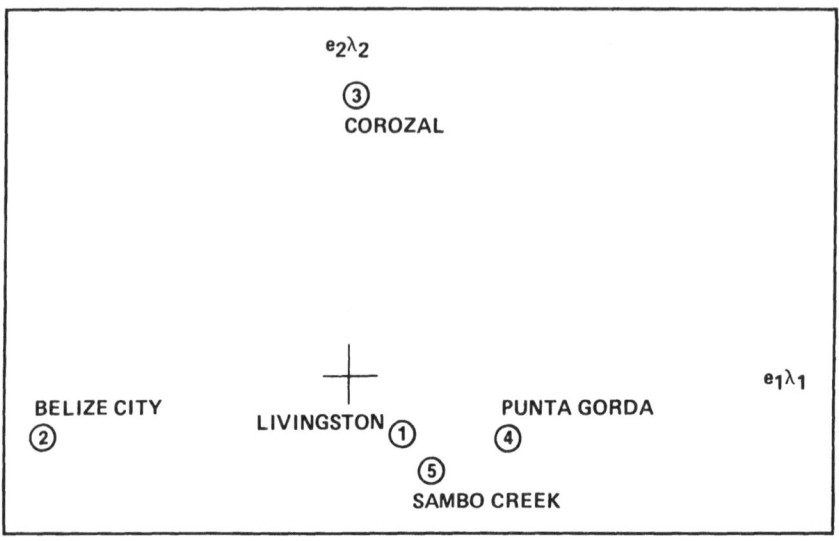

FIGURE 5. Two-dimensional least-squares representation of five female Black Carib populations.

measures were also computed by the Mahalanobis D^2 method (Table 7), these distances were also compared to geographical distance, with similar results (Fig. 7). Again Punta Gorda is divergent from the other four populations in dermatoglyphic traits, and the correlation between males and geography is almost the same (0.363), while the female correlation is even higher (0.714).

Similar eigenvectorial reduction plots (Figs. 8 and 9) were constructed including other potential representatives of the parental gene pools that con-

Table 8. *Distance Measures Calculated from Frequencies of Pattern Types per Digit*[a]

	Livingston	Belize City	Corozal	Punta Gorda	Sambo Creek
Livingston	–	0.082	0.055	0.079	0.049
Belize City	0.029	–	0.044	0.152	0.059
Corozal	0.025	0.035	–	0.091	0.038
Punta Gorda	0.012	0.038	0.027	–	0.054
Sambo Creek	0.023	0.035	0.029	0.022	–

[a] Males, upper triangle; females, lower triangle.

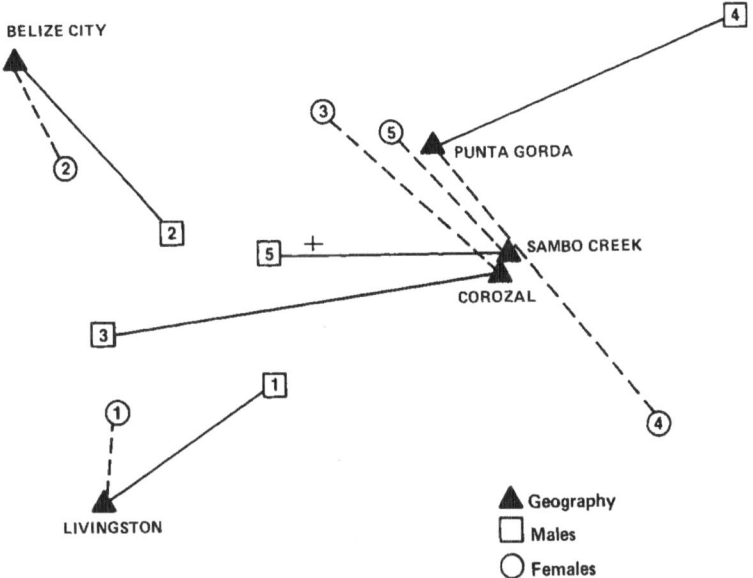

FIGURE 6. Fitting of matrices based upon Euclidean distance from pattern frequencies with geography.

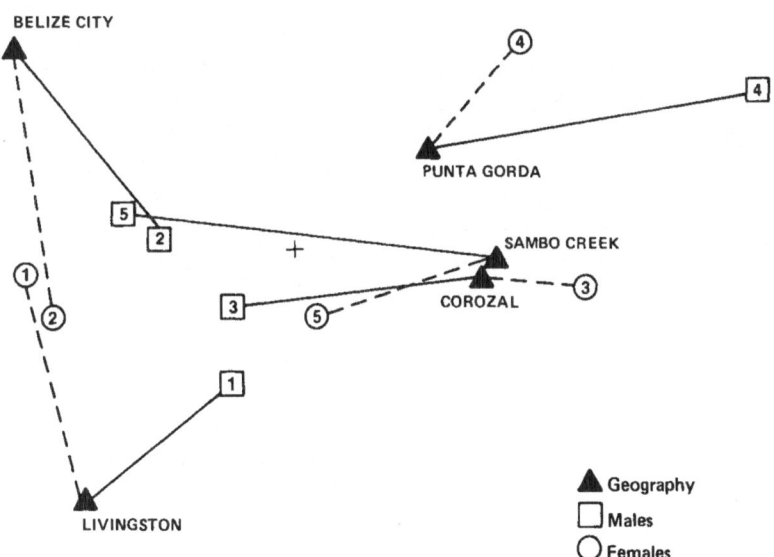

FIGURE 7. Fitting of matrices based upon D^2 from 40 ridge counts with geography.

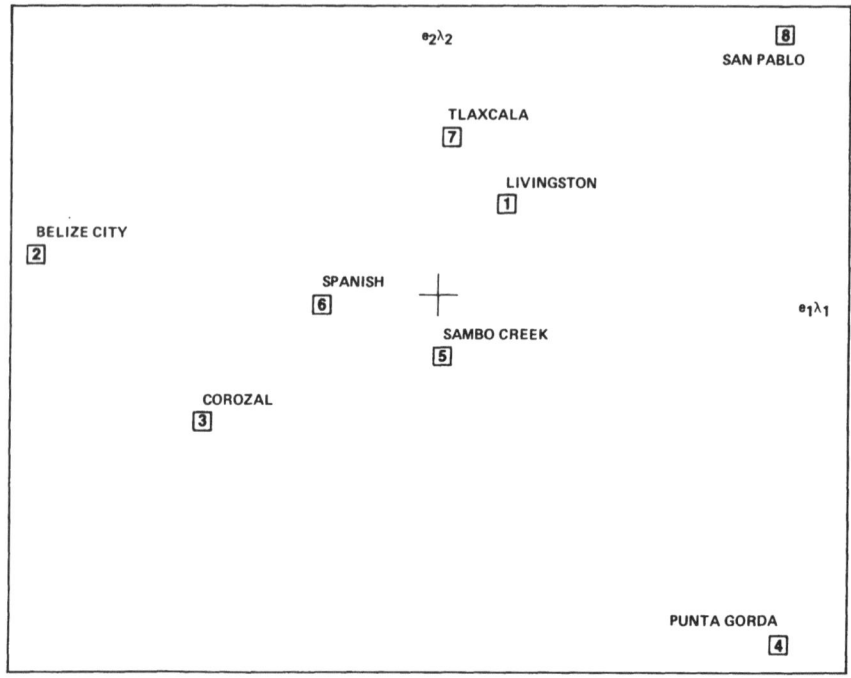

FIGURE 8. "Genetic map" of eight male Black Carib and parental representative groups based upon dermatoglyphic traits.

tributed to the Black Caribs. For lack of more appropriate samples, San Pablo and Tlaxcala from central Mexico are being utilized as representative of pure and admixed Amerindian populations. The Spanish sample is made up of individuals from different parts of Spain and represents the European component. The male Black Carib populations (see Fig. 8) are distributed along the first axis, which accounts for 41% of the variation, with Punta Gorda at one end and a Creole sample (Belize City) at the other end of the axis. The second axis, which accounts for 20% of the variation, apparently reflects a gradient of Amerindian and African admixture. Thus San Pablo, which has been shown to be entirely Indian, forms one extreme, while Punta Gorda's gene pool has a high proportion of African genes. Again this first axis reflects the PII, which is lowest in Belize City (11.9) and highest in San Pablo (14.5), contrasting whorls and arches, especially on digit I. The second axis reflects the divergence of whorls versus ulnar loops in digit V. While the third eigenvector contributes only 12%, it separates the Spanish from the other populations.

The female samples provide a similar picture (Fig. 9), but with San Pablo and Tlaxcala clearly separated from the other populations along the first axis, which accounts for 36% of the observed variation. The second axis subsumes

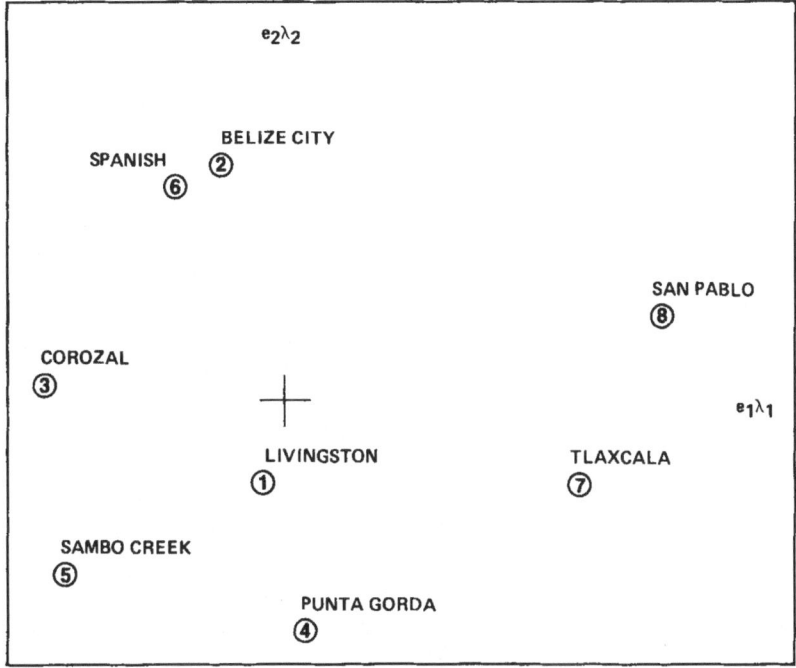

FIGURE 9. "Genetic map" of eight female Black Carib and parental representative groups based upon dermatoglyphic traits.

19% of the variation and separates Belize City Creoles from the cluster of Black Carib communities. The third axis (15%) contrasts Belize City from the Spanish samples. Again females show less variability; $\bar{r}_{ii}$ is equal to 0.016, versus an $\bar{r}_{ii}$ of 0.31 for the males. This greater male dermatoglyphic variability probably reflects the greater migration mobility of the males in the matrilocal social structure of the Black Caribs.

5. Discussion

It is apparent from these two-dimensional representations that the five Black Carib populations are dermatoglyphically homogeneous. For most of the comparisons, Belize City and Punta Gorda are at opposite ends of axis 1, which in general reflects pattern size of PII, especially for males. Female samples, however, exhibit a different pattern of populational affinities than do the males. There is probably less differentiation between dermatoglyphic pattern frequencies of females than of males. Historically, Black Carib males have been more mobile and have formed liaisons with females widely distributed along the coast. Given such a population structure, one would expect to find greater variability in male samples for any Black Carib community.

The addition of three more distantly related populations to the comparison indicates that, at least for males, Livingston is deviating in the direction of the direction of increased Indian admixture. Punta Gorda may also tend toward the Amerindian component, but is probably distinct from all the others due to its reproductive and geographical isolation. Unfortunately, the sample size for Punta Gorda males is small ($N = 25$), and its apparent differentiation is enhanced by sampling error.

The fitting of the genetic distance matrices to geography by the MATFIT method indicates that female dermatoglyphics represent a better reflection of the geographical relationship than do the male. Again, Punta Gorda appears to be distinct dermatoglyphically in both males and females, thus diverging from other Black Carib groups, whose dermatoglyphics tend to converge. It is interesting to note that similar patterns of dermatoglyphic relationship emerge irrespective of whether distances are computed from the percentage occurrence of digital pattern types or through the use of sophisticated multivariate distance measure based upon 40 dermatoglyphic traits.

The total interpopulational comparison of the Black Carib dermatoglyphics indicates that Punta Gorda is distinct in digital ridge counts, TRC, and frequency of pattern types, and in the comparison of dermatoglyphics with geography. Population differences in affinities between male and female samples may reflect migration patterns. However, it must be remembered that four of the samples used in this study, Belize City, Corozal, Sambo Creek, and Punta Gorda, consist of children from schools and should reflect the similar genetic composition of stationary families. Three different types of analyses, the PII/TRC correlations, the distance measures from pattern frequencies, and multivariate distance measures, all suggest that the females provide better fit to the expected geographical positions than males. Whatever developmental forces are acting on male dermatoglyphics, they may actually obscure the patterns of interpopulational relationships.

Ideally, these Black Carib populations should fall in the intermediate range between their parental groups: African, Indian, and European. When Spanish data are included in the analysis, they do not separate from the Black Carib populations. The Amerindian sample (San Pablo) sometimes is distinct, but this may be due to its isolated situation. Tlaxcala, which is an admixed Indian/Spanish population but with different contributions from the parent populations, frequently neither clusters with the Black Caribs nor appears intermediate between San Pablo and the Spanish. Some attempt was made to use Black African data for comparison, but the variation among tribes and regions was so great that no clear gradient appeared. Some of the "noise" in this admixture model may be due to the inappropriateness of some of the parental samples. Unfortunately, data representing Carib Indians are not available.

6. Conclusions

This chapter examines dermatoglyphic variation among the Black Caribs and Creoles on two different levels of analysis, within the population and between populations. These two forms of analysis are closely interrelated; for example, the variation associated with sexual dimorphism affects the observed affinities between populations.

The results of intrapopulational analyses of the Black Carib and Creole dermatoglyphics support our view of the existence of eigenstructures that underlie the qualitative and quantitative features observed in human populations. This underlying structure, observed in Mexican Indians (Crawford *et al.*, 1976*a*), Spanish, a Black Carib group (Lin *et al.*, 1979), and New Guinea communities (Lin *et al.*, 1983) appears to be universal in humans. Previous investigations have documented racial and sex differences in dermatoglyphics but found some discordance between genetics and dermatoglyphically measured affinities between populations. There is some question, however, as to whether the traits that have traditionally been utilized in dermatoglyphic studies represent the genotype of the organism.

The analysis described in this chapter illustrates the usefulness of certain dermatoglyphic traits in measuring the genetic architecture of human populations. The relationship between dermatoglyphics and geography, measured by MATFIT, is a respectable 0.64 for females but a lower 0.38 for males. This differential is probably the result of greater male migration among the Black Caribs. Our unpublished results reveal a high correlation between dermatoglyphics and blood-group-based genetic distances in Mexican Indian populations. Thus, dermatoglyphics should be utilized together with blood genetic markers, anthropometrics, and dental traits for the measure of genetic structure in human populations.

ACKNOWLEDGMENTS

The authors acknowledge the UCLA Health Sciences Computing Facility for providing program BMDP7M with the support of the National Institutes of Health Special Research Resources Grant RR-3.

This research was supported in part by NIH grant DEO4115 and Biomedical Science Research Grants 4349-5706, 4309-5706, and 4932-x706. One of the authors (MHC) was on a PHS Research Career Development Award, NIH KO4 DEO28-01.

We thank Marcia Early and Laura Porascsky for their help in the preparation of this manuscript.

References

Crawford, M. H. (ed.), 1976, *The Tlaxcaltecans: Prehistory, Demography, Morphology and Genetics*, University of Kansas Publications in Anthropology, no. 7, Lawrence, Kansas.

Crawford, M. H., Lin, P. M., and Thippeswamy, G., 1976*a*, Quantitative analysis of dermato-glyphics of four Tlaxcaltecan populations, in *The Tlaxcaltecans: Prehistory, Demography, Morphology and Genetics* (M. H. Crawford, ed.), pp. 120–144, University of Kansas Publications in Anthropology, no. 7, Lawrence, Kansas.

Crawford, M. H., Workman, P. L., McLean, C., and Lees, F. C., 1976*b*, Admixture estimates and selection in Tlaxcala, in *The Tlaxcaltecans: Prehistory, Demography, Morphology and Genetics* (M. H. Crawford, ed.), pp. 161–168, University of Kansas Publications in Anthropology, no. 7, Lawrence, Kansas.

Crawford, M. H., Gonzalez, N. L., Schanfield, M. S., Dykes, D. D., Skradski, D., and Polesky, H. F., 1981, The Black Caribs (Garifuna) of Livingston, Guatemala: Genetic markers and admixture estimates, *Hum. Biol.* **53**:87–104.

Cummins, H., and Midlo, C., 1943, *Finger Prints, Palms and Soles: An Introduction to Dermatoglyphics*, Blakiston, Philadelphia.

Dixon, W. J., and Brown, M. B., 1979, *BMDP Biomedical Computer Programs P-Series*, University of California Press, Berkeley.

Friedlaender, J. S., 1975, *Patterns of Human Variation: The Demography, Genetics, and Phenetics of Bougainville Islanders*, Harvard University Press, Cambridge.

Froehlich, J. W., and Giles, E., 1981, A multivariate approach to finger print variation in Papua, New Guinea: Perspectives on the evolutionary stability of dermatoglyphic markers, *Am. J. Phys. Anthropol.* **54**:93–106.

Harpending, H., and Jenkins, T., 1973, Genetic distance among Southern African populations in *Methods and Theories of Anthropological Genetics* (M. H. Crawford, ed.), pp. 177–199, University of New Mexico Press, Albuquerque.

Harpending, H., and Jenkins, T., 1974, !Kung population structure, in *Genetic Distance* (J. F. Crow and C. Denniston, eds.), pp. 137–165, Plenum, New York.

Holt, S. B., 1968, *The Genetics of Dermal Ridges*, Charles C. Thomas, Springfield, Illinois.

Kendall, M. G., 1970, *Ranking Correlation Methods*, Griffin, London.

Lalouel, J. M. 1973, Topology of population structure, in *Genetic Structure of Populations* (N. E. Morton, ed.), University Press of Hawaii, Honolulu.

Lin, P. M., n.d., MSGP: Multivariate statistical and graphic computer programs, Unreleased.

Lin, P. M., Crawford, M. H., and Oronzi, M., 1979, Universals in dermatoglyphics, in *Dermatoglyphics – Fifty Years Later* (V. Wertelecki, and C. C. Plato, eds.), pp. 63–84, Birth Defects: Original Article Series, Vol. XV, No. 6.

Lin, P. M., Enciso, V. B., and Crawford, M. H., 1983, Dermatoglyphic inter- and intra-populational variation among indigenous New Guinea groups, *J. Hum. Evol.*, **12**: 103–123.

Plato, C. C., Cerighino, J. J., and Steinberg, F. S., 1975, The dermatoglyphics of American Caucasians, *Am. J. Phys. Anthropol.* **42**:195–210.

Quazi, Q. H., Mapa, H. C., and Woods, J., 1977, Dermatoglyphics of American Blacks, *Am. J. Phys. Anthropol.* **47**:483–488.

Roberts, D. F., and Coope, E., 1975, Components of variation in multifactorial characters: A dermatoglyphic analysis, *Hum. Biol.* **47**:169–188.

Sokal, R. R., and Friedlaender, J., 1982, Spatial autocorrelation analysis of biological variation on Bougainville Island, in *Current Developments in Anthropological Genetics*, Vol. 2, *Ecology and Population Structure* (M. H. Crawford and J. H. Mielke, eds.), pp. 205–227, Plenum, New York.

Steinberg, F. S., Cereghino, J. J., and Plato, C. C., 1975, The dermatoglyphics of American Negroes, *Am. J. Phys. Anthropol.* **42**:183–194.

PART III

GENETIC SECTION

14

Genetic Structure of the Garifuna Population in Belize

HAZEL WEYMES and HENRY GERSHOWITZ

1. Introduction

The Garifuna community is of particular interest to students of population genetics because it represents a group of people who have been relatively isolated, culturally and genetically, for the last 200 years. Their demographic and migratory patterns can be traced and a genetic profile constructed from examination of hemoglobins, red cell enzymes, and serum proteins.

The ancestors of the Garifuna are (1) Island (or Red) Carib from St. Vincent and Dominica, Windward Islands, and (2) West Africans brought to the area as slaves (see Fig. 1). Members of these groups intermarried from the early 17th century (Taylor, 1951), and it was adult individuals of both groups together with offspring with varying degrees of mixed blood who were transported to Roatan in 1797. Today there are estimated to be about 35,000– 40,000 Garifuna living along the eastern coast of Central America from the southern Yucatan to Nicaragua (see Fig. 2). Environmental forces such as malaria, endemic along the coast until the 1950s, resulted in differential survival of resistant individuals. Other virulent diseases, such as yellow fever and black water fever, may also have acted as selective agents. The other important influence in the formation of a specific Garifuna genome has been drift, since we can reasonably assume mutation to have been negligible within the time available, and migration to have been random with respect to the proteins under consideration.

HAZEL WEYMES • Department of Anthropology, University College London, London WC1E 6BT, England.   HENRY GERSHOWITZ • Department of Human Genetics, University of Michigan, Ann Arbor, Michigan 48104.

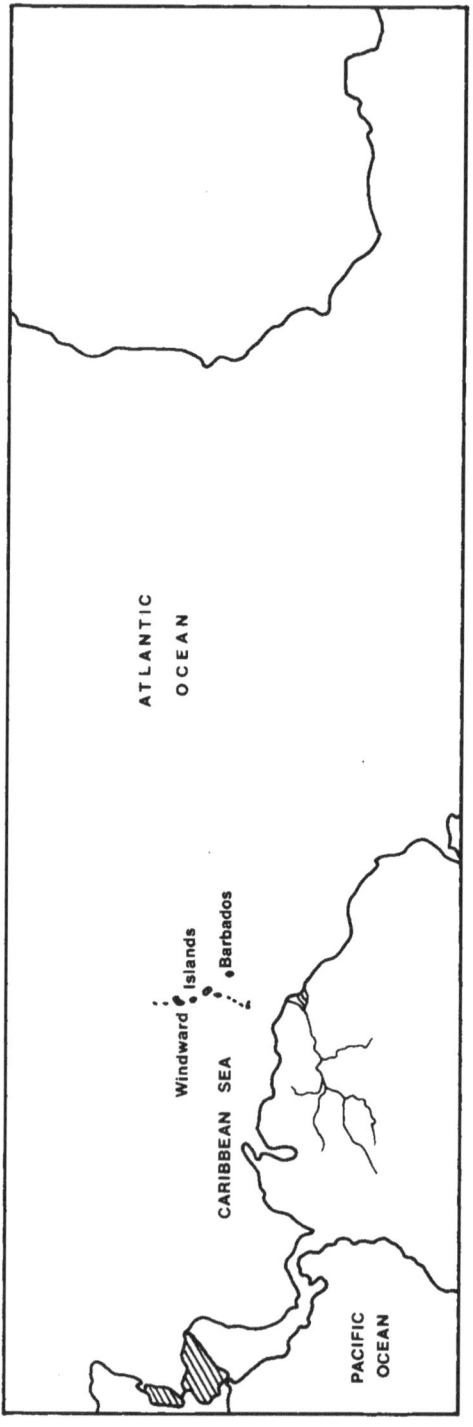

FIGURE 1. Origins of the Carib Indians, ancestors of the Garifuna.

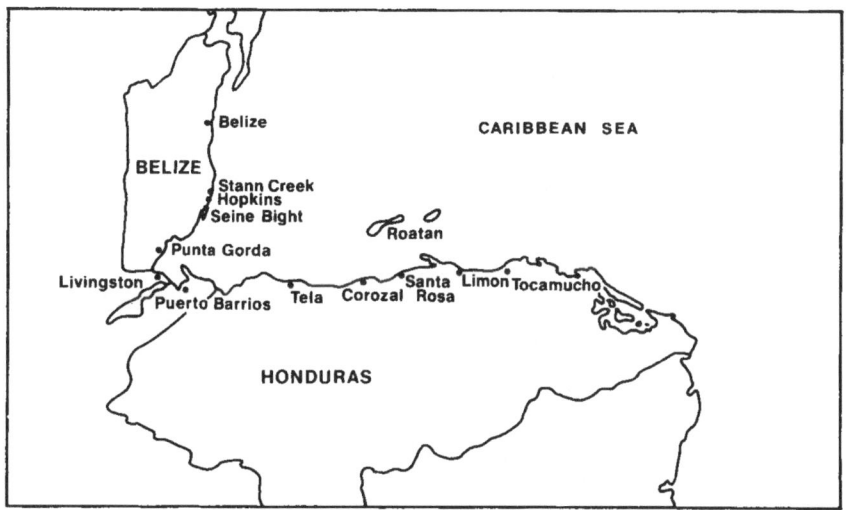

FIGURE 2. Garifuna towns and villages.

2. Material and Methods

The village of Hopkins was selected for a detailed study of the genetic structure of a Garifuna community; it can serve as a suitable starting point for a larger study of Garifuna populations throughout Central America.

Blood specimens from 284 individuals were collected from volunteers and from school children over the age of 7 in Hopkins. A breakdown by age and sex of the sample is given in Table 1. The village has an estimated population of 1000 people, of whom up to one-third may be absent at any one time. Seasonal labor draws men of working age away periodically, and there is a constant movement of young adults away from the village to join relatives in distant towns, either to complete their education or to find work. Often people send their young children back to the village to be cared for by older female relatives, and this swells the number of young children, making them a very large proportion of the community.

The blood was collected by venipuncture, using vacutainers containing acid–citrate–dextrose solution. The samples were immediately placed in a polystyrene box containing wet ice and were transported to Belize City the following day. They were prepared for subsequent analysis by Dr. H. Gershowitz and his assistant at Ann Arbor, Michigan, and put into deep freeze storage within 5 days of being drawn.

Immunoglobulin allotypes were tested under conditions described by Gershowitz and Neel (1978). In brief, sera to be typed were diluted 1:30 in saline and tested for inhibiting capacity on microtiter plates. All sera were

Table 1. Breakdown of the Sample
from Hopkins by Age and Sex

Age interval	Number
Males	
0–15	85
16–44	22
45 +	15
Total	122
Females	
0–15	92
16–44	39
45 +	31
Total	162
Total	284

tested for the specificities Glm(a, x, f), G3m(b0, b1, b3, c3, t, g), Km(1), and Km(3). An inability to test for G3m(s) precluded the identification of $Gm^{a;b0,3,5}$ black phenotype when heterozygous with either $Gm^{a;b0,1,3}$ or $Gm^{f;b}$.

In addition, 114 samples of hemolysate and 212 samples of whole blood from Stann Creek were sent to me in 1975 by Dr. R. Custodio and Dr. R. Huntsman. In 1978 I returned to Belize and collected 138 samples of whole blood from schoolchildren at Punta Gorda and 24 samples from individuals at Hopkins whose blood proved in the initial analysis to be of some specific interest.

Tables 2–4 give the phenotypes and gene frequencies in the three settlements from which samples were drawn, along with results reported elsewhere.

Estimation of gene frequencies may be subject to inaccuracy if a large proportion of the sample is of closely related individuals. The sample from Hopkins necessarily contained several sibships and some parent–child combinations. Many of the individuals in the sample could trace some relationship to others, usually as cousins, aunts, and nephews and nieces or second cousins. However, no one of the several large extended families was represented more than any other, and the sample is probably representative of the whole population since the proportion of related subjects in it corresponds to the incidence of related persons in the population as a whole.

2.1. Hemoglobins

Hemolysate was run at full strength, about 10% hemoglobin (Hb), on starch gels at pH 3.6 using the tris–borate–EDTA system (Huehns and Shooter,

Table 2. Phenotype Distribution of Black Carib Red-Cell Enzyme Markers

	Distribution	
System and phenotype	Hopkins	Stann Creek
Red cell enzymes		
Glucose-6-phosphate dehydrogenase		
A	23	23
A⁻	19	20
AB	17	22
B	190	247
AB	3	3
Total	257	328
6-Phosphogluconate dehydrogenase		
AA	247	320
AC	7	8
Total	254	328
Adenosine deaminase		
1-1	252	321
1-2	5	7
Total	257	328

1964). This system allows the main components, HbA, HbS, and HbC, to remain compact and well separated from each other. Slices from the gels were stained with *o*-toluidine to show heme components.

2.1.1. HbS

Samples that showed a component at the HbS position were rerun alongside a standard sample of HbAS obtained from the Department of Haematology, University College Hospital, London. In order to differentiate those hemoglobins that run to the same position in the gel, a sickledex solution was used for a solubility test. A buffer containing 197.3 g/liter KH_2PO_4 and 174 g/liter K_2HOP_4 was made up. An amount of 0.59 g sodium dithionite and 0.1 g saponin was added to 10 ml of this buffer immediately before testing the specimens. Then 0.02 ml of hemolysate was mixed with 2 ml of the above solution and allowed to stand for 15–30 min at room temperature. Where the blood contained HbS, the solution became turbid. On only one occasion was there a negative result, and this sample was later identified as HbG.

The distribution of HbS is shown for age and sex at Hopkins in Table 5. There are more female than male heterozygotes under 15 years of age, but the difference is not significant at the 0.05% level.

Table 3. *Phenotypic Distribution of Black Carib Serum Protein and Hemoglobin Markers*

	Distribution		
System and phenotype	Hopkins	Stann Creek	Punta Gorda
Hemoglobins			
AA	243	269	127
AS	13	56	9
AC	1	2 (+ 1 AG)	2
Total	257	328	138
Serum proteins			
Transferrin			
CC	246	208	134
CD	19	3	4
DD	1	1	0
Total	266	212	138
Albumin			
Normal	264	202	–
Bisalbum	2	10	–
Total	266	212	–
Haptoglobin			
1-1	52	58	32
2-1	121	90	55
2-2	55	44	27
2-1M	7	11	6
0	32	9	13
Total	267	212	133

2.1.2. HbC

The occurrence of HbC in all of the settlements suggests that much of the ancestral population must have come from a region west of the Niger River, since this river acts as a barrier to the spread of HbC to the east (Lehmann and Nwokolo, 1959).

2.1.3. HbG

This variant is uncommon but widespread in its occurrence. The most likely origin in this instance is from Ghana (Lehmann and Huntsman, 1974).

2.2. Phosphoglucomutase (PGM)

Horizontal starch-gel electrophoresis using a phosphate buffer system (Spencer *et al.*, 1964) was used to examine this enzyme. No variation was

Table 4. Red Cell and Serum Protein Gene Frequencies of Black Carib in Belize

System and alleles	Hopkins	Stann Creek	Punta Gorda
Red cell proteins			
Phosphoglucomutase			
PGM_1^1	0.840	0.890	–
PGM_1^2	0.160	0.110	–
6-Phosphogluconate dehydrogenase			
PGD^A	0.970	0.990	–
PGD^C	0.030	0.010	–
Adenosine deaminase			
ADA^1	0.990	0.990	–
ADA^2	0.010	0.010	–
Serum proteins			
Albumin			
Al^A	0.995	0.980	–
$Al^{VARIANT}$	0.005	0.020	–
Haptoglobin			
Hp^1	0.500	0.530	0.520
Hp^2	0.500	0.470	0.480
Transferrin			
Tf^C	0.970	0.990	0.990
Tf^D	0.030	0.010	0.010

Table 5. Distribution of Variant Hemoglobins at Hopkins, Subdivided by Age Cohorts and Sex

	Distribution			
Age	HbAA	HbAS	HbAC	Total
Male				
0–15	75	2	0	77
16–45	16	0	1	17
45 +	13	0	0	13
Total	104	2	1	107
Female				
0–15	79	7	0	86
16–45	34	3	0	37
45 +	26	1	0	27
Total	139	11	0	150

detected in the PGM2 bands, but all the communities had similar gene frequencies for the alleles PGM_1^1 and PGM_1^2. Table 6 shows the distribution of the phenotypes (genotypes) at Hopkins.

A χ^2 test for homogeneity of the distribution of the phenotypes by sex

Table 6. Distribution of Phosphoglucomutase (PGM) Phenotypes at Hopkins, by Age and Sex

Sex and age	PGM1	PGM2-1	PGM2	Total
Male <15	58	8	2	68
Male >15	22	6	1	29
Female <15	43	33	2	78
Female >15	46	13	4	63
Total	169	60	9	238

Table 7. Distribution of 6-Phosphogluconate Dehydrogenase (6PGD) Phenotypes at Hopkins

Sex and age	A +	A +	A −	B	0^a	Total
Males <15	12	12	15	47	3	77
Males 15–45		3	3	10	1	17
Males >45		2	1	9	1	13
Total		17	19	66	5	107

^{a} No G6PD activity.

shows that there is an unexpectedly high frequency of heterozygotes in females although the alleles are distributed proportionately between the sexes. A χ^2 test for goodness of fit to the Hardy−Weinberg distribution of the phenotypes for the total sample shows that these do not differ significantly from the expected frequencies, yet a breakdown by age and sex shows a slight excess of female heterozygotes under the age of 15 years. The frequencies of the alleles PGM_1^1 and PGM_1^2 at Stann Creek (1975) are similar to those found at Hopkins, but unfortunately no record of age and sex is available for a comparison to be made.

2.3. Glucose-6-phosphate Dehydrogenase (G6PD) and 6-Phosphogluconate Dehydrogenase (6PGD)

These enzymes were examined together on a single gel using a phosphate buffer system suggested by C. W. Parr (personal communication). The gel buffer consists of a 0.016 M phosphate and 10^{-5} M NADP solution, while the bridge buffer includes 0.2 M phosphate and the same molarity of NADP. The distribution of G6PD phenotypes is shown for Hopkins in Table 7. The frequency of G6PD-deficient males is similar to that seen in some West African populations (Mourant, 1976), and this might be expected because the same environmental conditions that favor the maintenance of the variant hemoglobins also favor the allele for G6PD deficiency. The maintenance of a high frequency of variant hemoglobins, particularly HbS, is usually explained by the heterozygote's relative resistance to malaria and/or by the differential fertility of female heterozygotes for this gene. According to Motulsky (1964), the selective mechanism for G6PD deficiency is based on the requirement of malarial parasites for the oxidative pathway in red-cell respiration. This requires the unimpaired production of G6PD. A diminished production of the enzyme is destructive to the parasites and increases the viability of the individual concerned.

The gene for G6PD has allelic forms PGD^A and PGD^C in addition to some rare variants. The frequency of the PGD^C allele is low in most populations, around 6% in West Africans (Parr, 1966; Tills et al., 1971), and either absent or at very low frequencies in Amerindian populations (Weitkapp and Neel, 1970; Harvey et al., 1969). The frequencies of this allele seen at Hopkins (0.03) and at Stann Creek (0.01) are lower than expected from the hemoglobin and G6PD results, which are similar to African frequencies (Table 4).

2.4. Adenosine Deaminase (ADA)

This enzyme was examined using the horizontal gel phosphate buffer system of Spencer et al. (1968).

Although this enzyme has not yet been extensively studied in many populations, it is a useful marker because of its stability and the polymorphic forms of its common alleles ADA^1 and ADA^2 in the populations where it has been investigated. The frequencies seen at Hopkins and Stann Creek (both 0.01) for ADA^2 are similar to those seen in Africans and American Negroes (Mourant, 1976). Higher frequencies are seen in other populations, but few data have been published on gene frequencies for this enzyme in Amerindian populations.

2.5. Serum Proteins

2.5.1. Haptoglobin (Hp)

Haptoglobins and transferrins were typed using horizontal starch gel electrophoresis, with the tris–borate discontinuous buffer system of Poulik (1957). For haptoglobin examination the sample was first saturated with hemoglobin.

The range of haptoglobins commonly seen in populations of African origin is present in the Carib population. Similar frequencies of the Hp^1 allele are seen at each of the three settlements where samples were examined for this protein: Hopkins 0.50, Stann Creek 0.53, and Punta Gorda 0.52. The Hp2-1M phenotype occurs in similar frequencies in all three populations (3, 4, and 5%, respectively) and is not unlike that found in Western African populations (Mourant, 1976). Several individuals were typed as Hp0, the highest frequency being at Hopkins. This is discussed in detail in the next section. The frequency of the Hp^1 allele in Carib-speaking Indians in South America is on average nearer to 0.6 and thus

Table 8. Haptoglobin Phenotypes at Hopkins

Sex and age	Hp1	Hp2-1	Hp2	Hp2-1M	Hp0	Total
Males < 15	16	29	18	1	20	84
Males > 15	4	15	8	2	0	29
Females < 15	17	43	17	1	11	89
Females > 15	15	33	12	3	1	64
Total	52	121	55	7	32	266

considerably higher than is seen in Belizean Caribs. A breakdown of the hapto-globin phenotypes at Hopkins by age and sex shows that 32 of 266 individuals were anhaptoglobinemic in 1974 (see Table 8). All of those typed as Hp0 were aged between 7 and 13 years, with the exception of one female aged 37. There appears to be no familial relationship between these individuals, and both sexes are equally represented. Two of the anhaptoglobinemic individuals are also G6PD-deficient, and two others are heterozygotes HbAS. In the total population at Hopkins, 12% of the sample are either G6PD-deficient or are heterozygotes HbAS. In the individuals with anhaptoglobinemia, there are 21% G6PD-deficient or with HbAS. It seems possible therefore that a connection exists between these conditions.

2.5.2. *Transferrin (Tf)*

The lithium–tris–borate buffer system of Ashton and Braden (1961) was used to separate the transferrins, and amido black was the protein stain. At Hopkins 19 transferrin variants (CD) and one homozygote (DD) were identified, and at Stann Creek three CD and one DD, using ^{59}Fe. It is not known yet whether the transferrin variant is D_{CHI} or D_1.

2.5.3. *Albumin*

Horizontal starch gel typing was performed using the lithium–tris–borate buffer system described by Ashton and Braden (1961). An electrophoretic slow-moving band running behind the usual albumin zone was seen in 12 samples. It was not possible to obtain a standard sample of a known slow-running variant with which to compare these. At present positive identification of these variants is not possible without access to standards, as there are several that migrate to a position within a small zone of the gel.

Slow-moving alloalbuminemia is known to occur in Amerindian populations, but little data are available on the occurrence of the variant in West African populations.

Table 9. Gene Frequencies of the Black Caribs at the Hemoglobin Locus

Population and date of fieldwork	Frequency		
	Hb^A	Hb^S	Hb^C
Hopkins 1957	0.870	0.130	0.00
Hopkins 1974	0.969	0.030	0.001
Stann Creek 1956	0.873	0.111	0.016
Stann Creek 1957	0.900	0.100	0.000
Stann Creek 1975	0.908	0.090	0.002
Punta Gorda 1978	0.965	0.030	0.005
Seine Bight 1956	0.872	0.116	0.012
Seine Bight 1957	0.718	0.236	0.046
Seine Bight 1975	0.915	0.075	0.010

3. Results and Discussion

3.1. The Hemoglobins

Variant hemoglobins have been of particular interest to population geneticists since the connection between their distribution and that of endemic malaria was detected (Allison, 1954). They are easily diagnosed in the field using paper electrophoresis and turbidity tests. For these reasons the hemoglobins provide the most complete data available on genetic polymorphisms in Belize.

It can be seen from Table 9 that there is still a considerable variety of hemoglobins in Belize. All the communities so far tested show the presence of two variants, and one other variant, identified as Hb^G, was found in Stann Creek in 1975. The presence of Hb^C as well as Hb^S in all of the communities indicates that the environment has been favorable for both these variants, and that some of the ancestral population came from an area west of the Niger Rivers, the only region in which Hb^C is commonly found in the Old World (Lehmann and Nwokolo, 1959). Malaria was endemic in the lowlands of Central America until the mid-1950s. It has since been eradicated from Belize, only to be reintroduced in 1977 and 1978 by migrant workers from Mexico and Guatemala. The disease may become reestablished because of the presence of vectors that have become resistant to insecticides due to the extensive spraying of cotton crops.

The variability seen in Belize in the frequency of the Hb^S gene calls for some comment. The gene frequencies for Hb^S at Punta Gorda and at Hopkins are very similar (see Table 9). The frequency of Hb^S reported by Firschein (1961) at Stann Creek and Seine Bight is similar and not significantly different from those reported by Custodio and Huntsman (1975). These four communities, however, present a very interesting contrast. Hopkins and Seine Bight are villages with very similar environments. Both are built along the seashore with swampland behind them, and all the inhabitants of both communities are Caribs.

In contrast, the two towns, Stann Creek and Punta Gorda, are cosmopolitan and are inhabited by Black Caribs (the numerical majority), Creoles, whites, and some Chinese. Stann Creek is very much larger than Punta Gorda (6000 versus 3000 inhabitants), but they are similar in many ways. Punta Gorda is the main crossing point for travelers to the Carib settlements of Livingston and Puerto Barrios in Guatemala and as such has a constant stream of people moving through it.

The towns are both served by sea, road, and air links and act as magnets, drawing people from nearby villages to attend the weekly markets and frequent dances and festivities. Many people from villages go to the towns to find work and to attend the hospitals or the high schools. Under these circumstances it could be expected that the villages would have gene frequencies considerably different from those in the towns, due to the degree to which village people are interrelated and the increased likelihood of drift. In the towns there is a wider choice of mates; thus, drift will have less effect, and admixture is more likely. However, as it turns out, each of the two villages has a different frequency of Hb^S, which is matched by one of the towns. The town of Punta Gorda has the same Hb^S frequency as the village of Hopkins (0.03), and the town of Stann Creek has the same frequency as the village of Seine Bight (0.11). Table 9 shows the gene frequencies of hemoglobins collected at the four settlements; two of them were taken in 1956 and 1957. A test for the significance of the difference of proportions (Chambers, 1952) shows the frequencies of Hb^S at Stann Creek and Seine Bight in 1956, 1957, and 1975 not to be statistically significantly different from one another. The samples at Hopkins, from 1974, are the same test not significantly different from those at Punta Gorda, from 1978. Firchein's high estimate (0.13) of Hb^S for Hopkins in 1957 was based on 59 individuals. The frequencies of Hb^S at one town—village pair are significantly different from those at the other pair. This finding is surprising, because the village samples are known to contain many distantly related individuals belonging to large extended families. The town samples consist mainly of schoolchildren from whom sibs were deliberately excluded.

3.2. The Haptoglobins

The haptoglobins (Hp) are of particular interest because of the variety of phenotypes that can be distinguished, and because they have been investigated in so many populations around the world that they can be used to make comparisons of population gene frequencies. They allow speculation on the function of polymorphisms and the mechanism by which these are maintained in a community.

Haptoglobin polymorphism occurs in every population so far studied, and most individuals belong to one of the phenotypes: Hp1, Hp2-1, and Hp2. In addition, there is a modified form of the 2-1 phenotype found principally in people of African ancestry and designated Hp2-1M (mod). In some communities there are individuals in whom no haptoglobin can be detected by electrophoresis. These are known as anhaptoglobinemic, with the phenotype Hp0.

3.2.1. Hp0

The cause of an apparent lack of haptoglobin is not clearly understood, but it seems likely that a small proportion of the individuals typed as Hp0 have a genetically caused deficiency of this protein. The majority of Hp0 individuals, however, have a low quantity of haptoglobin present in the plasma, even though they produce a normal amount; i.e., there is no suppression of haptoglobin production, but for some reason what is there is used up. There has been much speculation as to the cause of haptoglobin depletion. There was reportedly an increased frequency of Hp0 phenotypes among those with the sickle cell trait (HbAS) (Mehta and Jensen, 1960). On investigation this was found not to be the case in adults, but a raised frequency of anhaptoglobinemia was seen in children with the sickle cell trait (Giblett and Steinberg, 1960). This could not be tested in the present study because the numbers involved are too small to be useful. However, two of the Hp0 individuals were also carriers of the sickle cell trait, and two others were G6PD-deficient.

The majority of the anhaptoglobinemic individuals are children, but the HbAS individuals are distributed evenly among all age groups. This seems to suggest that there is no increased incidence of Hp0 among HbAS individuals in this community. Very young children, particularly under 1 year of age, are frequently found to be Hp0 phenotypes, but subsequently they develop a normal haptoglobin concentration. Other factors suggested as predisposing to low haptoglobin levels are female sex (Barnicot et al., 1960), pregnancy, and G6PD deficiency (Giblett et al., 1966). Since the majority of anhaptoglobinemics are found in malarious regions of Africa, it was thought that this or another hemolytic disease might be the cause of the depletion. However, finding Hp0 in regions where there is no malaria makes this assumption only one of several possible explanations.

The genetic basis for depressed production of haptoglobin is also not yet clear. Studies so far indicate that the children of parents who themselves have Hp2-1M or Hp0 phenotypes are more likely to be anhaptoglobinemic than are children of other haptoglobin phenotypes. It is well known that the Hp1 phenotype produces more haptoglobin than the other phenotypes, and this is therefore the least likely parental phenotype of an Hp0 child. The 2-1M phenotype is commonly found in parents of Negro children and Hp0 (Giblett and Steinberg, 1960).

The most likely explanation to date for the occurrence of genetically caused anhaptoglobinemia is given by Cann and West (1966). It implicates the existence of an allele Hp^0 with no demonstrable gene product, which, when partnered with the Hp^1 or Hp^2 allele, sometimes leads to the suppression of the normal allele. For example, 3–5% of American Negro adults and about 12–15% of American Negro children have undetectable levels of haptoglobin in the plasma, and this cannot be correlated with malarial infection (Giblett, 1959). Two of the three Garifuna communities studied in Belize show levels of anhaptoglobinemia similar to those of North American Negroes: Hopkins with 12% and Punta Gorda with 9%. At Stann Creek a surprisingly low incidence was observed, considering the geographical proximity of the communities and the similarity of their environments.

The phenotype designated 2-1M is found predominantly in people of African ancestry and occurs in the majority of African populations with a frequency of between 2 and 6% (Kirk, 1968). The samples from Belize fall within this range, being 3, 4, and 5%. It is interesting to note that the frequency of 2-1M in North American Negroes is said to be around 10%. Some populations in West Africa have a higher frequency of this phenotype than the majority of African populations; for instance, 13% is reported for a group in Liberia and 11% for another community in Senegal (Kirk, 1968). However, the ancestors of the Garifuna who came from Africa were most probably from the same tribal groups as the ancestors of the American Negroes, so this finding is puzzling. American Negroes have a higher number of 2-1M phentotypes than Garifuna or West Africans in general and an incidence of Hp0 much lower than West African populations but similar to Garifuna populations.

In order to clarify the situation in Hopkins, fresh samples were drawn in 1978 from 10 of the 32 anhaptoglobinemic individuals in Hopkins. Thirty-one of these 32 individuals were aged between 8 and 13 years, and both sexes were represented equally. Four years had elapsed since the previous sampling, and of the 10 samples, only one was classified as anhaptoglobinemic on the second occasion. The others were typed as follows: two as Hp1, two as Hp2, two as Hp2-1, and three as Hp2-1M. These findings support the generally accepted hypothesis concerning the environmental basis for the majority of anhaptoglobinemics but do nothing to elucidate the cause of this phenomenon.

3.3. Immunoglobulins

The immunoglobulin allotype frequencies among the Garifuna of Hopkins are summarized in Table 10. Since the G3m(s) were not tested, it was not possible to identify the $Gm^{a;b0,3,s}$ black haplotype when heterozygous with either $Gm^{a;b0,1,3}$ or $Gm^{f;b}$. All sera lacked G3m(t) specificity; thus the Mongoloid haplotype $Gm^{a;b0,3,s,t}$ is *not* present, and all instances of $Gm^{a;b}$ haplotypes can be presumed to be black in origin. The total black contribution to this population is estimated to be 75.6%.

The Caucasian gene contribution can be estimated from the frequency of $Gm^{f;b}$, assuming that the Mongoloid $Gm^{a,f;b}$ is absent and that instances of

Table 10. Immunoglobulin Allotype
Frequencies among the Garifuna of
Hopkins[a]

Number	Phenotype
Gm system	
90	a; b0,1,3,c3
56	a; b0,1,3
46	a; g, b0,1,3
34	ax; g, b0,1,3
28	a; b0,1,c3
18	a; g, b0,1,c3
14	ax; g, b0,1,c3
8	ax; g, b0,3
8	ax; g
6	a; g
2	a; g, b0,3
1	a, f; b0,1,3
1	a, f; b0,1,3,c3
312	Total
Km system	
21	1 + 3 −
106	1 + 3 +
186	1 − 3 +
313	Total

[a] All sera were tested at 1:30 dilutions for
the Glm specifities (a, x, f) and for the
G3m specifities (b0,b1,b3,c3,t,g).

admixture were multiple and random. The parent admixing Caucasian population can be presumed to have been composed of approximately 0.65 $Gm^{f;b}$ and 0.35 ($Gm^{a;g} + Gm^{ax;g}$). Thus, the present finding of a $Gm^{f;b}$ frequency of 0.003 leads to a Caucasian contribution of 0.005 and, by simple subtraction, an Indian contribution of 0.239 (see Table 11).

In general, the ethnic contributions to the various Garifuna populations of Belize seem to be very similar. Hopkins occupies a middle position, both geographically and numerically, and provides the key to what seems to be a slight cline in the frequency of the black contribution, ranging from 0.79 in Stann Creek to 0.71 in Livingston (see Schanfield et al., this volume, Chapter 18). The Caucasian contribution to the Garifuna population of Hopkins is some 10 times lower than to the other communities. This difference may have been caused by genetic drift maintained by the relative isolation of this community.

In order to elucidate the genetic structure (relationships) of the Carib communities for which gene frequencies are available, Euclidean genetic distances between the populations were computed using the gene frequencies,

Table 11. Immunoglobulin Gene Frequencies
among the Garifuna of Hopkins

System		Frequency
Gm haplotype:		
Glm	G3m	
a;	b0,1,3	0.422
a;	b0,1,c3	0.287
a;	b0,3	0.047
a;	g	0.134
ax;	g	0.106
f;	b	0.003
		$\chi^2_{10} = 21.9$
	Km system:	
Km^1		0.236
Km^3		0.764
		$\chi^2 = 1.2$

and these distances were used to produce a hierarchical clustering of the populations according to the methods of Ward (1963) and Wishart (1969). As can be seen from Fig. 3, the populations are grouped in a two-pair manner similar to the pattern seen in the distribution of the variant hemoglobins; Hopkins is

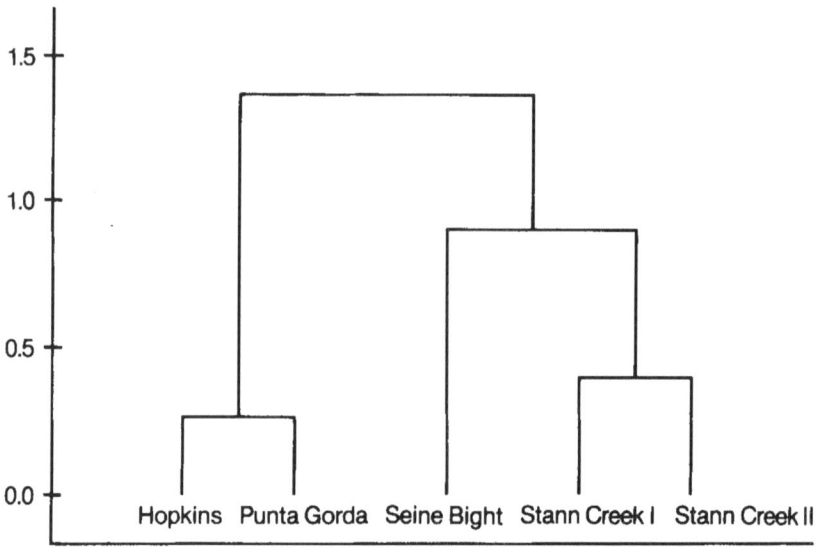

FIGURE 3. CLUSTAN diagram representing genetic distances among populations of Garifuna in Belize based on gene frequencies of eight genetic markers.

closely linked to Punta Gorda, and Stann Creek to Seine Bight. Since the clusters were based on eight gene frequencies (although all eight are not available for every community), this is a strong indication that the gene pools at each of the pairs of settlements are much more similar to each other than the pools between the pairs of settlements.

4. Conclusion

The distributions of hemoglobin, red cell enzyme, and serum protein gene frequencies at four Garifuna settlements in Belize are given. Four other red cell enzyme systems were examined at Hopkins (LDH, MDH, AP, and PHI) and showed no variability. The distribution of PGM2-1 females under the age of 15 years was seen to be high at Hopkins. Ten of the individuals whose haptoglobin levels had been undetectably low in 1974 were reexamined in 1978, and nine of them were successfully typed. These data support the environmental hypothesis of haptoglobin depletion. The genetic distances between the four settlements calculated on the basis of eight genetic markers showed the town Punta Gorda and the village of Hopkins to be similar and the town of Stann Creek to be like the village of Seine Bight. This unexpected similarity of pairs is also seen in the distribution of the variant hemoglobins.

ACKNOWLEDGMENTS

This study was made with the aid of a grant from the Central Research Fund, University of London. The cooperation of the chief Medical Officers in Belize, Dr. L. Pike and Dr. R. Hoy, was of great assistance. I am grateful to Dr. Miranda of Stann Creek and Dr. Castillo von Henkel of Punta Gorda for their help and kind hospitality. A special thank you is due to Mrs. Janes, of the ice shop in Dangriga, and to Sister Anna Marie.

References

Allison, A. C., 1954, Protection afforded by sickle cell trait against subtertian malarial infection, *Br. Med. J.* i:290.

Ashton, G. C., and Braden, A. W. H., 1961, Serum a globin polymorphism in mice, *Aust. J. Biol. Sci.* 14(2):248–263.

Barnicot, N. A., Garlick, J. P., and Roberts, D. F., 1960, Haptoglobin and transferrin inheritance in Northern Nigerians, *Ann. Hum. Genet.* 24:174.

Cann, H. M. and van West, B., 1966, Atypical segregation of haptoglobin types, *Int. Congr. Hum. Genet.*, Chicago, abstract no. 47.

Chambers, E. G., 1952, *Statistical Calculation for Beginners*, Cambridge University Press, Cambridge.

Firschein, I. L., 1961, Population dynamics of the sickle cell trait in the Black Caribs of British Honduras, Central America, *Am. J. Hum. Genet.* **13**:233.

Gershowitz, H., and Neel, J. V., 1978, The immunoglobulin allotype (Gm and Km) of twelve Indian tribes of Central and South America, *Am. J. Phys. Antrhopol.* **49**:289–301.

Giblett, E. R., Hickman, C. G., and Smithies, O., 1959, Haptoglobin types in American Negroes, *Nature (London)* **183**:192.

Giblett, E. R., and Steinberg, A. G., 1960, The inheritance of serum haptoglobin types in American Negroes: Evidence for a third allele, Hp^{2M}, *Am. J. Hum. Genet.* **12**:160.

Giblett, E. R., Motulsky, A. G., and Fraser, G. R., 1966, Population genetics in the Congo IV. Haptoglobin and transferrin serum groups in the Congo and in other African populations, *Am. J. Hum. Genet.* **18**:553.

Harvey, R. G., Godber, M. J., Kopec, A. C., Mourant, A. E., and Tills, D., 1969, Caribs of Dominica, *Hum. Biol.* **41**(3):342–364.

Huehns, E. R. and Shooter, E. M., 1964, Human haemoglobins, *J. Med. Genet.* **2**(1):48.

Kirk, R. L., 1968, *The Haptoglobin Groups in Man*, S. Karger, New York.

Lehmann, H., and Nwokolo, C., 1959, The river Niger as a barrier in the spread eastwards of haemoglobin C: A survey of haemoglobins in the Ibo, *Nature* **183**:1587.

Lehmann, H., and Huntsman, R. G., 1974, *Man's Haemoglobins*, North-Holland, Oxford.

Mehta, S. R., and Jensen, W. N., 1960, Haptoglobins in haemoglobinopathy: A genetic and clinical study, *Br. J. Haematol.* **6**:250.

Motulsky, A. G., 1964, Hereditary red cell traits and malaria, *Am. J. Trop. Med. Hyg.* **13**:147.

Motulsky, A. G., 1972, Metabolic polymorphisms and the role of infectious diseases in human evolution, in *Human Populations Genetic Variation and Evolution* (Morris, L. N., ed.), International Textbook Co., London.

Mourant, A. E., 1976, *The Distribution of the Human Blood Groups*, Oxford University Press, Oxford.

Parr, C. W., 1966, Erythrocyte phosphogluconate dehydrogenase polymorphism, *Nature* **210**:487–489.

Poulik, M. D., 1957, Starch gel electrophoresis in a discontinuous system of buffers, *Nature* **180**:1477.

Spencer, N., Hopkinson, D. A., and Harris, H., 1964, Phosphoglucomutase polymorphism in man, *Nature* **204**:742–745.

Taylor, D. M., 1951, *The Black Carib of British Honduras*, Viking Fund Publications in Anthropology, no. 17, Wenner-Gren Foundation, New York.

Tills, D., van den Branden, J. L., Clements, V. R., and Mourant, A. E., 1970, The distribution in man of genetic variants of 6-phosphogluconate dehydrogenase, *Hum. Hered.* **20**:523–529.

Ward, J. H., 1963, Hierarchical grouping to optimize an objective function, *J. Am. Stat. Assoc.* **58**:236–244.

Weitkamp, L. and Neel, J. V., 1970, Gene frequencies and microdifferentiation among the Makiritare Indians (iii), Nine erythrocyte systems, *Am. J. Hum. Genet.* **22**:533.

Wishart, D., 1969, An algorithm for hierarchical classifications, *Biometrics* **25**:165–170.

15

Blood Group, Hemoglobin, and Plasma Protein Polymorphisms in Black Carib Populations

RAMON CUSTODIO, R. G. HUNTSMAN,
R. M. NEWTON, D. TILLS, HAZEL WEYMES,
A. WARLOW, A. C. KOPEČ, and J. M. LORD

1. Introduction

On emigration of a proportion of a population, three factors exert an effect on altering the genetic composition of the emigrant group from that of the native gene pool from which it originated: founder effect, genetic drift, and changed environmental conditions.

The founder effect is inversely proportional to the number of founders: the smaller the number of founders, the greater the effect. It is the rarer genes that probably are most affected; usually these are missing from a small group, but when they are present in a small group, the frequency is almost always higher than it was in the original population; this high frequency may be further increased by genetic drift or, conversely, drift may result in these genes

RAMON CUSTODIO • Laboratorio Custodio, S. de R. L. Pathologia Clínica y Anatomia Pathologica, 1229 Tegucigalpa, D. C., Honduras.   R. G. HUNTSMAN and R. M. NEWTON • Canadian Red Cross, Blood Transfusion Services, St. Johns, Newfoundland, Canada A1B 4A4.   D. TILLS, A. WARLOW, and J. M. LORD • British Museum (Natural History), Sub-Department of Anthropology, London SW7, England.   HAZEL WEYMES • Department of Anthropology, University College London, London WC1E 6BT, England. A. C. KOPEČ • Serological Population Genetics Laboratory, London, England.

disappearing from the group's descendants. In some respects genetic drift is similar to the founder effect, as it will be most effective in a small group. The drift may be in either direction; it may cause rare alleles to increase in frequency. This differs from the founder effect in that only the succeeding generations are subject to it, and it has recognized limitations in that only genes present in the group are subject to it. In retrospective studies it is often impossible to ascribe measurable changes in gene frequencies between the native gene pool and the emigrant population derived from that pool to one or the other of these factors.

Superimposed upon the results of these factors are altered selective pressures resulting from the different environment in which the emigrant group has settled. Again it is very difficult to unravel the effects of the three agents, all of which may be in opposition or may act synergistically.

This chapter provides a brief account of investigations carried out in three Black Carib communities of Belize and Honduras during 1978. These investigations focus particularly on those systems of the blood that may provide some resistance against malaria and are an example of the action of natural selection.

2. Methods

Blood was collected from Punta Gorda, Belize, and Limon, Honduras, and dispatched in vacuum containers to London. The tests on these two populations were performed in the subdepartment of Anthropology, British Museum of Natural History, London. The samples collected in Roatan, Honduras, were tested in the Canadian Red Cross (Blood Transfusion Service) Centre, St. John's, Newfoundland.

In London the blood grouping tests were performed by the micromethod of Warlow and Tills (1978). The hemoglobin, haptoglobin, and transferrin phenotypes were determined using methods and modifications recommended by Tills (1977).

In Newfoundland the blood group tests were performed as recommended by the Canadian Red Cross Blood Transfusion Service (Moore, 1980).

3. Results

The phenotypic distributions and gene frequencies for the ABO, MNSs, Rhesus, Lutheran, Kell, Duffy, P, Kidd, and Diego blood group systems for Black Caribs from Punta Gorda, Limon, and Roatan are summarized in Tables 1–4. Haptoglobin and transferrin phenotypes and gene frequencies for two of these three communities are presented in Table 5.

Table 1. ABO Phenotypes Observed and Gene Frequencies of Three Populations of Black Caribs

		Honduras	
	Punta Gorda, Belize	Limon	Roatan
A_1	10	30	
A_{int}	8	5	41
A_2	3	3	
B	26	23	27
A_1B	2	1	
$A_{int}B$	0	0	1
A_2B	0	0	
O	89	101	99
Total	138	163	168
p_1	4.44	10.04	
p_{int}	3.08	1.73	13.47
p_2	1.19	1.06	
q	10.73	7.69	8.76
r	80.56	79.48	77.77

3.1. ABO

South American Indians are practically all group O; however, up to 5% of ABO genes in different populations of the area are A. The Black Caribs have a lower frequency of gene B and a higher frequency of gene O than do West African Blacks. The data suggest an admixture of about 10% Red Carib genes; the A-gene frequency is essentially unchanged, which would fit well with a Red Carib A-gene frequency of 5%.

3.2. Rhesus

The West African Black and Black Carib frequencies match extremely well, except for the frequency of the three haplotypes R_0, r', and r. Haplotype R_0 is reduced, while r' and r compensate for this reduction in the Black Caribs. Both r' and r are practically absent in Amerinds; therefore, the differences in this blood group system between the Black Caribs and Blacks must be due to founder effects, genetic drift, natural selection, or any combination thereof.

It is not possible to estimate the genetic contribution of the Red Caribs from these data, but it would appear to be close to zero.

3.3. MNSs

The haplotype *NS* is completely absent from West African Blacks and has only a low frequency in Amerinds; the frequency in the Black Caribs is higher

Table 2. MM^gNSsS^uHe Phenotypes Observed and Gene Frequencies of Three
Populations of Black Caribs

	Punta Gorda, Belize	Honduras	
		Limon[a]	Roatan[b]
MMSS	4	10.53	–
MM^{g}SS	–	2.78	1.04
M^{g}M^{g}SS	–	–	–
MMSs	15	9.47	–
MM^{g}Ss	1	11.13	7.27
M^{g}M^{g}Ss	–	–	–
MMss	29	14	–
MM^{g}ss	–	1.09	18.69
M^{g}M^{g}ss	–	–	–
MMS^{u}S^u	1	–	–
MNSS	4	9.33	4
M^{g}NSS	–	–	–
MNSs	17	29.13	8
M^{g}NSs	–	3.33	–
MNss	37	36.54	–
M^{g}Nss	–	1.67	21
MNS^{u}S^u	1	–	–
NNSS	–	2.19	4
NNSs	11	7.68	23
NNss	15	24.13	55
NNS^{u}S^u	3	–	–
Total	138	163	142
MS	11.86	20.54	6.12
M^{g}S	0.36	4.46	–
Ms	39.51	27.93	24.52
M^{g}s	–	1.67	–
MS^u	5.88	–	–
NS	7.92	8.86	13.72
Ns	26.55	36.54	55.64
NS^u	7.92	–	–
Henshaw			
He+	2	3	Not tested
He–	136	160	–
Total	138	163	–
He+	1.45%	1.84%	–

[a] One MMS, three MM^{g}S, and three MNS not tested with anti-s. One MM^g, five MN, two M^{g}N, and three NN not tested with either anti-S or anti-s. These are distributed throughout by proportion.
[b] One MM not tested with either anti-S or anti-s and distributed in the ratio of those tested. Anti-M^g not available for testing these samples. No S^u samples found.

Table 3. Rhesus Phenotypes and Haplotype Frequencies for Three Populations of Black Caribs

| | Punta Gorda, Belize | Honduras | |
		Limon	Roatan
CCDEe	–	–	1
CCDee	1	5	4
CCddee	–	1	–
CcDEe	5	1	8
CcDee	35	48	39
C^wcDee	–	–	1
Ccddee	10	9	10
ccDEE	1	2	3
ccDEe	15	6	15
ccDee	65	71	74
ccddee	6	20	13
Total	138	163	168
CDE	–	–	1.17
CDe	6.41	13.81	10.55
Cde	12.43	7.66	8.22
C^wDe	–	–	0.30
cDE	7.97	3.37	7.76
cDe	51.00	40.14	43.41
cde	22.19	35.02	28.59

than that of the Red Caribs. If this haplotype did enter the former from the latter, which is almost certain, then either genetic drift or natural selection has been responsible for the increased frequency. Genetic drift is most suspected in this case. In either event no estimate of degree of admixture is possible from these data.

The frequency of *Ms* is essentially the same in West African Blacks and Amerinds, but *Ms* is reduced in the Black Caribs; again this leads to the suspicion that genetic drift has been the most effective agent of change in this blood group system.

3.4. Lutheran

The data suggest a massive influx of Amerind genes into the Black Caribs, as these have an Lu^a frequency of only 25% that of West African Blacks. It would appear that the founder effect, genetic drift, and natural selection have all acted synergistically on this gene in the Black Caribs.

Any gene flow from the Red Caribs would act in the same direction to decrease the frequency of Lu^a in the Black Caribs.

Table 4. Lutheran, Kell, Duffy, P, Kidd, and Diego Blood Groups

| | Punta Gorda, Belize | Honduras | |
		Limon	Roatan
Lutheran blood groups			
Lu(a + b −)	−	−	−
Lu(a + b +)	2[a]	1[b]	Not tested
Lu(a − b +)	136	162	−
Total	138	163	−
Lu^a	0.72	0.31	−
Lu^b	99.28	99.69	−
Kell blood groups			
KK	−	−	−
Kk	1	4[c]	Not tested
kk	136	147	−
Total	137	151	−
K	0.36	1.32	−
k	99.64	98.68	−
Js(a + b −)			−
Js(a + b +)	17	20[c]	Not tested
Js(a − b +)	119	124	−
Total	136	144	−
Js^a	6.25	6.94	−
Js^b	93.75	93.06	−
Duffy blood group system			
Fy(a + b −)	25	10.56[d]	9
Fy(a + b +)	4	8.44	3
Fy(a − b +)	4	23	4
Fy(a − b −)	103	108	126
Total	136	150	142
Fy^a (Fy^1)	11.23	11.57	4.30
Fy^b (Fy^2)	2.97	10.57	2.48
Fy (Fy^4)	85.80	77.69	93.22
P Blood groups			
P_1 +	123	135	Not tested
P_1 −	15	27	−
Total	138	162	−
P_1	67.03	59.18	−
$P_2 + p$	32.97	40.82	−

Table 4. (Continued)

| | Punta Gorda, Belize | Honduras | |
		Limon	Roatan
Kidd blood groups			
Jk(a + b −)	−	−	49
Jk(a + b +)	Not tested	Not tested	70
Jk(a − b +)	−	−	23
Total	−	−	142
Jk^a	−	−	59.16
Jk^b	−	−	40.84
Diego blood groups			
Di^a +	35[e]	75[e]	0
Di^a −	101	66	142
Total	136	141	142

[a] Two Lu^a + and 66 Lu^a − not tested with anti-Lu^b and assumed to be Lu^b +.
[b] Seventy-three Lu^a − not tested with anti-Lu^b and assumed to be Lu^b +.
[c] One k + not tested with anti-K and assumed to be K−; four K− not tested with anti-k and assumed to be k +. Two Js^a − not tested with anti-Js^b and assumed to be Js^b +.
[d] One Fy^a + not tested with anti-Fy^b has been proportioned according to the ratio of those tested.
[e] These results are probably incorrect, as we have reason to suspect that the anti-Di^a serum used for these studies was giving nonspecific positive reactions.

3.5. Kell

The Kell gene *K* is almost completely lacking in West African Blacks; it is present at about the same frequency in Red and Black Caribs. This gene in the Black Caribs must be derived from the Amerinds and has since been elevated by genetic drift, natural selection, or both. The gene Js^a is lacking in Amerinds and is reduced in the Black Caribs compared with the West African Blacks. If the reduction is entirely due to gene flow from Red to Black Caribs, it would suggest that approximately 3% of Black Carib genes are of Amerind origin.

3.6. Kidd

Black Caribs lack the gene *Jk*, and this is present in West African Blacks only in low frequency. This difference between the two groups may be an example of a founder effect, or a founder effect and genetic drift.

3.7. P

The data clearly demonstrate that either genetic drift or natural selection or both have been operative here in the Black Caribs.

*Table 5. Haptoglobin and Transferrin Phenotypes and Gene Frequencies in
Three Populations of Black Caribs*

		Honduras	
	Punta Gorda, Belize	Limon	Roatan
Haptoglobin			
Hp1	32	45	Not tested
Hp2-1	55	65	
Hp2-1M[a]	6	10	
Hp2	27	21	
Hp0	13	15	
Total	133	156	
Hp^1	52.08	58.51	
Hp^2	47.92	41.49	
Hp^0	9.77	9.62	
Hp^{2-1M}	4.51	6.41	
Transferrin			
TfC	126	144	
TfCD	4	8	
TfD	0	0	
Total	130	152	
Tf^c	98.46	97.37	
Tf^D	1.54	2.63	

[a] To calculate gene frequencies the Hp2-1M numbers are added to the Hp2-1 phenotype
and the Hp0 phenotype is omitted.

3.8. Diego

Unfortunately, the conflicting results given by the two different examples
of anti-Di[a] prevent any conclusions from being drawn in this system. This is
most unfortunate, as this is the system in which gene flow from Amerinds to
the Black Caribs should have been most obvious.

3.9. Duffy

The Fy^a is almost completely lacking in West African Blacks; therefore,
its appearance in the Black Caribs depends upon gene flow from Amerinds. The
frequency in the Black Caribs suggests an admixture of about 8%.

In the area inhabited by the Black Caribs, two types of malaria, that
caused by *P. falciparum* and that caused by *P. vivax*, exist. Hence, both the Fy^a
and Fy^b genes will be selected against. The existence of Fy^b but not Fy^a in West

Africans suggests that the Fy^a gene is more strongly selected against. It is therefore possible, even probable, that the estimate of 8% is too low.

3.10. Hemoglobin, Haptoglobin, Transferrin

Data for haptoglobin and transferrin are available only for the Punta Gorda and Limon samples. The classically African variants HbS and HbC were both present in the former sample, but only HbS was found in Limon. A surprising finding was of HbSS homozygotes in Limon. The frequency of the HbS gene in Limon is very high (see Chapter 17), suggesting some adaptive significance. In view of the existence of *Plasmodium falciparum* in the area, this high frequency of HbS is not very surprising.

The frequencies of the haptoglobin alleles Hp^1 and Hp^2 are similar in both West Africans and Amerinds, so that little information can be gained from these. The Hp2-1M phenotype, however, has not been found in Amerinds, and the frequencies in the Black Caribs are very similar to those of West African populations.

The transferrin variant allele Tf^D is present in both West African Black and Amerind populations, and it is not possible to comment on the origin of this gene in the Black Caribs.

3.11. Other Genes

A_{int} occurs in Blacks and the Black Caribs; unfortunately, it appears that no Amerind population has been tested with anti-H, so the existence of this gene in Amerinds is at this time a matter of conjecture.

$S^ü$ occurs in Black populations; some blood samples react with neither anti-S nor anti-s and are termed S^u. This allele is extremely rare in other populations; it is present in the Punta Gorda population but not in samples from Honduras. This is surprising; presumably the absence in these populations of this allele is due to a founder effect, or genetic drift, or both.

Henshaw (*He*) is part of the MNSs system and is practically confined to Blacks. In West Africans it is present in about 5%; in Punta Gorda the frequency was 1.5%, and in Limon 1.8%. Samples from Roatan were not tested for this antigen. Amerinds have so far been shown to lack this antigen.

The antigen M^g, which is expressed via an allele at the MN locus of the MNSs system, was discovered by Allen *et al.* (1958). Mourant *et al.* (1976) list 40 populations as having been tested for this antigen, a total of 52,470 persons, of whom 15 were positive. Only three populations have been shown to have this antigen: 0.15% in Switzerland (Metaxes *et al.*, 1966), 0.79% in Greek Cypriots (Plato *et al.*, 1964), and 0.80% in a population from Boston (Allen *et al.*, 1958).

The antigen M^g was found in 20 persons from Limon (12.27%) and one from Punta Gorda (0.72%); the number of M^g-positives in these two Black Carib populations is greater than the total for the rest of the world. No M^g-positives have been found in Amerind populations, but some M^g data appear to have been published on Africans. Although Tills *et al*. (1979) did not find any M^g-positives among Nigerians, they did find one positive in samples from Egyptians.

It is not possible at this time to account for this extremely high frequency in the Black Caribs, or indeed for its presence at all. More Amerind and African populations need to be tested for the presence of this antigen, after which the position of the Black Caribs may be clarified. Further work on this interesting antigen is in progress in Newfoundland at this time.

4. Discussion

Two of the few genes in human populations for which we know of selective pressures for and against are the hemoglobin genes Hb^A and Hb^S. In endemic malarious areas where *Plasmodium falciparum* is the major parasite, heterozygotes HbAS have a selective advantage over both the "wild" homozygote HbAA and the homozygous mutant HbSS. The heterozygote is more resistant to malaria than the HbAA homozygote, and this increased viability is not offset by the mild effects, if any, of the Hb^S gene in a single dose. The HbSS homozygote is inferior to both HbAA and HbAS due directly to the deleterious effects of the Hb^S gene in a double dose, where it results in severe anemia and frequently in childhood death.

Hence, if a subpopulation in which both genes were present emigrated from Central Africa to a nonmalarious area of the New World, the founder effect, genetic drift, and natural selection would all be operative. Due to the selective pressure against the HbSS homozygote, the frequency of the Hb^S gene would be expected to decrease in each generation. The founder effect and genetic drift may temporarily negate the full effects of natural selection, but would not do so over several generations. The American Black has been exposed to this, but here the situation is further complicated by a degree of miscegenation. The maintenance of sickle cell hemoglobin in the Black Caribs who remain under malarial pressure is discussed in Chapter 17.

The Duffy blood group system is also involved in susceptibility and resistance to malaria, but in this case malaria is due to the parasite *Plasmodium vivax*. The antigens Fy^a and Fy^b appear to act as the portals through which the parasite gains entry to the erythrocyte (Miller *et al.*, 1975). The genotype *FyFy*, which produces neither of the above antigens, confers resistance to this type of malaria. The natural selection of this gene *Fy* appears to be a biologically efficient and "cheap" process (Mourant *et al.*, 1978), cheap in that it seems to have no selective disadvantage compared with the other genotypes of the system, in distinction to the situation regarding Hb^S. In West African Blacks the incidence of the *FyFy* genotype is 90–95%, while the present data demonstrate an incidence of 80% in the Black Caribs. It is, however, known that there has been some admixture with Amerinds, in whom the *Fy* gene is extremely rare.

In all blood group systems in which the maternal antibody produced in response to fetomaternal immunization is completely or partially composed of immunoglobulin G (IgG), hemolytic disease of the newborn (HDN) is the most obvious selective agent. In all cases it is the rarer gene (haplotype) that is selected against; however, it is only in the ABO system that it is theoretically possible for this process to reduce the level of the *A* and *B* genes to zero. This is due to the fact that in group O mothers the causative antibodies are present prior to the first pregnancy and are at least partially composed of IgG. The antibodies are not produced as a result of fetomaternal immunization, although the titer is frequently increased following pregnancy with an ABO incompatible child.

In all other systems in which "naturally occurring" antibodies are found (for example, the Lewis blood group system), these antibodies are composed entirely of IgM and cannot cause HDN. In those systems in which the "naturally occurring" antibodies are absent, the first incompatible child, though frequently acting as the immunizing agent, usually escapes unscathed, rendering total eradication of the causative antigen impossible to achieve.

At this point our knowledge of the selective agents leading to development and maintenance of the balanced genetic polymorphisms in human populations throughout the world is insufficient to permit any explanation of how these developed and continue to exist.

The Red Caribs have an incidence of about 14% Diego (Di^a)-positive individuals; the present data indicate levels of 25% for Punta Gorda and 53% for Limon of Di^a-positive individuals. In Roatan 142 individuals were tested with anti-Di^a, of whom none were positive. There is reason to suspect that in the case of the two former groups, the antiserum used was giving nonspecific positive reactions. This is very disappointing, since an accurate estimate of the frequency of *Di^a* in Black Caribs would give a very good estimate of the degree of admixture with the Red Caribs. A different antiserum was used for the third group, and it is felt that these results are accurate, since all controls included gave the expected reactions.

In situations where a population survey is being performed and the area is difficult to reach or the continued cooperation of the population over a long period of time is improbable, it would appear essential to check all results with at least two antisera having the same specificity. This would enable discrepancies to be investigated immediately. If two antisera of the required specificity are not available, it is advisable that aliquots of the red cell samples be frozen for a check when a second example of that antibody is available.

An area of considerable interest is the study of gene flow from one population to another, especially in those cases where the two populations have remained reasonably distinct from each other, a situation existing for the Red and Black Caribs.

Table 6. Gene Frequencies of West African Blacks (WA), Black Caribs (BC),
and Amerinds (AI)

Gene	WA	BC	AI	Gene	WA	BC	AI
O	72.07	78.50	95.00	R_1	10.60	10.58	56.00
A	13.83	12.23	5.00	R_2	7.68	8.74	41.55
B	14.10	9.27	0.00	R_0	60.11	43.00	2.04
				R_z	0.00	0.00	0.41
MS	4.17	12.70	24.67	r'	1.88	8.84	0.00
Ms	51.39	34.84	50.33	r''	0.00	0.00	0.00
NS	0.00	9.26	6.62	r^y	0.00	0.00	0.00
Ns	44.44	43.20	18.38	r	19.73	28.84	0.00
Lu^a	3.57	0.75	0.51	K	0.00	0.87	0.88
Lu^b	96.43	99.25	99.49	k	100.00	99.13	99.12
				Js^a	8.06	6.61	0.00
Fy^a	0.00	6.01	78.03	Js^b	91.94	93.39	100.00
Fy^b	5.56	5.25	21.97				
Fy	94.44	88.74	0.00	Jk^a	76.98	59.16	41.85
				Jk^b	16.94	40.84	33.62
Di^a	0.00		4.12	Jk	6.08	0.00	24.53
Di^b	100.00		95.88				
P_1	76.41	88.17	51.42				
$P_2 + p$	23.59	11.83	48.58				

An assessment of the gene flow from the Red to the Black Caribs is difficult, as the gene pool of the latter has been subject to a founder effect, genetic drift, and natural selection in a "new" environment. In addition to this and compounding the inherent difficulties of such a task are the facts that the native population from which the Black Caribs descend has not been adequately defined and that blood group data for this putative group and for the Red Caribs are incomplete.

In the assessment of the proportion of Red Carib genes in the Black Caribs, blood group gene frequencies are needed for the original Black population and for the Red Caribs. The data for Red Caribs and for Nigerian Negroes have been used where available; if such data have not been available, the geographically closest population for which the required data exist were used. The data were obtained from collected data on blood group frequencies (Mourant *et al.*, 1976).

Despite the less than satisfactory data available, we feel that it is possible to draw tentative conclusions as to the proportion of Red Carib genes in the Black Caribs, and this has been performed for each blood group system as follows. Blood group gene frequencies for Amerinds, West African Blacks, and Black Caribs are listed in Table 6. From these data it is obvious that the Black Caribs are intermediate in most of the gene frequencies between Amerindians and West Africans. Small founding populations and the action of natural selection may have contributed to the unique frequencies of a few alleles that are not intermediate between the parental values. Chapters 18 and 19 discuss more fully the proportion of Amerindian and West African genes present in the Black Carib gene pools.

ACKNOWLEDGMENTS

We wish to thank the many colleagues who have kindly provided antisera used in this study; the Blood Group Reference Laboratory, London; The Canadian Red Cross Blood Transfusion Service, Toronto; Fay Boyce, Ortho; Dr. T. Cleghorn, North London Blood Transfusion Centre; Dr. Marie Crookston, Toronto General Hospital; Dr. P. D. Issitt, University of Cincinnati; Dr. Layrisse, Instituto Venezolano de Investigaciones Cientificas; Miss Julia Mann, Pfizer; Dr. M. Metaxes, Swiss Blood Transfusion Service: and J. Moulds, Gamma.

We are grateful to Dr. Ruth Sanger and the Staff of the Medical Research Council's Blood Group Research Unit, London for confirming some of the M^g results.

References

Allen, F. H., Corcoran, P. A., Kenton, H. B., and Breare, N., 1958, M^g, A new blood group antigen in the MNS system, *Vox Sang.* (n.s.) 3:81–91.

Metaxas, M. N., Metaxas-Bühler, M., and Roamski, Y., 1966, Studies on the blood group antigen M^g. i. Frequency of M^g in Switzerland and family studies, *Vox Sang.* 11: 157–69.

Miller, L. H., Mason, S. J., Dvorak, J. A., McGinniss, M. H., and Rothman, I. K., 1975, Erythrocyte receptors for (*Plasmodium knowlesi*) malaria: Duffy blood group determinants, *Science* 189:561–563.

Moore, B. P. L., 1980, *Serological and Immunological Methods*, 8th ed., Canadian Red Cross Society.

Mourant, A. E., Kopeč, A. C., Domaniewska-Sobczak, K., 1976, *The Distribution of the Human Blood Groups and Other Polymorphisms*, 2nd ed., Oxford University Press.

Mourant, A. E., Kopeč, A. C., Domaniewska-Sobczak, K., 1978, *Blood Groups and Diseases*, Oxford University Press.

Plato, C. C., Rucknagel, D. L., and Gershowitz, H., 1964, Studies on the distribution of glucose-6-phosphate dehydrogenase deficiency, thalassemia, and other genetic markers in the coastal and mountain villages of Cyprus, *Am. J. Hum. Genet.* 16:267–283.

Tills, D., 1977, Red cell and serum proteins of the Irish, *Ann. Hum. Biol. H.* 1977:25–42.

Tills, D., Warlow, A., and Lord, J. M., 1979, Unpublished observations.

Warlow, A., and Tills, D., 1978, Micromethods in blood group serology, *Vox Sang.* 35:354–356 (1977).

16

Blood Group, Serum Protein, and Red Cell Enzyme Polymorphisms, and Admixture among the Black Caribs and Creoles of Central America and the Caribbean

MICHAEL H. CRAWFORD, DALE D. DYKES,
K. SKRADSKY, and H. F. POLESKY

1. Introduction

With rapid innovations in transportation during the last two centuries, systematic evolutionary pressures in the form of migration, population movement, and gene flow have increased exponentially. Populations of the New and Old World have been amalgamated in various combinations, resulting in unique hybrid aggregates. For example, Amerindian groups interbred with Spanish conquistadores and other Hispanic settlers to produce biologically and culturally hybrid entities termed *Mestizo* or *Ladino* in Mexico and much of Central America.

MICHAEL H. CRAWFORD ● Laboratory of Biological Anthropology, University of Kansas, Lawrence, Kansas 66045. DALE D. DYKES, K. SKRADSKY, and H. F. POLESKY ● Minneapolis War Memorial Blood Bank, Minneapolis, Minnesota 55404.

304 M. H. CRAWFORD *ET AL.*

In addition, African slaves that were brought to the New World interbred with both Hispanic colonists and indigenous populations on the west and east coasts of Mexico to form triracial hybrids.

This chapter examines the blood group, serum, and red blood cell protein variation among several hybrid populations of Central America and St. Vincent Island in the Caribbean. Two groups, the Black Caribs and the Creoles, apparently share a similar ancestral West African genetic component while differing in the presence of either European or Amerindian genes in their composite gene pools. In addition, all of the Carib populations share common historical roots, which were initially planted on St. Vincent Island and eventually relocated to Central America (see Chapter 2). The precise ethnohistorical reconstructions for the Black Caribs permit the study of evolutionary changes, both systematic and nonsystematic pressures, on the distribution of gene frequencies of the blood.

A number of Black Carib populations of Central America described in this chapter have been surveyed genetically by several investigators spanning at least two to three generations. It is unusual in anthropological genetics to be able to compare allelic frequencies of the same populations obtained through sequential sampling over a number of generations. Such comparison not only may aid in establishing the reliability of sampling procedures, but may contribute to our understanding of gross evolutionary changes. Undoubtedly, similar samples representing different temporal points over many generations will be available in the future for the monitoring of evolutionary change. However, at present, genetic sampling representing two or even three generations is unique.

2. Methods and Material

During the summers of 1975, 1976, and 1978, a total of 1327 blood specimens were collected from Black Carib and Creole populations of Belize, Guatemala, and St. Vincent Island. This sample was obtained from four Central American and three Caribbean communities (see Table 1). The majority of the participants in this study were Black Caribs ($N = 1044$), with 283 Creoles included for comparative purposes.

The blood specimens were drawn by venipuncture in vacutainers containing ACD preservative. These specimens were immediately packed in ice and shipped for analysis, within 10 days of collection, to the War Memorial Blood Bank of Minneapolis. These blood samples were tested with the following antisera: MNSs (M, N, S, s), Rhesus (C, c, D, E, e), Kell (K, k), ABO (A, A_1, B), Diego (Di^a), Duffy (Fy^a and Fy^b, as available), and Kidd (Jk^a). The red cell typings were performed in microtiter (U) plates using 2% suspension of washed cells by modification of the method of M. N. Crawford *et al.* (1970). Antisera were diluted to obtain optimal reactivity. Typings were incubated for 1 hr at room temperature (20°C). The typing plates were centrifuged in a Sorvall GLC-1

Table 1. Sample Sizes in This Study

Population	N
Mainland samples	
Caribs	
Livingston	205
Stann Creek (Dangriga)	354
Punta Gorda	239
Total Caribs	798
Creoles	
Belize City	129
Dangriga	78
Total	207
St. Vincent samples	
Caribs	
Sandy Bay	161
Owia	85
Creole	
Fancy	76
Total in study	1327

centrifuge for 2 min at 500 rpm prior to reading. Antiglobulin testing was also done in microtiter plates, after washing three times, using a 12-channel saline dispenser (antiglobulin test rinser) and centrifuged subsequent to the addition of antiglobulin reagent and reading.

The serum protein phenotypes for transferrin (Tf), albumin (Al), and group-specific component (Gc) were determined by acrylamide slab electrophoresis and stained with amido black (Polesky *et al.*, 1975). Subtypes of transferrin were ascertained using two different buffer systems (H. E. Sutton, personal communication). Haptoglobin (Hp) and ceruloplasmin (Cp) phenotypes were determined simultaneously by electrophoresis on acrylamide slabs (McComb and Bowman, 1969). The vitamin D-binding globulin Gc was also phenotyped by isoelectric focusing (IEF), and Gc subtypes were identified on acrylamide at a pH gradient of pH 4–6 as described by Dykes and Polesky (1981*b*).

Serum protein properdin factor B (Bf) was phenotyped by means of standard agarose gel electrophoresis followed by immunofixation to identify variants (Dykes and Polesky, 1980).

Stroma-free hemolysates for determining erythrocyte enzyme phenotypes were obtained by washing cells three times in saline, diluting 1:1 in distilled water, and centrifuging at high speed. Specimens were stored at −20°C until tested.

Adenylate kinase (AK), adenosine deaminase (ADA), 6-phosphogluconate dehydrogenase (6PGD), and acid phosphatase (AcP) were electrophoresed simultaneously on a single horizontal starch slab (Dykes and Polesky, 1976). Esterase D (EsD) was phenotyped on starch using the citrate phosphate buffer system, pH 5.9, of Karp and Sutton (1967). Phosphoglucomutase (PGM) was tested utilizing the original technique of Spencer *et al.* (1964) and subsequently subtyped using IEF on agarose according to the method of Dykes and Polesky (1981a). Hemoglobin variants were screened electrophoretically by the method described by Yunis (1969).

   Allelic frequencies for the blood group systems are maximum likelihood estimates computed by the MAXLIK computer program of Reed and Schull (1968).

2.1. Admixture Estimates

   Gene flow and genetic hybridization measures have been based either upon a single locus or allele in a population with biracial ancestry or through combining information from various loci for the computation of a composite proportion of admixture. The single allelic estimates are based upon Bernstein's formula, which may be expressed as follows:

$$m = \frac{q_x - Q}{q - Q} \tag{1}$$

where m is the proportion of admixture, Q and q are the allelic frequencies in two parental populations, and q_x is the frequency of the same allele in the hybrid group.

   Methods for the estimation of admixture based upon multiple loci include those of Roberts and Hiorns (1962, 1965), Kreiger *et al.* (1963), Chakraborty (1975), and Crawford *et al.* (1976). The Roberts and Hiorns method is a least-squares measure of m, which assumes a parental population with known gene frequencies, and no selection or drift. Krieger and his colleagues have utilized a maximum likelihood solution to the estimation of m. Chakraborty (1975) estimated racial admixture on the basis of the probability of gene identity. Crawford *et al.* measured m through a weighted multiple regression analysis and through the summation of individual locus m values weighted by variance. All of these methods provide similar results, although the maximum likelihood estimates tend to slightly overestimate the Amerindian component (Crawford *et al.*, 1976).

2.2. Genetic Heterozygosity

   Mean per-locus heterozygosity $\bar{d}$ was computed by the method of Harpending and Chasko (1976),

$$\bar{d}_i = 1 - \sum_{k=1}^{t} p_k^2$$

where t is the number of alleles at this ith locus. The overall or absolute hetero-zygosity D is computed as the mean for all loci,

$$D = (1/N) \sum_{i=1}^{N} d_i$$

3. Results and Discussion

Tables 2–7 summarize the phenotypic distributions and frequencies for blood groups, serum proteins, and red cell enzymes observed in the blood samples from Livingston, Belize City, Stann Creek, Punta Gorda, and three communities from St. Vincent Island (Sandy Bay, Owia, and Fancy). Genetic variation at polymorphic levels ($q \geqslant 0.01$) is observed at all loci tested, with the exception of PGM_2 and the Diego blood group system in the Stann Creek Creole. In addition, none of the genetic loci deviate significantly from Hardy–Weinberg expectations.

3.1. Blood Group Systems

The gene frequencies for the erythrocytic antigens are contained in Tables 8 and 9. The A_1 allele varies between 3.3% in Owia and 12.1% in Fancy, St. Vincent Island. The observed genetic variation in three adjoining villages on St. Vincent Island is equal to the variation at the ABO locus found in Black Carib and Creole villages widely dispersed along the coast of Central America. The A_2 allele is more frequent on St. Vincent Island than on the mainland African derived populations. The incidences of A and B blood group alleles are intermediate between observed West African and Amerindian frequencies.

One of the most reliable marker genes used to identify West African ancestry is the R_0 (cDe) haplotype of the Rhesus blood group system. Sandy Bay, a Carib village on St. Vincent Island, exhibits by far the lowest incidence of the cDe chromosomal segment (0.247 versus a range of 0.418–0.566 among the remaining populations). The Gm frequencies (see Chapter 18) indicate that this low incidence of cDe is reflective of the high Amerindian gene flow into the Sandy Bay gene pool. Fancy Creoles and Livingston Caribs have the highest incidence of cDe and most closely resemble the African cDe pattern.

The CDe (R_1) and cDE (R_2) are common Rhesus chromosomal segments among the indigenous Amerindian populations. Similarly, the Black Caribs reflect their Amerindian ancestry by exhibiting high to medium frequencies of these gene complexes. Sandy Bay Black Caribs, as expected, have the highest

Table 2. Distribution of Blood Group Phenotypes in Belizean and Guatemalan Populations[a]

	Belize													Guatemala	
	Belize City Creole		Stann Creek				Punta Gorda Carib		Total Carib		Total Creole		Livingston Carib	
			Carib		Creole									
System and phenotype	N	P	N	P	N	P	N	P	N	P	N	P	N	P
ABO														
A₁	15	0.127	64	0.194	15	0.192	32	0.148	96	0.176	30	0.153	23	0.113
A₂	3	0.025	13	0.039	6	0.077	8	0.037	21	0.038	9	0.046	9	0.044
B	22	0.187	65	0.197	9	0.115	34	0.157	99	0.181	31	0.158	55	0.270
A₁B	1	0.008	4	0.012	1	0.013	0	0.000	4	0.007	2	0.010	2	0.010
A₂B	2	0.017	11	0.033	1	0.013	4	0.018	15	0.027	3	0.015	3	0.015
O	75	0.636	173	0.525	46	0.590	139	0.640	312	0.571	121	0.618	112	0.549
Total	118	1.000	330	1.000	78	1.000	217	1.000	547	1.000	196	1.000	204	1.000
Rhesus														
CCDEE	0	0.000	1	0.003	0	0.000	0	0.000	1	0.002	0	0.000	0	0.000
CCDEe	0	0.000	1	0.003	0	0.000	1	0.004	2	0.003	0	0.000	9	0.044
CCDee	2	0.017	4	0.012	3	0.039	0	0.000	4	0.007	5	0.026	4	0.019
CcDEE	0	0.000	3	0.009	0	0.000	2	0.009	5	0.009	0	0.000	0	0.000
CcDEe	5	0.042	17	0.050	6	0.079	12	0.052	29	0.051	11	0.056	26	0.127
CcDee	34	0.286	74	0.216	14	0.184	29	0.127	103	0.180	48	0.246	49	0.239
ccDEE	3	0.025	19	0.055	1	0.013	8	0.035	27	0.047	4	0.020	2	0.010
ccDEe	20	0.168	65	0.189	10	0.132	61	0.266	126	0.220	30	0.154	38	0.185
ccDee	45	0.378	132	0.385	35	0.461	92	0.402	224	0.392	80	0.410	68	0.332
Ccdee	3	0.025	6	0.017	2	0.026	8	0.035	14	0.024	5	0.026	0	0.000
ccdee	7	0.059	21	0.061	5	0.066	16	0.070	37	0.065	12	0.062	9	0.044
Total	119	1.000	343	1.000	76	1.000	229	1.000	572	1.000	195	1.000	205	1.000

	N	P	N	P	N	P	N	P	N	P	N	P	N	P
MNSs														
MMSS	0	0.000	6	0.018	1	0.014	10	0.044	16	0.029	1	0.005	3	0.015
MMSs	7	0.059	26	0.078	4	0.055	30	0.131	56	0.100	11	0.058	17	0.084
MMss	12	0.102	48	0.145	9	0.123	24	0.105	72	0.128	21	0.110	20	0.099
MNSS	4	0.034	23	0.069	0	0.000	11	0.048	34	0.061	4	0.021	5	0.025
MNSs	46	0.390	48	0.145	11	0.151	33	0.144	81	0.144	57	0.298	27	0.134
MNss	30	0.254	88	0.265	22	0.301	62	0.271	150	0.267	52	0.272	59	0.292
MNSᵘSᵘ	0	0.000	0	0.000	2	0.027	0	0.000	0	0.000	2	0.011	0	0.000
NNSS	0	0.000	4	0.012	0	0.000	3	0.013	7	0.012	0	0.000	5	0.025
NNSs	10	0.085	21	0.063	7	0.096	8	0.035	29	0.052	17	0.089	18	0.089
NNss	9	0.076	67	0.202	17	0.233	48	0.209	115	0.205	26	0.136	48	0.238
NNSᵘSᵘ	0	0.000	1	0.003	0	0.000	0	0.000	1	0.002	0	0.000	0	0.000
Total	118	1.000	332	1.000	73	1.000	229	1.000	561	1.000	191	1.000	202	1.000
Duffy														
Fy(a+)	47	0.398	62	0.186	28	0.384	78	0.341	140	0.249	75	0.393	—	—
Fy(a−)	71	0.602	271	0.814	45	0.616	151	0.659	422	0.751	116	0.607	—	—
Total	118	1.000	333	1.000	73	1.000	229	1.000	562	1.000	191	1.000	NT	NT
Diego														
Di(a+)	1	0.008	9	0.027	1	0.015	7	0.030	16	0.029	2	0.011	8	0.040
Di(a−)	117	0.992	319	0.973	65	0.985	223	0.970	542	0.971	182	0.989	193	0.960
Total	118	1.000	328	1.000	66	1.000	230	1.000	558	1.000	184	1.000	201	1.000
Kell														
Kk	2	0.017	0	0.000	2	0.027	6	0.026	6	0.011	4	0.021	0	0.000
kk	116	0.983	328	1.000	72	0.973	223	0.974	551	0.989	188	0.979	202	1.000
Total	118	1.000	328	1.000	74	1.000	229	1.000	557	1.000	192	1.000	202	1.000
Kidd														
Jk(a+)	107	0.922	321	0.976	72	0.986	—	—	—	—	179	0.947	—	—
Jk(a−)	9	0.078	8	0.024	1	0.014	—	—	—	—	10	0.053	—	—
Total	116	1.000	329	1.000	73	1.000	NT	NT	NT	NT	189	1.000	NT	NT

a N, Number; P, proportion.
b NT, Not tested

Table 3. Distribution of Blood Group Phenotypes in St. Vincentian Populations[a]

System and phenotype	Sandy Bay Carib		Owia Carib		Owia Creole		Fancy Carib		Fancy Creole		Total Carib		Total Creole	
	N	P	N	P	N	P	N	P	N	P	N	P	N	P
ABO														
A₁	17	0.1030	5	0.0543	5	0.2083	0	0.0000	14	0.2258	22	0.0786	22	0.2178
A₂	27	0.1636	11	0.1196	1	0.0417	5	0.2174	5	0.0806	43	0.1536	6	0.0594
B	25	0.1515	16	0.1739	4	0.1667	0	0.0000	7	0.1129	41	0.1464	16	0.1584
A₁B	1	0.0061	1	0.0109	0	0.0000	0	0.0000	0	0.0000	2	0.0071	0	0.0000
A₂B	1	0.0061	2	0.0217	0	0.0000	0	0.0000	4	0.0645	3	0.0107	5	0.0495
O	94	0.5697	57	0.6196	14	0.5833	18	0.7826	32	0.5161	169	0.6036	52	0.5149
Total	165	1.0000	92	1.0000	24	1.0000	23	1.0000	62	1.0000	280	1.0000	101	1.0000
Rhesus														
CCDEE	0	0.0000	0	0.0000	0	0.0000	0	0.0000	0	0.0000	0	0.0000	0	0.0000
CCDEe	1	0.0061	1	0.0109	0	0.0000	0	0.0000	0	0.0000	2	0.0071	0	0.0000
CCDee	3	0.0182	1	0.0109	0	0.0000	0	0.0000	0	0.0000	4	0.0143	0	0.0000
CcDEE	0	0.0000	1	0.0109	0	0.0000	0	0.0000	0	0.0000	1	0.0036	0	0.0000
CcDEe	19	0.1152	7	0.0761	0	0.0000	3	0.1304	2	0.0323	29	0.1036	2	0.0198
CcDee	29	0.1758	12	0.1304	4	0.1667	4	0.1739	9	0.1452	45	0.1607	14	0.1386
ccDEE	12	0.0727	10	0.1087	1	0.0417	5	0.2174	4	0.0645	27	0.0964	7	0.0693
ccDEe	61	0.3697	26	0.2826	3	0.1250	5	0.2174	17	0.2742	92	0.3286	24	0.2376
ccDee	29	0.1758	32	0.3478	16	0.6667	5	0.2174	28	0.4516	66	0.2357	50	0.4950
Ccdee	0	0.0000	0	0.0000	0	0.0000	0	0.0000	0	0.0000	0	0.0000	0	0.0000
ccdee	11	0.0667	2	0.0217	0	0.0000	1	0.0435	2	0.0323	14	0.0500	4	0.0396
Total	165	1.0000	92	1.0000	24	1.0000	23	1.0000	62	1.0000	280	1.0000	101	1.0000

	N	P	N	P	N	P	N	P	N	P	N	P	N	P
MNSs														
MMSS	0	0.0000	1	0.0109	0	0.0000	0	0.0000	0	0.0000	1	0.0036	0	0.0000
MMSs	4	0.0242	6	0.0652	2	0.0833	2	0.0870	1	0.0161	12	0.0429	3	0.0297
MMss	14	0.0848	8	0.0870	5	0.2083	3	0.1304	8	0.1290	25	0.0893	14	0.1386
MMs^{u}s^u	0	0.0000	0	0.0000	0	0.0000	0	0.0000	0	0.0000	0	0.0000	0	0.0000
MNSS	6	0.0364	1	0.0109	0	0.0000	0	0.0000	1	0.0161	7	0.0250	2	0.0198
MNSs	17	0.1030	13	0.1413	4	0.1666	2	0.0870	7	0.1129	32	0.1143	11	0.1089
MNss	86	0.5212	30	0.3261	9	0.3750	11	0.4783	33	0.5323	127	0.4536	48	0.4752
MNs^{u}s^u	0	0.0000	0	0.0000	0	0.0000	0	0.0000	0	0.0000	0	0.0000	1	0.0099
NNSS	3	0.0182	4	0.0435	0	0.0000	1	0.0435	0	0.0000	8	0.0286	0	0.0000
NNSs	7	0.0424	14	0.1522	1	0.0417	2	0.0870	3	0.0484	23	0.0821	6	0.0594
NNss	28	0.1698	15	0.1630	3	0.1250	2	0.0870	9	0.1452	45	0.1607	16	0.1585
NNs^{u}s^u	0	0.0000	0	0.0000	0	0.0000	0	0.0000	0	0.0000	0	0.0000	0	0.0000
Total	165	1.0000	92	1.0000	24	1.0000	23	1.0000	62	1.0000	280	1.0000	101	1.0000
Kell														
Kk	3	0.0182	0	0.0000	0	0.0000	0	0.0000	1	0.0161	3	0.0107	1	0.0099
kk	162	0.9818	92	1.0000	24	1.0000	23	1.0000	61	0.9839	277	0.9893	100	0.9901
Total	165	1.0000	92	1.0000	24	1.0000	23	1.0000	62	1.0000	280	1.0000	101	1.0000
Diego														
Di(a+)							0	0.0000	0	0.0000				
Di(a−)							23	1.0000	62	1.0000				
Total							23	1.0000	62	1.0000				
Henshaw														
He⁺							1	0.0435	2	0.0322				
He⁻							22	0.9565	60	0.9678				
Total							23	1.0000	62	1.0000				

[a] N, Number; P, proportion.

Table 4. Serum Protein Phenotypic Frequencies from Populations of Belize and Guatemala[a]

System and phenotype	Belize								Guatemala	
	Belize City Creole		Stann Creek				Punta Gorda Carib		Livingston Carib	
			Carib		Creole					
	N	P	N	P	N	P	N	P	N	P
Albumin										
AA	124	0.976	341	0.977	76	0.987	230	0.975	203	0.990
AMe	3	0.024	8	0.023	1	0.013	6	0.025	2	0.010
Total	127	1.000	349	1.000	77	1.000	236	1.000	205	1.000
Haptoglobin										
1-1	29	0.238	101	0.291	25	0.342	70	0.303	73	0.358
2-1	57	0.467	162	0.467	36	0.493	110	0.476	97	0.475
2-1M	14	0.115	17	0.049	2	0.028	9	0.039	4	0.020
2-2	22	0.180	66	0.190	10	0.137	42	0.182	30	0.147
0	0	0.000	1	0.003	0	0.000	0	0.000	0	0.000
Total	122	1.000	347	1.000	73	1.000	231	1.000	204	1.000

	N	P	N	P	N	P	N	P	N	P
Transferrin										
CB	0	0.000	2	0.006	0	0.000	0	0.000	0	0.000
CC	110	0.873	324	0.934	71	0.888	229	0.966	195	0.947
CD	16	0.127	21	0.060	9	0.112	8	0.034	11	0.053
Total	126	1.000	347	1.000	80	1.000	237	1.000	206	1.000
Group-specific component										
1-1	97	0.764	270	0.778	63	0.829	175	0.738	43	0.210
2-1	30	0.236	71	0.205	12	0.158	60	0.253	161	0.790
2-2	0	0.000	6	0.017	1	0.013	2	0.009	0	0.000
Total	127	1.000	347	1.000	76	1.000	237	1.000	204	1.000
Ceruloplasmin										
AA	2	0.016	2	0.006	0	0.000	0	0.000	0	0.000
AB	12	0.097	25	0.073	4	0.055	13	0.055	9	0.044
BB	109	0.879	315	0.915	69	0.945	223	0.941	196	0.956
BC	1	0.008	1	0.003	0	0.000	1	0.004	0	0.000
AC	0	0.000	1	0.003	0	0.000	0	0.000	0	0.000
Total	124	1.000	344	1.000	73	1.000	237	1.000	205	1.000

[a] N, Number; P, proportion.

Table 5. Phenotype Distributions of Serum and Red Cell Proteins among Communities of St. Vincent Island

System and phenotype	Sandy Bay				Owia				Fancy			
	Carib		Creole		Carib		Creole		Carib		Creole	
	N	P	N	P	N	P	N	P	N	P	N	P
Albumin												
AA	158	1.000	15	1.000	79	1.000	21	1.000	20	1.000	69	1.000
Group-specific component												
standard electrophoresis												
1-1	128	0.806	14	0.933	44	0.579	13	0.813	15	0.789	60	0.810
2-1	28	0.176	1	0.067	26	0.342	3	0.187	2	0.105	11	0.148
2-2	1	0.006	0	0.000	3	0.040	0	0.000	1	0.053	0	0.000
1-Ab	1	0.006	0	0.000	1	0.013	0	0.000	1	0.053	1	0.014
2-Ab	0	0.000	0	0.000	2	0.026	0	0.000	0	0.000	1	0.014
Ab-Ab	1	0.006	0	0.000	0	0.000	0	0.000	0	0.000	1	0.014
Total	159	1.000	15	1.000	76	1.000	16	1.000	19	1.000	74	1.000
isoelectric focusing												
$1_S 1_S$	35	0.267	0	0.000	10	0.156	0	0.000	3	0.166	4	0.055
$1_S 1_F$	49	0.374	4	0.286	12	0.188	3	0.231	5	0.278	22	0.306
$1_F 1_F$	18	0.137	9	0.643	13	0.203	7	0.538	6	0.333	33	0.458
2-1_S	10	0.076	0	0.000	10	0.156	0	0.000	0	0.000	0	0.000
2-1_F	16	0.122	1	0.071	13	0.203	3	0.231	2	0.111	10	0.139
2-2	1	0.008	0	0.000	3	0.047	0	0.000	1	0.056	0	0.000
1_S-Ab	1	0.008	0	0.000	0	0.000	0	0.000	0	0.000	1	0.014
1_F-Ab	0	0.000	0	0.000	1	0.016	0	0.000	1	0.056	0	0.000
2-Ab	0	0.000	0	0.000	2	0.031	0	0.000	0	0.000	1	0.014
Ab-Ab	1	0.008	0	0.000	0	0.000	0	0.000	0	0.000	1	0.014
Total	131	1.000	14	1.000	64	1.000	13	1.000	18	1.000	72	1.000

	N	P	N	P	N	P	N	P	N	P	N	P
Transferrin												
CC	159	1.000	15	1.000	72	0.948	18	0.947	22	1.000	74	0.987
CD$_1$	0	0.000	0	0.000	4	0.052	1	0.053	0	0.000	1	0.013
Total	159	1.000	15	1.000	76	1.000	19	1.000	22	1.000	75	1.000
Haptoglobin												
1-1	30	0.462	2	0.250	22	0.297	6	0.333	7	0.368	17	0.246
2-1	29	0.446	6	0.750	21	0.284	4	0.222	8	0.421	23	0.333
2-1M	0	0.000	0	0.000	19	0.257	3	0.167	3	0.158	13	0.189
2-2	6	0.092	0	0.000	12	0.162	5	0.278	1	0.053	16	0.232
Total	65	1.000	8	1.000	74	1.000	18	1.000	19	1.000	69	1.000
Properdin factor B												
SS	39	0.265	7	0.467	22	0.290	2	0.133	4	0.200	8	0.109
SF	47	0.320	4	0.267	27	0.355	7	0.467	8	0.400	30	0.411
SF$_1$	22	0.150	0	0.000	6	0.079	1	0.067	2	0.100	4	0.055
FF$_1$	13	0.088	3	0.200	5	0.066	0	0.000	4	0.200	10	0.137
FF	17	0.116	1	0.066	14	0.184	5	0.333	2	0.100	21	0.288
F$_1$F$_1$	5	0.034	0	0.000	1	0.013	0	0.000	0	0.000	0	0.000
S$_{07}$F	1	0.007	0	0.000	1	0.013	0	0.000	0	0.000	0	0.000
SS$_{07}$	3	0.020	0	0.000	0	0.000	0	0.000	0	0.000	0	0.000
Total	147	1.000	15	1.000	76	1.000	15	1.000	20	1.000	73	1.000

[a] N, Number; P, proportion.

Table 6. Red Blood Cell Phenotypic Frequencies in Population Samples from Belize and Guatemala[a]

System and phenotype	Belize							Guatemala	
	Belize City Creole		Stann Creek				Punta Gorda Carib		Livingston Carib	
			Carib		Creole					
	N	P	N	P	N	P	N	P	N	P
Hemoglobin										
AA	114	0.898	292	0.836	66	0.857	211	0.890	172	0.851
AS	11	0.087	54	0.155	11	0.143	25	0.106	29	0.143
AC	2	0.015	2	0.006	0	0.000	1	0.004	0	0.000
SS	0	0.000	1	0.003	0	0.000	0	0.000	1	0.006
Total	127	1.000	349	1.000	77	1.000	237	1.000	202	1.000
Acid phosphatase										
AA	4	0.031	10	0.028	2	0.026	5	0.021	6	0.030
AB	41	0.323	107	0.306	26	0.338	58	0.245	58	0.286
BB	81	0.638	224	0.640	46	0.597	165	0.696	122	0.601
CB	0	0.000	0	0.000	0	0.000	1	0.004	0	0.000
AR	1	0.008	1	0.003	1	0.013	1	0.004	1	0.005
BR	0	0.000	8	0.023	2	0.026	7	0.030	16	0.079
Total	127	1.000	350	1.000	77	1.000	237	1.000	203	1.000
Phosphoglucomutase (locus 1)										
1-1	80	0.661	240	0.694	43	0.573	169	0.716	154	0.774
2-1	37	0.306	100	0.289	29	0.387	63	0.267	42	0.211
2-2	4	0.033	6	0.017	3	0.040	4	0.017	3	0.015
Total	121	1.000	346	1.000	75	1.000	236	1.000	199	1.000

	N	P	N	P	N	P	N	P	N	P
Phosphoglucomutase (locus 2)										
1-1	122	1.000	345	0.997	71	1.000	219	0.986	200	1.000
2-1	0	0.000	0	0.000	0	0.000	3	0.014	0	0.000
2-2	0	0.000	1	0.003	0	0.000	0	0.000	0	0.000
Total	122	1.000	346	1.000	71	1.000	222	1.000	200	1.000
6-Phosphogluconate dehydrogenase										
AA	111	0.881	331	0.957	70	0.921	219	0.924	198	0.966
AC	15	0.119	15	0.043	5	0.066	17	0.072	7	0.034
CC	0	0.000	0	0.000	1	0.013	1	0.004	0	0.000
Total	126	1.000	346	1.000	76	1.000	237	1.000	205	1.000
Adenosine deaminase										
1-1	126	0.992	343	0.977	76	0.987	235	0.983	204	0.997
2-1	1	0.008	8	0.023	1	0.013	4	0.017	0	0.000
2-2	0	0.000	0	0.000	0	0.000	0	0.000	1	0.003
Total	127	1.000	351	1.000	77	1.000	239	1.000	205	1.000
Adenylate kinase										
1-1	120	0.945	333	0.948	70	0.909	226	0.946	198	0.975
2-1	7	0.055	15	0.043	7	0.091	12	0.050	5	0.025
2-2	0	0.000	1	0.003	0	0.000	1	0.004	0	0.000
3-1	0	0.000	2	0.006	0	0.000	0	0.000	0	0.000
Total	127	1.000	351	1.000	77	1.000	239	1.000	203	1.000
Esterase D										
1-1	119	0.922	308	0.875	58	0.784	208	0.875	166	0.834
2-1	10	0.078	44	0.125	15	0.203	30	0.126	31	0.156
2-2	0	0.000	0	0.000	1	0.013	0	0.000	2	0.010
Total	129	1.000	352	1.000	75	1.000	238	1.000	199	1.000

[a] N, Number; P, proportion.

Table 7. Red Cell Protein Phenotype Distribution among Communities of St. Vincent Island[a]

System and phenotype	Sandy Bay Carib N	Sandy Bay Carib P	Sandy Bay Creole N	Sandy Bay Creole P	Owia Carib P	Owia Carib N	Owia Creole P	Owia Creole N	Fancy Carib P	Fancy Carib N	Fancy Creole P	Fancy Creole N
Adenylate kinase												
1-1	161	0.994	15	1.000	87	1.000	25	1.000	21	1.000	74	0.974
2-1	1	0.006	0	0.000	0	0.000	0	0.000	0	0.000	2	0.026
Total	162	1.000	15	1.000	87	1.000	25	1.000	21	1.000	76	1.000
6-Phosphogluconate dehydrogenase												
AA	162	0.994	14	0.933	45	0.978	14	0.933		NT	4	1.000
AC	1	0.006	1	0.067	1	0.022	1	0.067	0	0.000	0	0.000
Total	163	1.000	15	1.000	46	1.000	15	1.000	0	0.000	4	1.000
Acid phosphatase												
AA	2	0.012	0	0.000	2	0.023	0	0.000	0	0.000	0	0.000
AB	42	0.258	4	0.267	22	0.250	10	0.435	10	0.370	10	0.149
BB	117	0.718	11	0.733	64	0.727	13	0.565	16	0.593	56	0.836
BR	2	0.012	0	0.000	0	0.000	0	0.000	0	0.000	1	0.015
BD	0	0.000	0	0.000	0	0.000	0	0.000	1	0.037	0	0.000
Total	163	1.000	15	1.000	88	1.000	23	1.000	27	1.000	67	1.000

	N	P	N	P	N	P	N	P	N	P	N	P
Esterase D												
1-1	127	0.825	12	0.857	66	0.930	24	1.000	13	0.650	72	0.972
2-1	24	0.156	2	0.143	4	0.056	0	0.000	7	0.350	1	0.014
2-2	3	0.019	0	0.000	1	0.014	0	0.000	0	0.000	1	0.014
Total	154	1.000	14	1.000	71	1.000	24	1.000	20	1.000	74	1.000
Phosphoglucomutase-1 (isoelectric focusing)												
1 + 1 +	34	0.211	7	0.411	22	0.259	6	0.240	1	0.048	22	0.290
1 + 1 −	55	0.342	4	0.235	27	0.318	4	0.160	9	0.428	22	0.290
1 − 1 −	22	0.137	1	0.059	12	0.141	3	0.120	3	0.143	1	0.013
1 + 2 +	16	0.099	2	0.118	11	0.129	8	0.320	5	0.238	14	0.184
1 − 2 +	16	0.099	1	0.059	9	0.106	0	0.000	2	0.095	8	0.105
1 + 2 −	5	0.031	1	0.059	1	0.012	1	0.040	0	0.000	1	0.013
1 − 2 −	8	0.050	1	0.059	1	0.012	0	0.000	0	0.000	3	0.039
2 + 2 +	3	0.019	0	0.000	2	0.023	1	0.040	1	0.048	3	0.039
2 + 2 −	2	0.012	0	0.000	0	0.000	1	0.040	0	0.000	2	0.027
2 − 2 −	0	0.000	0	0.000	0	0.000	1	0.040	0	0.000	0	0.000
Total	161	1.000	17	1.000	85	1.000	25	1.000	21	1.000	76	1.000
Hemoglobin												
AA	159	0.976	10	0.714	85	0.966	23	1.000	19	0.905	51	0.689
AS	2	0.012	2	0.143	3	0.034	0	0.000	2	0.095	19	0.257
AC	2	0.012	2	0.143	0	0.000	0	0.000	0	0.000	4	0.054
Total	163	1.000	14	1.000	88	1.000	23	1.000	21	1.000	74	1.000
MDH												
1-1	163	1.000	15	1.000	46	1.000	14	1.000	NT		NT	

[a] N, Number; P, proportion. NT, Not tested.

Table 8. Blood Group Gene Frequency Distribution among Belizean and Guatemalan Populations[a]

		Belize					Guatemala
		Stann Creek					
System and allele	Belize City Creole	Carib	Creole	Punta Gorda Carib	Total Carib	Total Creole	Livingston Carib
ABO							
A_1	0.070	0.110	0.108	0.077	0.097	0.085	0.064
A_2	0.023	0.042	0.052	0.030	0.037	0.034	0.032
B	0.112	0.129	0.073	0.092	0.114	0.097	0.160
O	0.795	0.719	0.767	0.801	0.752	0.784	0.744
Rhesus							
CDE	0.000	0.016	0.000	0.016	0.016	0.000	0.034
CDe	0.153	0.119	0.154	0.000	0.090	0.146	0.091
cDE	0.130	0.172	0.115	0.189	0.179	0.125	0.145
cDe	0.427	0.418	0.469	0.456	0.421	0.435	0.508
CdE	0.000	0.000	0.000	0.000	0.000	0.000	0.000
Cde	0.040	0.028	0.051	0.099	0.038	0.044	0.121
cdE	0.000	0.000	0.000	0.000	0.000	0.000	0.000
cde	0.250	0.247	0.256	0.240	0.256	0.250	0.101
MNSs							
MS	0.097	0.136	0.091	0.189	0.158	0.126	0.110
Ms	0.403	0.346	0.339	0.322	0.336	0.348	0.314
NS	0.203	0.108	0.078	0.071	0.092	0.125	0.108
Ns	0.297	0.410	0.492	0.418	0.414	0.401	0.468
Duffy							
Fy^a	0.224	0.098	0.215	0.188	0.133	0.221	NT
$Fy^b + Fy$	0.776	0.902	0.785	0.812	0.867	0.779	NT
Diego							
Di^a	0.004	0.014	0.008	0.015	0.014	0.005	0.020
Di^b	0.996	0.986	0.992	0.985	0.986	0.995	0.980
Kell							
K	0.008	0.000	0.013	0.013	0.005	0.010	0.000
k	0.992	1.000	0.987	0.987	0.995	0.990	1.000
Kidd							
Jk^a	0.722	0.844	0.883	NT	NT	0.770	NT
$Jk^b + JK$	0.278	0.156	0.117	NT	NT	0.230	NT

[a] NT, Not tested.

Table 9. Blood Group Gene Frequency Distribution among St. Vincentian
Populations[a]

System and allele	Sandy Bay Carib	Owia		Fancy		Total Carib	Total Creole
		Carib	Creole	Carib	Creole		
ABO							
A_1	0.056	0.033	0.111	0.000	0.121	0.044	0.117
A_2	0.095	0.076	0.024	0.115	0.086	0.090	0.064
B	0.086	0.109	0.088	0.000	0.092	0.086	0.110
O	0.763	0.782	0.777	0.885	0.700	0.780	0.710
Rhesus							
CDe	0.166	0.112	0.083	0.152	0.000	0.147	0.000
cDE	0.314	0.286	0.104	0.391	0.218	0.312	0.198
CdE	0.004	0.019	0.000	0.000	0.000	0.008	0.000
Cde	0.000	0.000	0.000	0.000	0.089	0.000	0.079
cde	0.269	0.134	0.000	0.186	0.128	0.220	0.148
cDe	0.247	0.450	0.813	0.217	0.566	0.313	0.575
MNSs							
MS	0.052	0.075	0.086	0.056	0.036	0.059	0.048
Ms	0.388	0.328	0.476	0.444	0.440	0.373	0.427
NS	0.087	0.170	0.060	0.118	0.069	0.118	0.073
Ns	0.473	0.438	0.378	0.382	0.455	0.450	0.452
Kell							
K	0.009	0.000	0.000	0.000	0.008	0.005	0.005
k	0.991	1.000	1.000	1.000	0.992	0.995	0.995
Diego							
Di^a	NT	NT	NT	0.000	0.000	NT	NT
Di^b	NT	NT	NT	1.000	1.000	NT	NT

[a] NT, Not tested.

incidence of CDe, 16.6%, while Fancy Creoles totally lack this chromosomal segment. Perplexing exceptions are the Punta Gorda Caribs, who also lack CDe despite the high proportion of Amerindian genes in their gene pool. The most likely explanation for this genetic omission from their gene pool revolves around the small-sized founder populations that migrated from Honduras to colonize the Belizian coast.

The MNSs system reflects the bi- or triracial origins of the Black Caribs and Creoles. The incidence of MS is lowest in West Africa, 8–12%, high in Europe, 25–27%, and relatively high among the Amerindians of South America, 17–33%. The Black Caribs and Creoles range between 4 and 19%, with the St. Vincent Island communities exhibiting lower MS frequencies and Punta Gorda Caribs possessing the highest frequencies. The NS haplotype is rare among West

African populations and is of intermediate incidence among South American populations. Yet the Black Carib populations exhibit an exceptionally high frequency of *NS*, with a range of 41–47%. In Chapter 15, Custodio *et al.* attribute a frequency of 55.64% to Roatan, well outside the observed Black Carib *NS* range. They explain these high frequencies of *NS* by invoking genetic drift as the most likely cause. A special case of genetic drift, founder effect, is the most probable cause of the gene frequency fluctuation. Roatan, in the Bay Islands, served as a stepping-stone for the forced transplantation of the Black Caribs from St. Vincent to Honduras. The deported Black Caribs may have numbered as few as 2000 persons. Thus, the founding population of Roatan may have been miniscule, since most of those deported from St. Vincent did not remain on the Bay Islands after 1800.

A few S^uS^u phenotypes were observed both on St. Vincent Island and in Central American populations. Two S^uS^u Creoles and one S^uS^u Black Carib from Stann Creek exhibit the rare African variant. In addition, one S^uS^u Black Carib was identified from Sandy Bay. In Chapter 15, Custodio and his colleagues note the detection of five subjects with the S^uS^u phenotype out of 138 sampled from Punta Gorda. Firschein (1961), while investigating differential fertility in HbAS females, identified a total of seven individuals with the S^uS^u phenotype from Stann Creek, Belize. In all of the studies reporting S^uS^u values to date (Mourant *et al.*, 1976), this phenotype is rare and apparently restricted to African groups or those who had originated in Africa.

Due to the unavailability of Duffy antisera and the poor condition of the specimens upon their arrival from St. Vincent Island, some of the populations were tested only by a single Duffy antiserum (Fy^a), while others were not phenotyped for the Duffy system. Only the blood specimens from Stann Creek Caribs and Belize City Creoles were tested for both Fy^a and Fy^b, thus revealing the African *Fy* allele. There is a significant difference in the presence of the *Fy* allele when Stann Creek Caribs are compared to Belize City Creoles (84.66 to 51.51%). The *Fy* percentage observed in Stann Creek closely approximates the 85.80% *Fy* allelic frequency in Punta Gorda (see Chapter 15). Custodio and his colleagues report considerable variation of the *Fy* allele in Honduras, from 77.69% in Limon to 93.22% in Roatan. The low incidence of *Fy* in Belize City could in part be a result of the eradication of mosquitoes in the urban area, thus reducing the selective pressures associated with malaria. In addition, the observed variation at this genetic locus may have been influenced by a founder effect or random fluctuations due to the small effective size of populations.

In the Diego blood group system, the Di^a allele is often used as a marker gene for the detection of Amerindian gene flow. As expected, the Black Carib communities exhibit higher frequencies of Di^a than do the Creole populations. It is interesting to note that although the Creole population is an amalgam of West African and European components, and that neither ancestral gene pool contains the Di^a allele, both the Belize City and Stann Creek Creoles exhibit low incidences of Di^a. This allele could have been introduced into these gene pools through marriage with either Black Caribs or Maya Indians from the surrounding mountainous regions of Belize.

The range of observed variability for the Kidd system (Jk^a allele) is relatively narrow, 72–88% among the Black Carib and Creole populations of Belize. Livingston and St. Vincent populations could not be tested. Roatan, as described in Chapter 15, falls outside the Belizean range, with a Jk^a incidence of 59.16%. The Jk^a frequencies observed in Belize are similar to those in West Africa. However, Dominican Caribs resemble the Roatan Black Caribs more closely than do the Caribs of Belize.

3.2. Serum Proteins

Albumin Mexico (Al^M) is found at low frequencies in the mainland Black Carib and Creole populations, but is absent in the St. Vincent communities. Apparently the presence of Al^M in Black Caribs of Belize is a result of gene flow from Central American Indian groups into the Carib gene pool. The Al^M variant could not have been introduced by the Carib or Arawak Indians, since this allele is a Central American marker and does not exist among South American indigenous groups. The economic and social contacts between Maya Indians and the Black Caribs and Creoles of Stann Creek, Punta Gorda, and Belize City has resulted in gene flow of low magnitude between the groups. The Livingston Black Carib community is more isolated geographically from Amerindian groups, a fact reflected in the extremely low incidence of Al^M. Weymes and Gershowitz in Chapter 14, describe albumin variants in Hopkins, an isolated Black Carib community of Belize. They detected only 0.5% of Al^M in a community that has little contact with Amerindians.

The presence of specific marker genes such as Al^M permits the critical examination of ethnohistorical controversies and questions concerning population dynamics. Thus Al^M allowed the resolution of the question concerning the reproductive isolation of the Black Carib gene pool *vis-à-vis* the Maya Indians. Firschein (1961) has argued that the Black Carib gene pool did not intermix with the surrounding Amerindian groups. Kerns (see Chapter 6) presented marital documentary evidence in support of the Black Carib more "catholic" mate selection patterns.

The haptoglobin-1 allele (Hp^1) is found at high frequency in West African populations south of the Sahara, but at lower frequencies among the Bushmen of the Kalahari. In this study, the Black Carib and Creole populations of Central American and St. Vincent Island exhibit an Hp^1 range of 51–69%. In addition, the African Hp^{1M} allele occurs at a high frequency of 12.8% among the Black Caribs of Owia. Surprisingly, the Hp2-1M phenotype was observed neither in Punta Gorda Caribs nor in Sandy Bay Caribs. Custodio *et al.* (Chapter 15) observed the Hp2-1M phenotype at 4.5% in Punta Gorda, Belize and 6.4% in

Table 10. *Allelic Frequencies of Serum Protein Polymorphisms in Population Samples from Belize and Guatemala*[a]

| System and allele | Belize | | | | | | Guatemala |
| | Belize City Creole | Stann Creek | | Punta Gorda Carib | Total Carib | Total Creole | Livingston Carib |
		Carib	Creole				
Albumin							
Al^A	0.988	0.989	0.993	0.987	0.988	0.991	0.995
Al^M	0.012	0.011	0.007	0.013	0.012	0.009	0.005
Haptoglobin							
Hp^1	0.464	0.531	0.563	0.561	0.554	0.531	0.596
Hp^2	0.476	0.446	0.418	0.439	0.446	0.469	0.394
Hp^{1M}	0.060	0.023	0.019	0.000	0.000	0.000	0.010
Transferrin							
Tf^B	0.000	0.003	0.000	0.000	0.002	0.000	0.000
Tf^C	0.936	0.967	0.944	0.983	0.973	0.947	0.973
Tf^D	0.064	0.030	0.056	0.017	0.025	0.053	0.027
Group-specific component							
Gc^1	0.882	0.880	0.908	0.865	0.874	0.890	0.895
Gc^2	0.118	0.120	0.092	0.135	0.126	0.110	0.105
Ceruloplasmin							
Cp^A	0.065	0.044	0.027	0.028	0.037	0.046	0.022
Cp^B	0.931	0.953	0.973	0.970	0.960	0.951	0.978
Cp^C	0.004	0.003	0.000	0.002	0.003	0.002	0.000
Properdin factor B (Bf)							
Bf^S	NT	0.523	0.537	0.471	0.470	0.537	0.385
Bf^F	NT	0.372	0.389	0.445	0.437	0.389	0.523
$Bf^{S0.7}$	NT	0.002	0.004	0.000	0.002	0.004	0.004
Bf^{F1}	NT	0.103	0.070	0.084	0.091	0.070	0.088

[a] NT, Not tested.

Limon, Honduras. Although Custodio *et al.* had sampled Punta Gorda in 1978 and the University of Kansas group studied the same community 2 years earlier, the gene frequency concordance was close. The Hp2-1M phenotype was observed in six out of 133 subjects during the 1978 sample and nine out of 231 during the 1976 field study. A comparison of the Hp^1 allele frequency indicates that the sampling error, despite different sample sizes, is not significant, 56 versus 52%.

The allelic variation in the group-specific component (Gc) of the Black Caribs and Creoles is intermediate in frequency between West African and Amerindian populations. The degree of observed genetic variation is relatively

Table 11. Serum Protein Gene Frequency Distribution among Communities of St. Vincent Island

System and allele	Sandy Bay		Owia		Fancy		Total Carib	Total Creole
	Carib	Creole	Carib	Creole	Carib	Creole		
Albumin								
Al^A	1.000	1.000	1.000	1.000	1.000	1.000	1.000	1.000
Group-specific component								
Gc^1	0.896	0.967	0.756	0.906	0.869	0.892	0.852	0.905
Gc^2	0.094	0.033	0.224	0.094	0.105	0.081	0.134	0.076
Gc^{Ab}	0.010	0.000	0.020	0.000	0.026	0.027	0.014	0.019
Gc^{1S}	0.496	0.143	0.328	0.115	0.306	0.215	0.430	0.192
Gc^{1F}	0.385	0.821	0.406	0.770	0.555	0.681	0.406	0.712
Gc^2	0.107	0.036	0.242	0.115	0.111	0.076	0.148	0.076
Gc^{Ab}	0.012	0.000	0.024	0.000	0.028	0.028	0.016	0.020
Transferrin								
Tf^C	1.000	1.000	0.974	0.974	1.000	0.993	0.992	0.991
Tf^{D1}	0.000	0.000	0.026	0.026	0.000	0.007	0.008	0.009
Haptoglobin								
Hp^1	0.685	0.625	0.439	0.445	0.579	0.413	0.557	0.437
Hp^{1M}	0.000	0.000	0.128	0.083	0.079	0.094	0.070	0.084
Hp^2	0.315	0.375	0.433	0.472	0.342	0.493	0.373	0.479
Properdin factor B								
S	0.510	0.600	0.507	0.400	0.450	0.342	0.504	0.388
F	0.323	0.300	0.401	0.567	0.400	0.562	0.354	0.525
F_1	0.153	0.100	0.086	0.033	0.150	0.096	0.132	0.087
S_{07}	0.014	0.000	0.007	0.000	0.000	0.000	0.010	0.000

narrow for this locus, with Gc^1 ranging between 75.6 and 90.8%. One interesting note is that the Gc Aborigine (Gc^{Ab}) variant was observed only on St. Vincent Island populations, with this variant occurring at 2.7% in Fancy. Considering the geographical distribution of this allele, it is likely that when the Black Carib gene pool was forceably subdivided by the British in 1797, with the major portion being deported, those individuals with Gc^{Ab} apparently escaped deportation and founded the communities of Sandy Bay, Owia, and Fancy.

Isoelectric focusing (IEF) of the group-specific component (Gc) expands the incidence of common alleles from two (Gc^1 and Gc^2) to three (Gc^{1S}, Gc^{1F}, and Gc^2) and enhances the identification of numerous rare alleles (see Tables 13 and 14). This increase in the number of alleles distinguishes most of the world populations by placing them into distinct clusters. Dykes *et al.* (1983), following the graphical representation method of Constans *et al.* (1978), plotted an assortment of world populations on the basis of the relative frequencies of Gc^{1S} and

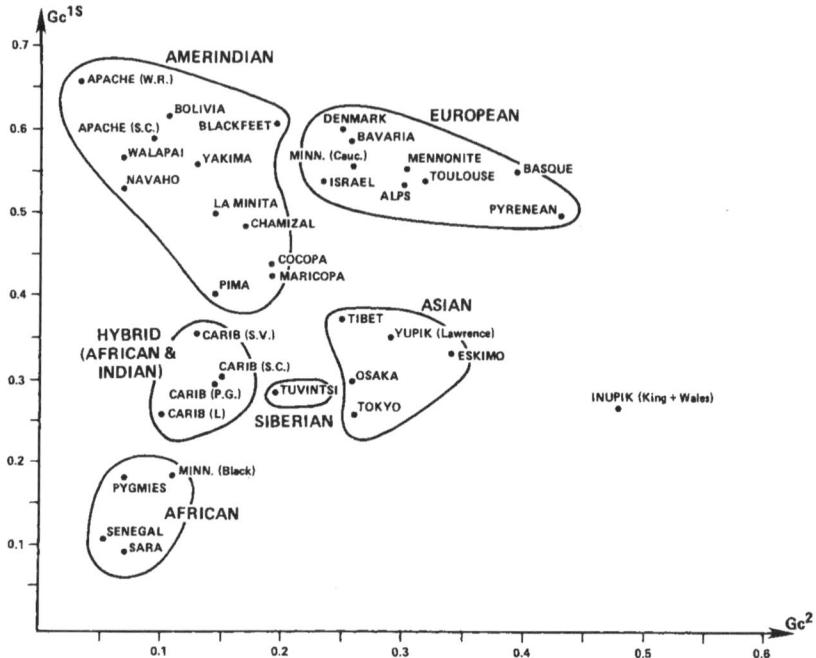

FIGURE 1. A plot of the frequencies of Gc^{1S} versus Gc^2 alleles for various human populations. After Dykes *et al.* (1983).

Gc^2 alleles. The Black Caribs form a tight cluster intermediate between the Amerindian and African groups. Within the Black Carib cluster, the St. Vincent populations gravitated toward the Amerindians, while Livingston Caribs more closely resembled the African grouping (see Fig. 1).

Although polymorphic, the ceruloplasmin locus does not appear to be informative with regard to population affinities. Although few data are available, the worldwide distribution for ceruloplasmin varies between 87 and 100% for the Cp^B allele. The five Black Carib and Creole communities tested for ceruloplasmin vary totally by only 5% (93–98%).

High Bf^S allelic frequencies, 95% and greater, identify the Amerindian populations of the New World. Similarly, frequencies of the Bf^F allele in the 50–60% range are observed in African groups. Thus, African–Amerindian hybrid groups should exhibit intermediate frequencies of both Bf^F and Bf^S. When the frequencies of these two alleles are plotted, a cluster of Black Carib and Creole populations is revealed, with their relative positions defined by the degree of African or Amerindian ancestry. Sandy Bay Caribs exhibit the highest incidence of Bf^{F1} alleles, although the other alleles at this locus better fit the Carib pattern. The Amerindian marker allele $Bf^{S0.45}$ has not been identified in any of these populations.

Table 12. Allelic Frequencies of Red Blood Cell Protein Polymorphisms in Population Samples from Belize and Guatemala

| System and allele | Belize | | | | | | Guatemala |
| | Belize City Creole | Stann Creek | | Punta Gorda Carib | Total Carib | Total Creole | Livingston Carib |
		Carib	Creole				
Hemoglobin							
Hb^A	0.949	0.917	0.929	0.945	0.928	0.941	0.923
Hb^S	0.043	0.080	0.071	0.053	0.069	0.052	0.077
Hb^C	0.008	0.003	0.000	0.002	0.003	0.007	0.000
Acid phosphatase							
p^A	0.197	0.183	0.201	0.146	0.167	0.190	0.175
p^B	0.799	0.804	0.779	0.836	0.817	0.799	0.783
p^C	0.000	0.000	0.000	0.002	0.001	0.000	0.000
p^R	0.004	0.013	0.020	0.017	0.015	0.011	0.042
Phosphoglucomutase							
PGM^1_1	0.814	0.838	0.767	0.850	0.843	0.812	0.879
PGM^2_1	0.186	0.162	0.233	0.150	0.157	0.188	0.121
PGM^1_2	1.000	0.997	1.000	0.993	0.996	1.000	1.000
PGM^2_2	0.000	0.003	0.000	0.007	0.004	0.000	0.000
Phosphogluconate dehydrogenase							
PGD^A	0.940	0.978	0.954	0.960	0.971	0.950	0.983
PGD^C	0.060	0.022	0.046	0.040	0.029	0.050	0.017
Adenosine diaminase							
ADA^1	0.996	0.989	0.993	0.992	0.990	0.996	1.000
ADA^2	0.004	0.011	0.007	0.008	0.010	0.004	0.000
Adenylate kinase							
AK^1	0.972	0.973	0.955	0.971	0.972	0.970	0.988
AK^2	0.028	0.024	0.045	0.029	0.026	0.030	0.012
AK^3	0.000	0.003	0.000	0.000	0.002	0.000	0.000
Esterase D							
ESD^1	0.961	0.938	0.885	0.937	0.937	0.935	0.912
ESD^2	0.039	0.062	0.115	0.063	0.063	0.065	0.088

3.3. Erythrocytic Protein Variation

Standard, electrophoretically based screening of the PGM_1 locus contains little information with regards to Black Carib population affinities. The PGM^1_1 allele ranges between 75 and 89% in Amerindian, European, and African populations. The incidence of this allele among the Black Caribs and Creoles of Central America and St. Vincent Island varies between 83 and 88%. Weymes and

Table 13. Red Cell Protein Gene Frequency Distribution among Communities of
St. Vincent Island

System and allele	Sandy Bay		Owia		Fancy		Total Carib	Total Creole
	Carib	Creole	Carib	Creole	Carib	Creole		
Acid phosphatase								
p^A	0.141	0.133	0.148	0.217	0.185	0.075	0.147	0.115
p^B	0.853	0.867	0.852	0.783	0.796	0.918	0.847	0.885
p^R	0.006	0.000	0.000	0.000	0.000	0.007	0.004	0.000
p^D	0.000	0.000	0.000	0.000	0.019	0.000	0.002	0.000
Esterase D								
ESD^1	0.903	0.929	0.958	1.000	0.825	0.980	0.912	0.978
ESD^2	0.097	0.071	0.042	0.000	0.175	0.020	0.088	0.022
Phosphoglucomutase-1								
PGM_1^{1+}	0.447	0.618	0.488	0.500	0.381	0.533	0.455	0.538
PGM_1^{1-}	0.382	0.235	0.359	0.200	0.405	0.230	0.376	0.225
PGM_1^{2+}	0.124	0.088	0.141	0.220	0.214	0.197	0.137	0.186
PGM_1^{2-}	0.047	0.059	0.012	0.080	0.000	0.040	0.032	0.051
Hemoglobin								
Hb^A	0.988	0.858	0.983	1.000	0.952	0.845	0.983	0.878
Hb^S	0.006	0.071	0.017	0.000	0.048	0.128	0.013	0.095
Hb^C	0.006	0.071	0.000	0.000	0.000	0.027	0.004	0.027
Adenylate kinase								
AK^1	0.997	1.000	1.000	1.000	1.000	0.987	0.998	0.991
AK^2	0.003	0.000	0.000	0.000	0.000	0.013	0.002	0.009
6-Phosphogluconate dehyrogenase								
6PGD	0.997	0.967	0.989	0.967	NT	1.000	0.995	0.971
$6PGD^C$	0.003	0.033	0.011	0.033	–	0.000	0.005	0.029

Gershowitz in Chapter 14 record a higher incidence of PGM_1^1 allele of 89% for
Stann Creek than the value reported in this chapter. Ferrell et al. (1978) similarly observed little variation at this locus for black populations of Panama with
PGM_1^1 varying from 78 to 84% (see Tables 12 and 13).

In contrast to the standard electrophoretically based phenotypes, isoelectric
forcusing (IEF) of the PGM_1 locus reveals greater variation. The IEF method
detects a total of four alleles instead of two, $1+$, $1-$, $2+$, and $2-$, as well as a
number of rare variants. Table 14 summarizes the frequencies of the four alleles
in selected Black Carib populations. A plot of the relative frequencies of PGM
$1+$ versus $1-$ and $2+$ versus $2-$ reveals a Black Carib cluster (see Dykes et al.,
1983; and Fig. 2). As expected, the Livingston Caribs show greater genetic
affinity toward the Old World populations, while the combined Black Caribs of
St. Vincent more closely resemble indigenous New World groups (see Table 14).

Table 14. Isoelectric Focusing Subtype Distribution in Black Carib and Creole Populations of Belize and St. Vincent

Population	Number tested	Gc Locus				PGM Locus			
		1S	1F	2	Rare variant	1 +	1 −	2 +	2 +
Livinston	215	0.256	0.637	0.107	0.01	0.645	0.230	0.122	0.003
Stann Creek	217	0.312	0.536	0.152	0.0	0.000	0.000	0.000	0.000
Punta Gorda	274	0.304	0.553	0.143	0.0	0.567	0.283	0.125	0.025
St. Vincent	311	0.360	0.498	0.126	0.016	0.479	0.330	0.158	0.033

The acid phosphatase locus p exhibits considerable variation among Black Carib and Creole groups. The p^A allele occurs from 7.5 to 20%, while p^B ranges from 78 to 92%. The West African marker p^R, normally observed from 1 to 4% in blacks, is either extremely rare or absent in St. Vincent Island populations. This low incidence may be due to the small numbers of St. Vincent Caribs who avoided the British deportation of 1797 and gave issue to the subsequent generations.

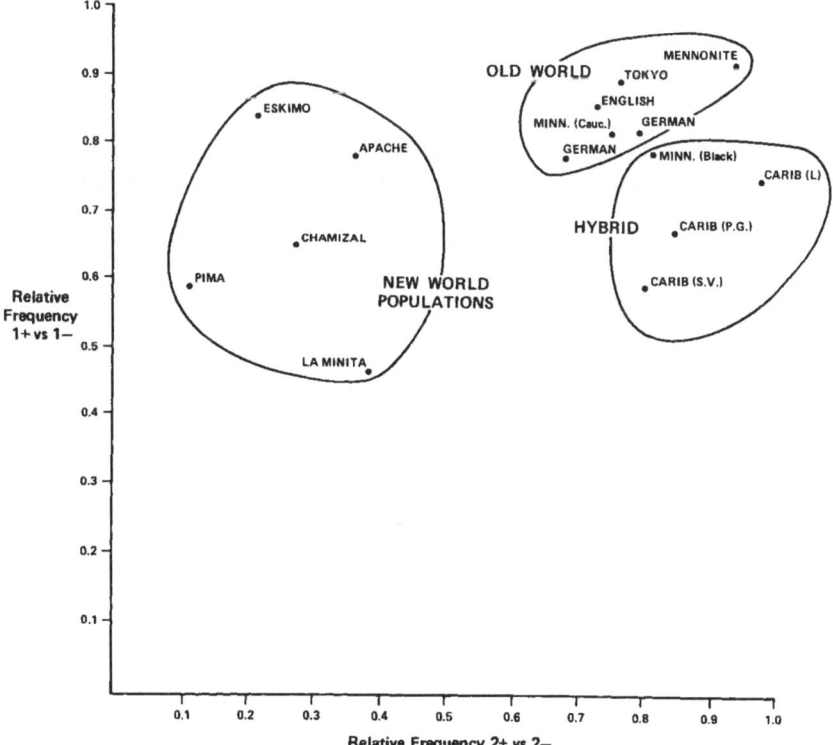

FIGURE 2. A plot of the relative frequencies of *PGM* 1 + versus 1 − alleles on the ordinate and the relative frequencies of *PGM* 2 + versus 2 − on the abscissa.

Table 15. Absolute Heterozygostiy D for the Gc and PGM
Loci Utilizing Conventional Electrophoresis and IEF

	D	
Carib populations	Conventional	IEF
St. Vincent	0.27	0.63
Livingston	0.21	0.52
Punta Gorda	0.25	0.58
Mean	0.24	0.58

The Caribs of Dominica described by Harvey *et al.* (1961) totally lack the p^R allele. However, the black Panamanians investigated by Ferrell *et al.* (1978) exhibit gene frequencies for p^A, p^B, and p^R comparable to those observed among Black Carib groups.

Although the genetic systems for adenylate kinase, esterase D, and 6-phosphogluconate dehydrogenase are polymorphic among the Black Caribs, these systems are not highly informative as to genetic affinities or degrees of admixture: EsD^1, AK^1, and PGD^C alleles occur close to unity among Black Caribs and Creoles.

3.4. Genetic Heterozygosity

Comparisons of absolute heterozygosity levels for St. Vincent, Livingston, and Punta Gorda for *Gc* and *PGM* loci based upon conventional electrophoresis versus IEF reveal more than a doubling of heterozygosity (see Table 15). The mean heterozygosity level for these two loci is 0.24 for standard electrophoretically based alleles and 0.58 for IEF-measured genetic variation. Thus, measures of heterozygosity and genetic variation computed by standard techniques should be reassessed if IEF is utilized.

3.5. Admixture Estimates

The ethnohistory of the Black Caribs suggests the existence of a biracial hybrid population. St. Vincent Island was an amalgam of Carib/Arawak Indians and West African slaves. The relative contributions of the two components cannot be ascertained from historical records. Phenotypically the Black Caribs of Central America closely resemble West African blacks. However, the Black Caribs on St. Vincent are less highly pigmented and exhibit some Amerindian as well as African morphological traits.

As a result, our first admixture estimates assumed a biracial model and were computed by the true least squares method. Eight genetic loci (ABO, Rhesus, MNSs, Duffy, Diego, Kell, Kidd, and hemoglobin) and 26 alleles were

Table 16. Proportion of African versus Carawak Admixture
in Black Carib Gene Pool

Carib population	Percent	
	African	Carawak
Livingston	75	25
Stann Creek	67	33
Punta Gorda	70	30
Sandy Bay	46	53
Owia	61	39
Limon	64	36

utilized in these estimates. The proportion of African versus Carawak (an average of gene frequencies of Arawak and Venezuelan Caribs) is given in Table 16.

These estimates of m indicate that Livingston has the highest proportion of African genes, while Sandy Bay has the lowest. These figures suggest that the founders of Sandy Bay, who escaped deportation, were much more Indian than those who were deported. Another explanation is that the original Black Carib gene pool of St. Vincent contained a high proportion of Amerindian alleles and that this proportion diminished as the population spread into Central America and interbred with the African colonies along the coast. This hypothesis is not contradicted by the Owia estimates, betause it is a hybrid Creole—Black Carib community with considerable gene flow between these ethnic groups.

The immunoglobulin typing of the sera from these communities revealed the presence of some European allotypes, such as Gm^{fb}. An attempt was made to estimate the proportion of European admixture by utilizing a triracial model. Unfortunately, the results failed to coincide with the estimates based upon Gms, and the European component was highly inflated at the expense of the Amerindian parental group.

4. Conclusions

The blood genetic markers clearly support the ethnohistorically based hypotheses that the Black Caribs are primarily an Amerindian—African amalgam while the Creoles are an African—European hybrid group. It is obvious from the genetic data that some gene flow occurred between these two groups and that Central American indigenous populations contributed genetically in the foundation of the Black Carib gene pool. It is likely that the Black Carib gene pool of St. Vincent Island contained a greater proportion of Amerindian genes at the time of British deportation. An alternative explanation for the observed gene frequency distributions is that the more "Indian" individuals escaped deportation while those of greater African ancestry were shipped to Roatan.

This chapter attests to the usefulness of isoelectric focusing (IEF) and immunoglobulins (*Gm* and *Km* loci) in disentangling problems of gene flow and ethnohistory. IEF almost doubles the observed genetic heterozygosity in protein systems screened by standard electrophoresis. This new method also exponentially increases the information on population affinities. Similarly, the *Gm* markers provide the most reliable basis for measuring gene flow of African, European, and Amerindian groups. This genetic locus is highly informative in that certain allotypes are unique to specific geographic populations. The combination of IEF with standard electrophoretic and serological techniques provides us with a powerful tool kit for measuring population affinities and gene flow.

References

Chakraborty, R., 1975, Estimation of race admixture – A new method, *Am. J. Phys. Anthropol.* **42**:507–512.

Constans, J., Cleve, H., Jaeger, G., Quilici, J. C., and Palisson, M. J., 1978, Analysis of the Gc polymorphism in human populations by isoelectric focusing on polyacrylamide gels. Demonstration of subtypes of the Gc^1 allele and of additional Gc variants, *Hum Genet.* **41**:53–60.

Crawford, M. H., Workman, P. L., Mclean, C., and Lees, F. C., 1976, Admixture estimates and selection in Tlaxcala, in *The Tlaxcaltecans: Prehistory, Demography, Morphology and Genetics* (M. H. Crawford, ed.), pp. 161–168, University of Kansas Publications in Anthropology, no. 17, Lawrence, Kansas.

Crawford, M. N., Gottman, F. E., and Gottman, C. A., 1970, Microplate system for routine use in blood bank laboratories, *Transfusion* **10**:258–263.

Dykes, D. D., and Polesky, H. F., 1976, The usefulness of serum protein and erythrocyte enzyme polymorphisms in paternity testing, *Am. J. Clin. Pathol.* **65**:982–986.

Dykes, D. D., and Polesky, H. F., 1980, Properdin factor B (Bf) as an exclusion determinate in parentage testing, *Hum. Genet.* **30**:286–290.

Dykes, D. D., and Polesky, H. F., 1981a, Isoelectric focusing of PGM (E.C. 2.7.5.1.) on agarose: Application to cases of disputed parentage, *Am. J. Clin. Pathol.* **75**:708–711.

Dykes, D. D., and Polesky, H. F., 1981b, Isoelectric focusing of Gc (vitamin D binding globulin) in parentage testing, *Hum. Genet.* **58**:174–175.

Dykes, D. D., Crawford, M. H., and Polesky, H. G., 1983, Population distribution in North and Central America of PGM_1 and Gc subtypes as determined by isoelectric focusing (IEF), *Am. J. Phys. Anthropol.* **62**:137–145.

Ferrell, R. E., Nunez, A., Bertin, T., La Barthe, D. R., and Schull, W. J., 1978, The blacks of Panama: Their genetic diversity as assessed by 15 inherited biochemical systems, *Am. J. Phys. Anthropol.* **48**:269–276.

Firschein, I. L., 1961, Population dynamics of the sickle-cell trait in the Black Caribs of British Honduras, Central America, *Am. J. Hum. Genet.* **13**:233–254.

Harpending, H. C., and Chasko, W. J., 1976, Heterozygosity and population structure in Southern Africa, in *The Measures of Man: Methodologies in Biological Anthropology.* (E. Giles and J. S. Friedlaender, eds.), pp. 214–229, Peabody Museum Press, Cambridge.

Harvey, R. G., Godber, M. J., Kopec, A. C., Mourant, A. E., and Tills, D., 1961, Frequency of genetic traits in the Caribs of Dominica, *Hum. Biol.* **41**:342.

Karp, G. W., and Sutton, H. E., 1967, Some new phenotypes of human red cell acid phosphatase, *Am. J. Hum. Genet.* **19**:54–62.

Kreiger, H., Morton, N. E., Mi, M. P., Azevedo, E., Freire-Maia, A., and Yasuda, N., 1963, Racial admixture in North-eastern Brazil, *Ann. Hum. Genet.* **29**:113–125.

McComb, M., and Bowman, B. H., 1969, Demonstration of inherited ceruloplasmin variants in human serum by acrylamide electrophoresis, *Texas Rep. Biol. Med.* **27**:769–772.

Mourant, A. E., Kopec, A. C., and Domanienska-Sobczak, K., 1976, *The distribution of the Human Blood Groups and Other Polymorphisms,* Oxford University Press, London.

Polesky, H. F., Rokala, D., and Huff, T., 1975, Serum proteins in paternity testing, in *Paternity Testing* (H. F. Polesky, ed.), pp. 30–44, Division of Educational Media Services, American Society of Clinical Pathologists, Chicago.

Reed, T. E. and Schull, W. J., 1968, A general maximum likelihood estimation program, *Am. J. Hum. Genet.* **20**:579–580.

Roberts, D. F., and Hiorns, R. W., 1962, The dynamics of racial admixture, *Am. J. Hum. Genet.* **14**:261–277.

Roberts, D. F., and Hiorns, R. W. 1965. Methods of analysis of genetic composition of a hybrid population, *Hum. Biol.* **37**:38–43.

Spencer, N., Hopkinson, D. A., and Harris, H., 1964, Phosphoglucomutase polymorphism in man, *Nature* **204**:742–745.

Yunis, J., 1969, *Biochemical Methods in Red Cell Genetics,* Academic, New York.

17

Abnormal Hemoglobins among the Black Caribs

RAMON CUSTODIO and R. G. HUNTSMAN

1. Introduction

The Black Caribs live in partially or completely isolated communities along the coast of Belize, Guatemala, and Honduras. The most numerous exist in Honduras, where there are at least 54 coastal settlements of Black Caribs (who are called Morenales) situated on the Atlantic Coast between the Motagua River to the west and the Tinto (or Negro) River to the east (Fig. 1).

Despite their move to the New World, these people have remained until recently under heavy malarial pressure both from *Plasmodium vivax* and *Plasmodium falciparum*. Despite attempts at malarial eradication, total elimination of this disease does not appear to have been attained.

Sickle-cell-trait heterozygote carriers have been shown to be more resistant to malarial infestation than "normal" homozygotes. In particular, children who are sickle cell carriers appear resistant to cerebral malaria — a lethal complication of falciparum malaria (Raper, 1956). The sickle cell carrier rate of the Black Caribs would clearly be of interest to compare with other black populations who have not been exposed to malaria since their arrival in the New World.

So far, three surveys of sickle cell carriers have been carried out. McGavack and German (1944) examined "Carib Indians" in San Juan, a village near Tela (Fig. 1) in Honduras and estimated the sickling rate to be 8% in a sample of 300. Firschein (1961) carried out a second survey. He reported that the sickling

RAMON CUSTODIO • Laboratorio Custodio, S. de R. L. Pathologia Clinica y Anatomia Pathologica, 1229 Tegucigalpa, D. C., Honduras. R. G. HUNTSMAN • Canadian Red Cross, Blood Transfusion Services, St. John's, Newfoundland, Canada A1B 4A4.

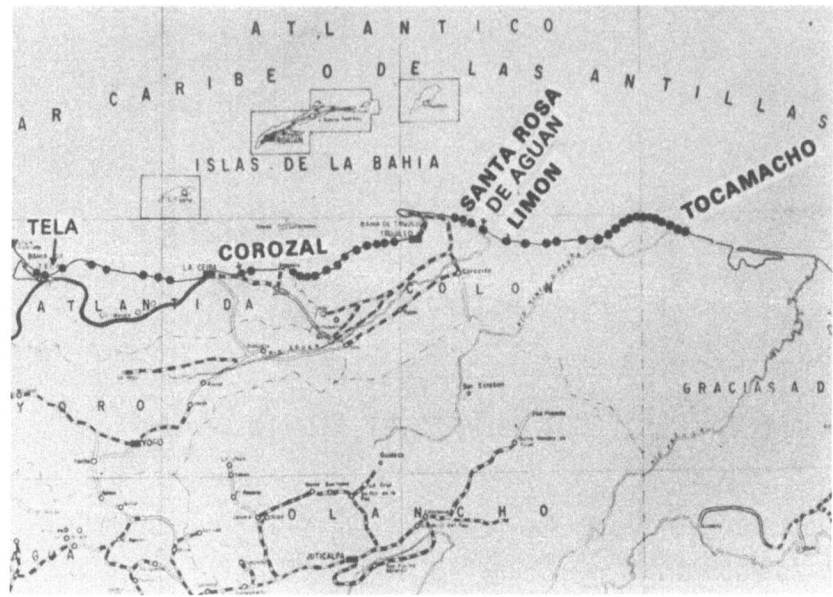

FIGURE 1. Black Carib settlements in Honduras.

rate in five Black Carib settlements in Belize was 24% in the 705 people he examined, "the highest sickle cell trait frequency yet found in the New World."

In addition to reporting the unexpectedly high sickle cell carrier rate, Firschein drew conclusions from demographic data concerning the maintenance of the sickle cell trait among the Black Carib communities. He found that mothers with sickle cell trait had significantly larger families than controls. He was then able to demonstrate that this difference in family size was sufficient to maintain the high sickle cell carrier rates in the communities that he studied. Firschein also found that sickle cell carrier females had more male children than the control group of normal mothers, and, as one would therefore expect, the sickle cell carrier rate in males was slightly but not significantly higher than that found in females in the communities that he studied. A third and smaller survey of Black Caribs in Livingston, Guatemala, by Tejada *et al.* (1965) showed an 18.3% sickling rate in the 82 people examined.

The purpose of the work reported in this chapter was as follows:

1. To investigate the sickle cell carrier rate in selected Black Carib communities, including communities surveyed in Belize by Firschein. The presence of sickle cell hemoglobin would be confirmed using both electrophoresis at alkaline pH and a solubility test (Lehmann and Huntsman, 1974) based on the Itano solubility test. Neither the survey by McGavack and German nor that of Firschein meets the present-day standard for the recognition of sickle cell hemoglobin, which demands the demonstration of both characteristic electrophoretic mobility

and insolubility in the reduced form (the latter being tested either by the classic sickling test or by a "solubility test"). The purpose of using the two techniques is to distinguish between sickle cell hemoglobin and other abnormal hemoglobins, such as the hemoglobins collectively called D or G, which have similar electrophoretic properties at alkaline pH but lack the insolubility of sickle cell hemoglobin in the reduced form.

2. To investigate the sickle cell carrier rate in isolated but geographically closely situated Black Carib communities in Honduras. During the community visits in Honduras, blood samples were examined by the National Service for the Eradication of Malaria in Honduras. The findings could be correlated with the sickle cell carrier rate found in these communities. Blood specimens were also examined for anemia, and appropriate therapeutic action was then offered.

3. To survey in particular the Black Carib community on the island of Roatan. This community is of special interest, as it was on this island that the Black Caribs landed, and from there they subsequently dispersed to form their mainland settlements.

4. To test the findings of Firschein that the sickle cell carrier women give birth to more males than did control women and that the sickle cell trait is therefore more common in the male.

5. To study the fertility of Black Carib sickle cell carrier women in further Black Carib communities and compare the results found with normal women in the same community.

2. Methods

The data discussed in this chapter were collected in four Black Carib communities in Honduras: Corozal, Santa Rosa de Aguan, Limon, and Tocamacho. In addition, the authors surveyed the community of Punta Gorda on Roatan, where the Black Caribs originated, and two communities in Belize, Stann Creek and Seine Bight, which had been included in Firschein's 1961 study.

Sampling was limited to Garifuna-speaking individuals, the majority being school children, although additional door-to-door sampling was undertaken (especially in Limon and Punta Gorda) in order to give us an opportunity to examine older people. During such house visits it was common to find only the women at home, and this is demonstrated in the sex ratio of the samples obtained in adults in those two communities. As one of the aims of this survey was to collect fertility data on older women, we did not consider this situation to be disadvantageous. Whereas Firschein obtained his fertility data in part from mothers attending a children's clinic (and admits to a bias toward "mothers"), we preferred to rely totally on door-to-door visiting in order to include an unbiased sample of sterile women or mothers with few children among those investigated. Whereas Firschein states that a special effort was made to secure information as to the children born to mothers with the sickle cell trait, all our questioning was carried out prior to the testing of the blood sample. Although the end result is clearly a much smaller sample size of sickle-cell-trait mothers, we wished to avoid bias, which we believe to be inevitable if the hemoglobin type were known to the investigator prior to the eliciting of information.

Both of the authors, being practicing clinicians, were surprised that information from older women regarding the sex of a child who had died in early life was thought by Firschein to be unreliable. Unless one were dealing with a patient who was so old as to be senile, one would expect in practice to find elderly multiparous women, even in unsophisticated environments, capable of accurately recalling the sexes of their live births. Requestioning participants on subsequent occasions gave us confidence that Black Carib women gave obstetric histories as reliable as others we have encountered. Indeed, we were sufficiently encouraged by the certainty with which the sex of a stillborn was given that we decided (perhaps naively) to collect at the same time data on abortions and still-births. They were subsequently grouped under a single heading, as the dividing line between them (500 g weight) is arbitrary and impossible to ascertain retrospectively in an interview situation.

3. Results and Discussion

3.1. The Sickle Cell Carrier Rate in the Black Carib Communities

Table 1 shows the results obtained from the abnormal hemoglobin survey carried out in Honduras on the four mainland Black Carib village settlements, the village of Punta Gorda in Roatan, and in two settlements also visited by Firschein in Belize.

The overall sickle cell carrier rate of this survey came to 12.1% in the 1750 people sampled. This total figure lies closer to the accepted black North American sickling rate of 8–9% than to the remarkably high figure of 24% found by Firschein. It is, however, of interest that the highest sickle rate found in the present survey (18.9%) was in the community of Seign Bight, which was examined in Firschein's original sampling of these people. In contrast, a survey limited to the community of Santa Rosa de Aguan would have found a figure (6.1%) lower than that ascribed to black North Americans. The sickle cell carrier rate for Punta Gorda, Roatan (13.1%), is intermediate between the extreme results obtained for Honduras–Limon and Santa Rosa de Aguan.

Carriers of hemoglobin C are unusually uncommon (1.1% of our total sample). This figure is lower than that obtained by Firschein, who found 18 examples in his sample 605 (2.9%). Firschein found a single example of sickle cell hemoglobin C in his sample, whereas we found two in ours.

Table 1. Frequency of Sickle Cell Trait (AS), Homozygous Sickle Cell Disease (SS), Hemoglobin C Trait (AC), and Sickle Cell Hemoglobin C Disease (SC) in Honduran and Belizean Communities

	Total number	AS	SS	AC	SC
Honduras					
Corozal	293	31 (10.6%)	0 (0%)	0 (0%)	0 (0%)
Santa Rosa de Aguan	342	21 (6.1%)	0 (0%)	6 (1.8%)	0 (0%)
Limon	457	74 (16.2%)	4 (0.9%)	8 (1.8%)	0 (0%)
Tocamacho	209	17 (8.1%)	1 (0.5%)	0 (0%)	0 (0%)
Punta Gorda, Roatan	130	17 (13.1%)	1 (0.8%)	1 (0.8%)	0 (0%)
Belize					
Stann Creek	192	28 (14.6%)	0 (0%)	2 (1.0%)	2 (1.0%)
Seine Bight	127	24 (18.9%)	0 (0%)	2 (1.6%)	0 (0%)
Total	1750	212 (12.1%)	6 (0.3%)	19 (1.1%)	2 (0.1%)

We found six examples of sickle cell anemia, four of them in the sample of 457 from the community of Limon, which had a relatively high sickle cell carrier rate of 16.2%. The cases were found in school children, which is not surprising, since they formed a large percentage of the sample size (Table 2). The apparent absence of the homozygous disease state in adults could be accounted for by sampling bias and did not therefore permit us to offer any conclusions on the clinical severity of this disease in the Black Carib, particularly with regard to childhood mortality.

3.2. Correlation of Sickle Cell Carrier Rate in Communities with Malarial Infestation

Figures for the province of Colon were made available to us by the Society for the Eradication of Malaria in Honduras (Table 3) and show that the people of the area surveyed have been subjected to malarial infestation primarily by *Plasmodium vivax* but also by *Plasmodium falciparum*. The vectors responsible are *Anopheles albinamus* and *Anopheles darlingii*.

It is of interest that the samples taken from our 1972 and 1975 surveys show that in 1972 the infestation in two neighboring communities appeared to show a considerably heavier infestation in Limon than in Santa Rosa de Aguan. Of these two communities, Limon showed the higher sickle cell carrier rate, which was the reason that this community was later selected for the study of the fertility of the sickle cell carrier woman.

3.3. Sex Distribution of the Sickle Cell Trait

In contrast to Firchein's results, we found the overall sickle cell carrier rate to be 10.4% in the male and 13.3% in the female. If male preponderance is the

Table 2. The Sickle Cell Trait Carrier Frequency in the Seven Communities Surveyed Examined for Age and Sex[a]

Age	Corozal Male N	AS	Corozal Female N	AS	St. Rosa de Aguan Male N	AS	St. Rosa de Aguan Female N	AS	Limon Male N	AS	Limon Female N	AS	Tocamacho Male N	AS	Tocamacho Female N	AS	Punta Gorda Male N	AS	Punta Gorda Female N	AS	Stann Creek Male N	AS	Stann Creek Female N	AS	Seine Bight Male N	AS	Seine Bight Female N	AS
0–10	102	14	73	6	99	4	109	8	92	14	107	20	64	2	54	7	4	0	15	2	30	3	25	6	27	6	30	4
11–20	56	5	61	6	48	3	46	4	45	6	57	5	43	4	48	4	19	1	41	7	33	4	57	8	4	1	25	3
21–30	0	0	0	0	2	0	8	1	2	1	48	8	0	0	0	0	1	0	18	3	3	0	4	1	5	1	4	3
31–40	0	0	0	0	1	0	12	1	0	0	47	5	0	0	0	0	1	0	8	0	1	0	7	1	1	0	3	0
41–50	0	0	0	0	2	0	3	0	1	1	20	3	0	0	0	0	1	0	7	3	3	0	10	3	2	0	6	0
51–60	1	0	0	0	0	0	2	0	2	0	12	1	0	0	0	0	0	0	6	1	1	0	4	1	2	0	10	2
61+	0	0	0	0	4	0	6	0	4	2	20	8	0	0	0	0	1	0	8	0	4	0	10	1	4	2	4	2
Total	159	19	134	12	156	7	186	14	146	24	311	50	107	6	102	11	27	1	103	16	75	7	117	21	45	10	82	14

Total males and females sampled 1750
Total males samples 715
Total females samples 1035

Total AS males and females sampled 212 (12.11%)
Total AS males sampled 74 (10.4%)
Total AS females samples 138 (13.3%)

[a] N, Total number; AS, sickle cell trait carriers.

Table 3. Malaria Infestation in the Province of Colon, Honduras[a]

		Positive	
Year	Total examined	P. vivax	P. falciparum
1973	9,094	1516 (16.7%)	78 (0.86%)
1974	12,713	917 (7.2%)	2 (0.02%)
1975	15,222	3969 (26.1%)	47 (0.31%)
1976	13,870	5198 (37.5%)	46 (0.33%)
1977	14,397	5398 (37.5%)	108 (0.75%)
1978	15,526	1753 (11.3%)	104 (0.67%)

[a] Data kindly supplied by the society for the Eradication of Malaria in Honduras.

Table 4. Sickle Cell Carrier Rate (Divided by Sex) in the Seven Communities Surveyed[a]

	Sickle cell carrier rate, %		
Community	Total	Male	Female
Seine Bight	18.9	22.2	17.1
Limon	16.2	16.4	16.1
Stann Creek	14.6	9.3	17.9
Punta Gorda	13.1	3.7	15.5
Corozal	10.6	11.9	9.1
Tocamacho	8.1	5.6	10.8
Santa Rosa de Aguan	6.1	4.5	7.5
Total	12.1	10.5	13.3

[a] Extracted from Table 2.

result of the sickle cell carrier women giving birth to more sons than the normal women, one might expect the sex disparity to be highest in the communities with the highest sickle cell carrier rate.

The figures we obtained (Table 4) do not support the hypothesis that the sickle cell carrier rate in the male is higher than in the female.

3.4. Fertility of Women with the Sickle Cell Trait Compared with Normal Women

Firschein based his finding that women who were sickle cell carriers had more children than normal women on a considerably larger sample (89 women with the sickle cell trait) than was available for this study (23 women with the sickle cell trait). Because we were unaware of the sickle cell status of the women being questioned, we were unable to specially select sickle cell carrier mothers for inclusion in this aspect of the survey.

Table 5. Live Births, Living Children, and Number of Abortions and Stillbirths in Normal and Sickle Cell Carrier Women

Age	Number	Live birth per woman (average)			Living per woman (average)[a]			Abortions/stillbirths per woman (average)
		Male	Female	Total	Male	Female	Total	
AA								
40+	57	3.0	3.14	6.14	2.5	2.8	5.3	0.82
30–39	38	3.0	2.3	5.3	2.6	2.0	4.6	0.34
29–	63	1.18	1.22	2.4	1.13	1.08	2.21	0.41
AS								
40+	11	2.1	2.9	5.0	1.5	2.4	3.9	0.73
30–39	2	1.0	3.0	4.0	1.0	3.0	4.0	0.00
29–	10	0.6	0.8	1.4	0.5	0.8	1.3	0.20

[a] Living = alive or survived to age of 6 (see text).

Firschein divided the women examined into two groups: (1) 30 years and over and (2) 29 years and under. The younger group was limited to those who commenced childbearing before 1946 (the observations being made during visits between 1955 and 1957). He concluded that the majority of the mothers in the younger group would be between 30 and 40 years of age. For this reason we divided our data into the ages 40 years and over and 30–39 years; we also included a third category of mothers of 29 and under, so that the results are comparable with those of Firschein. Again, to allow comparison with Firschein's data, the total live births were recorded (living and dead) as well as those children who were living at the time of the survey or had died after reaching the age of 6, the latter group being categorized as "living." In addition, all women were questioned as to their number of abortions and stillbirths. Our data as submitted in Table 5 fail to demonstrate in our relatively small sample that the sickle cell trait carrier is more fertile. This is true whether fertility is measured as total live births, as children alive at the time of survey, or as those who survived to the age of 6.

Although all women, irrespective of marital status, were asked to cooperate in the fertility survey, single women were subsequently excluded. There were nine childless single women over the age of 18 who were tested and excluded. Six of these were between the ages of 19 and 23, and two of these were sickle cell trait carriers. The remaining three single childless women were aged 40, 50, and 75, and all carried normal adult hemoglobin. The authors did not feel it was reasonable to further question them to establish whether their marital status had any relation to infertility. No single women were found to have children, and, with the exception of one girl of 17, the youngest married women encountered were 18 years of age. Eight married women of age 30 and older out of a total of 108 had had no live births and might be considered sterile. One of these eight was a sickle cell trait carrier. Eight of 73 married women ranging in age from 17 to 29 had had no children, and four of these were sickle cell trait carriers. The majority of these young women were recently married, and, indeed, some were pregnant at the time of the survey.

3.5. The History of Abortions and Stillbirths

In the case of the more mature stillbirths, the sex was often known, and of the 95 abortions and stillbirths, 24% were stated to have been male and 23% to have been female. The normal mothers (85 stillbirths and miscarriages) reported 25% males and 21% females, and the sickle cell trait mothers (10 stillbirths and abortions) reported 20% males and 40% females.

4. Conclusion

We would like to emphasize the importance of the Black Carib communities to epidemiologists, geneticists, clinicians, and anthropologists. These people offer unique opportunites to collect data that may well throw further light on the complex factors responsible for maintaining the sickle cell carrier rate. The terrain and the isolation make malarial eradication extremely difficult. Other additional and perhaps subtle differences in the environment, as well as the influence of a founder effect and genetic drift, may all be playing a complex and yet to be elucidated role in producing the results descibed in this survey. We fully appreciate that, whatever results are subsequently obtained, the pioneering work of Firschein in the 1950s was primarily responsible for drawing our attention to the potential for further investigation that exists in this area of Central America.

References

Firschein, I. L., 1961, Population dynamics of the sickle-cell trait in Black Caribs of British Honduras, Central America. *Am. J. Hum. Genet.* **13**:233–254.

Lehmann, H., and Huntsman, R. G., 1974, *Man's Haemoglobins*, rev. ed., North-Holland, Amsterdam.

McGavack, T. H., and German, W. M., 1944, Sicklemia in the Black Carib Indian, *Am. J. Med. Sci.* **208**:350–355.

Tejada, C., Gonzalez, N. L. S., and Sanchez, M., 1965, El factor Diego y el gene de celulas Falciformes entre los Caribes de raza Negra de Livingston, Guatemala, *Reimpreso Rev. Col. Med. Guatem.* **16**(2):83–86.

Raper, A. B., 1956, Sickling in relation to morbidity from malaria and other diseases, *Br. Med. J.* **1**:965–966.

18

Immunoglobulin Allotypes in the Black Caribs and Creoles of Belize and St. Vincent

MOSES S. SCHANFIELD, REBECCA BROWN, and MICHAEL H. CRAWFORD

1. Introduction

The genetic markers *Gm* and *Am* on the heavy chains of human immunoglobulins are anthropologically useful genetic polymorphisms because of the presence of unique haplotypes in certain populations and marked differences in frequencies in others. These genetic determinants are inherited in groups that have been referred to as "alleles," "phenogroups," "allogroups," or "haplotypes"; the latter is now the accepted term (WHO Committee on Human Immunoglobulin Allotypes, 1976). These haplotypes provide an extremely sensitive assay for the detection of admixture or gene flow and a set of labels that can be used to demonstrate population affinities. The genetically less complex *Km* (formerly *Inv*) genetic markers, on the kappa light chains, exhibit some differences between populations, but are less informative than the *Gm–Am* markers.

The historical interpretations, presented in Chapter 1 of this volume, indicate that the Garifuna or Black Caribs (hereafter referred to as Black Caribs) are Subsaharan African in origin, with Amerindian admixture subsequent to their

MOSES S. SCHANFIELD and REBECCA BROWN • American National Red Cross, Bethesda, Maryland 20814; present address for Dr. Schanfield: Genetic Testing Institute, Atlanta, Georgia 30308.   MICHAEL H. CRAWFORD • Laboratory of Biological Anthropology, University of Kansas, Lawrence, Kansas 66045.

arrival in the western hemisphere. The Black Creole (hereafter referred to as Creoles) have been characterized historically as a hybrid European and African group, speaking English or Creole languages. The original African population and the Caucasian and Amerindian admixing populations can be identified by the presence of unique $Gm-Am$ haplotypes or by markedly different haplotype distributions. These haplotype frequencies can be used to calculate estimates of African, Caucasian, and Amerindian components in the Black Carib and Creole populations studied. This is the first publication of immunoglobulin allotypes in Black Carib or Creole populations from Belize and St. Vincent (except for Chapter 14 in this volume, which reports immunoglobulin allotype frequencies from Hopkins, Belize). To this end, allotyping was done to characterize these populations, and the haplotype frequencies were used to estimate the proportions of African, European, and Amerindian genes in these populations.

2. Methods and Materials

All specimens were tested for Glm (f,a, and x), G3m (b0,b1,b3,b5,c3,s, and t), and Km (1) using the reagents listed in Table 1. All specimens from Belize and selected specimens from St. Vincent were tested for Glm(z). All Belize specimens except the Belize City Creoles were tested for G3m(v). Only St. Vincent specimens were tested for both G3m(c3-v) and G3m(c3-Br), the new allotypic determinant G3m(g5), and A2m(1 and 2). Selected specimens were variously tested with G3m(b4), G3m(c5), and G3m(c3 + 5). All specimens were tested at a dilution of 1:20 in microtiter plates using previously described methods (Schanfield, 1971; Schanfield and Fudenberg, 1975) with appropriate controls. Any specimen demonstrating direct agglutinating activity was heat-inactivated at 65°C for 10 min and retested. Frequencies of Gm and $Gm-Am$ haplotypes were estimated by gene counting. For the St. Vincent samples, which were not tested for G3m(c5), the frequency of $Gm^{z,a;b0,1,c3,5}$ was estimated from the square root of the Gm(a;b0,1,c3) phenotype frequency and from the frequency of $Gm^{\bar{a};b0,1,c3,5}$ heterozygotes. The Km^1 frequency was estimated from the square root of the Km(1−) frequency. No attempt was made to correct for the interrelationships of the individuals tested.

The estimates of ethnic composition were done as follows. The African component was estimated directly from the combined frequency of all African haplotypes: percent African = total frequency of African haplotypes. Estimates of the European component were based on the detection of $Gm^{f;b0,1,3,4,5,u,v}$ (hereafter referred to as $Gm^{f;b}$). As there is little information concerning the origin of hybridizing Europeans, a weighted frequency for $Gm^{f;b}$ was calculated from data available for English and Spanish populations, with $Gm^{f;b} = 0.654 \pm 0.002$ (Brazier and Goldsmith, 1968; Gallango and Arends, 1965; Lawler and Lele, 1961; Schanfield et al., 1981; Stevenson and Schanfield, 1981). European

Table 1. Reagents Used for Immunoglobulin Allotyping

	Notation[a]			
	Alphameric	Numeric	Agglutinator	Coat
Glm	f	3	Sta	Dan
	f	3	Pri[b]	Dan
	z	17	Pon[c] or Reed[c,d,e]	Dwi or Pet
	a	1	Pan	Dwi
	x	2	Dev or Max	Psn
	x	2	Ale[b,d]	Pet
G2m	n	23	R120[c,d,e]	Kop
G3m	b0	11	Tol	Hun or Puh
	b0/4	11/14	R-61[b]	Hun
	b0	11	Kek[b,d]	Puh
	b1	5	Ble or Tol	Hun
	b1	5	Tol[b,d]	Ada
	b1	5	Wat[b]	Hun
	b3	13	Rea[b] or Log[c]	Hun
	b3/5	10/13	Pla[c,d,e]	Hun
	b4	14	G84[d,e]	Hun
	b4	14	Goe[b,d,e]	Hun
	b4	14	Kek[b,d]	Hun
	b5	10	Fie[b,d]	Hun
	b5	10	Mol[b,d,e]	Hun
	b5	10	Let[b,d,e]	Hun
	c3 (v)	6	Alf	522
	c3 (Br)	6	Hen	522
	c3	6	3200[c,d,e]	522
	c3/5	6/24	And[d,e]	522 or Adams
	c3/5	6/24	Haw[b]	522
	c5	24	Hod[c,d]	522
	g	21	R-Hu	Sul
	g	21	R-68[b] or Leh[c]	Sul
	g5	28	Bro[b]	Sul
	g5	28	Lla[b,d,e]	Sul
	s	15	Rey[b] or Gai[c]	Puh
	t	16	Cra[b] or Ros[c]	Puh
	v	27	Ray[c,d]	Sul
A2m	1	1	Far	Sch, Bet, or Duv[e]
	2	2	Tay	Spe or Map[e]
Km	1	1	Sim	511 or 560
	1	1	Rut[b]	560
	1	1	Cla[c]	560

[a] Notation recommended by WHO Committee on Human Immunoglobulin Allotypes, (1976). Alphameric notation will be used throughout.
[b] Only St. Vincent specimens tested with this reagent.
[c] Only Belize specimens tested with this reagent.
[d] Only selected specimens tested with this reagent.
[e] Reagents generally provided by A. G. Steinberg, M. Blanc, L. Rivat, D. Brazier, S. Litwin, E. van Loghem, and R. Wistar.

admixture estimates were calculated separately for the Black Caribs, assuming either direct gene flow from Europeans or indirect flow through the Creoles. For the latter hypothesis, the Belize and St. Vincent Creole frequencies of $Gm^{f;b}$ were used rather than the English–Spanish estimate. The Amerindian components were more difficult to estimate, as there are no unique haplotypes. Three methods were used. The first method was Amerindian percent $= 1 - M_{African} - M_{European}$. The second method consisted in using the European admixture estimates based on $Gm^{f;b}$ to estimate the European contribution of $Gm^{z,a;g,u,v}$ and $Gm^{z,a,x;g,u,v}$ (hereafter referred to as $Gm^{z,a;g}$ and $Gm^{z,a,x;g}$, respectively). This was then subtracted from the observed freqencies to obtain an estimate of the Amerindian $Gm^{z,a;g}$ and $Gm^{z,a,x;g}$ frequencies. In order to calculate the total Amerindian contribution, this in turn was divided by an estimate of the Amerindian frequencies of $Gm^{z,a;g}$ and $Gm^{z,a,x;g}$, which were obtained from a sample of Carib Indians from Dominica corrected for European and African gene flow. The estimated original Amerindian frequencies are $Gm^{z,a;g} = 0.569 \pm 0.03$ and $Gm^{z,a,x;g} = 0.413 \pm 0.03$. The third method was based on the hypothesis that the European genes entered the Black Caribs through the Creole population. Corrections for Eurpean $Gm^{z,a;g}$ and $Gm^{z,a,x;g}$ frequencies were based on the estimates of Creole admixture and Creole $Gm^{z,a;g}$ and $Gm^{z,a,x;g}$ frequencies, rather than on European frequencies.

There is evidence based upon the presence of albumin Mexico (Al^{M}) (see Chapter 16) that additional Amerindian gene flow has entered the Belize Black Carib gene pool from resident Amerindians. No correction for this possibility has been attempted.

The Gm haplotype frequencies and ethnic proportions were tested by the z-test of proportions (Fleiss, 1973, p. 18), while the Km^{1} distributional differences were tested by contingency table χ^{2}.

2.1. Analytic Methods

Population structure analyses of these Black Carib groups is based upon the method of Harpending and Jenkins (1973). Haplotype frequencies from each population are used to construct a relationship matrix R of $L \times L$ dimension, where L is the number of populations sampled. The ijth element of R is

$$r_{ij} = \frac{1}{k} \sum_{i=1}^{k} \frac{(P_{iL} - \bar{P}_L)(P_{jL} - \bar{P}_L)}{\bar{P}_L(1 - \bar{P}_L)}$$

where k is the number of haplotypes. A second matrix A of $K \times K$ dimension describes the variation and covariation of K haplotype frequencies over all L populations (Harpending and Jenkins, 1973).

Least squares approximations of these two matrices R and A are utilized to graphically represent relative genetic relationships between populations and to assess the contribution of specific haplotypes to the dispersal of these populations in the reduced space. The R matrix is reduced by an eigenvectorial representation of haplotype distribution, which produces a two-dimensional map. In order to equalize the scale of projection eigenvector axes of the "genetic maps" are multiplied by the root of their corresponding eigenvalues (Lalouel, 1973). The eigenvectorial representation of the A matrix provides a two-dimensional plot of the haplotypes that contribute to the separation of the populations in the R-matrix genetic map.

3. Results and Discussion

3.1. Gene Frequency Data

The distribution of immunoglobulin phenotypes for the Belize and St. Vincent populations are presented in Tables 2 and 3; the haplotype frequencies are presented in Tables 4 and 5. For comparative purposes, immunoglobulin haplotype frequencies for selected African, European, and Amerindian populations are presented in Table 6.

All of the Black Carib and Creole specimens tested have polymorphic frequencies of all common black African haplotypes: $Gm^{z,a;b0,1,3,4,5,u,v}$ (hereafter referred to as $Gm^{z,a;b}$), $Gm^{z,a;b0,1,c3,5,u}$ (hereafter referred to as $Gm^{z,a;b,c3,5}$), $Gm^{z,a;b0,1,4,5,c3,u,v}$ (hereafter referred to as $Gm^{z,a;b,c3}$), and $Gm^{z,a;b0,3,5,s,v}$ (hereafter referred to as $Gm^{z,a;b,s}$). Although G3m(u = 26) was not tested, its distribution is known from previous studies (van Loghem and Grobbelaar, 1971; Steinberg, 1977). In addition, $Gm^{f;b}$, $Gm^{z,a;g}$, and $Gm^{z,a,x;g}$ were detected at polymorphic frequencies. The haplotype $Gm^{f;b}$ is a Caucasian marker haplotype, while $Gm^{z,a;g}$ and $Gm^{z,a,x;g}$ occur in both Caucasian and Amerindians, albeit with markedly different frequency distributions (see Table 6).

Due to the large array of phenotypes, only the St. Vincent Black Carib sample was large enough to attempt to calculate $Gm-Am$ haplotype frequencies. The $Gm-Am$ phenotype and haplotype distributions are presented in Table 7.

Though there is little comparative data on the distribution of $Gm-Am$ haplotypes, the previously reported relationships exist (Schanfield and Fudenberg, 1975). The African haplotypes are more often associated with A2m(2) than A2m(1). The European $Gm^{f;b}$ haplotype was uniformly A2m(1)-positive. The increased incidence of $Gm^{z,a;g}$, $A2m^2$, and $Gm^{z,a,x;g}$ $A2m^2$ associated with Amerindian or northern Asiatics was also observed. Therefore, the previously reported associations of $A2m$ allotypes and Gm haplotypes were found, although the exact frequencies differ (Schanfield and Fudenberg, 1975).

All the specimens from St. Vincent were tested for the new allotypic determinant G3m(g5 = 28) (van Loghem et al., 1977; Rivat et al., 1978). This marker usually is found in all European and Asiatic G3m(g)-positive sera, but

Table 2. Immunoglobulin Phenotypes in Black Caribs and Creoles from Belize[a]

	Caribs			Creoles			
Phenotype[b]	Stann Creek	Punta Gorda	Total	Belize City	Stann Creek	Punta Gorda	Total
G1m; G3m							
z,a;b,v	102	56	158	28	15	4	47
z,a;b,c3,5,v	43	29	72	24	8	2	34
z,a;b,c3,v	15	11	26	5	–	1	6
z,a;b,s,v	4	3	7	3	1	–	4
f,z,a;b,v	4	6	10	14	5	4	23
z,a;g,b,v	28	24	52	6	6	–	12
z,a,x;g,b,v	35	25	60	8	2	3	13
z,a,b0,1,c3,5	3	2	5	3	2	–	5
z,a;b0,1,4,5,c3,5,v	4	1	5	3	–	–	3
z,a;b0,1,3,5,c3,5,s,v	2	1	3	2	2	–	4
f,z,a;b,c3,5,v	1	1	2	2	1	2	5
z,a;g,b0,1,c3,5,v	3	8	11	1	–	–	1
z,a,x;g,b0,1,c3,5,v	10	7	17	–	–	1	1
z,a;b0,1,4,5,c3,v	3	–	3	–	–	–	–
z,a;b,c3,s,v	2	–	2	1	1	–	2
f,z,a;b,c3,v	–	–	–	1	–	–	1
z,a;g,b0,1,4,5,c3,v	1	2	3	–	–	–	–
z,a,x;g,b0,1,4,5,c3,v	1	4	5	1	–	–	1
z,a;b0,3,5, s,v	–	1	1	–	–	1	1
z,a;g,b0,3,5,s,v	3	–	3	–	–	–	–
z,a,x;g,b0,3,5,s,v	1	2	3	–	1	–	1
f;b,v	1	–	1	–	2	1	3
f,z,a;g,b,v	–	4	4	5	–	4	9
f,z,a,x;g,v	3	2	5	3	1	2	6
z,a;g,v	5	2	7	3	1	–	4
z,a,x;g,v	3	11	14	1	–	–	1
Total	277	202	479	114	48	25	187
Km (1 +)	155	116	271	59	23	9	91
Km (1 −)	122	87	209	56	26	16	98
Total	277	203	480	115	49	25	189

[a] Excluded phenotypes: Stann Creek Creole Gm(z,a,x;b0,1,3,4,5,v), Belize City Creole
  Gm(z,a;b0,1,3,4,5,c3,g,v).
[b] b = b0,1,3,4,5.

occurs in the absence of G3m(g) in Africans. Among those sera negative for G3m(g) and positive for one or more African haplotypes, 51 or 94 (54%) were positive for G3m(g5), while all G3m(g)-positive sera were G3m(g5)-positive (166/166). This is similar to the results reported by Rivat *et al*. (1978) for other African populations. Interestingly, three sera that might be expected to be G3m(g,g5)-positive on the basis of their phenotypes [Gm(f,a,x;b)] were

Table 3. Distribution of Immunoglobulin Phenotypes of Caribs and Creoles on St. Vincent[a]

	Caribs				Creoles			
Phenotype[b]	Sandy Bay	Owia	Fancy	Total	Sandy Bay	Owia	Fancy	Total
Glm; G3m								
a;b	15	15	–	30	3	3	16	22
a;b,c	11	4	1	16	8	9	7	24
a;b,s	1	4	–	5	1	–	–	1
a;g,b	9	7	2	18	–	–	8	8
a,x;g,b	15	16	4	35	–	2	1	3
f,z,a;b	11	1	2	14	–	3	10	13
a,b0,1,c	1	–	–	1	–	1	3	4
a;b0,1,4,5,c	4	–	–	4	3	2	2	7
a,b0,c,s	–	1	–	1	–	–	3	3
a;g,b0,1,c	5	1	–	6	–	–	4	4
a,x;g,b0,1,c	2	4	–	6	–	–	–	–
f,a;b,c	1	3	2	6	–	1	3	4
a;g,b0,1,4,5,c	4	1	–	5	–	–	–	–
a,x,g,b0,1,4,5,c	5	–	–	5	–	–	–	–
a;g,b0,3,5,s	1	–	–	1	–	–	–	–
a,x;g,b0,3,5,s	1	–	–	1	–	1	–	1
f,z,a;b,s	1	–	–	1	–	–	–	–
a;g	8	1	1	10	–	1	–	1
a,x;g	33	8	1	42	–	–	–	–
f,a;g,b	4	1	–	5	–	–	2	2
f,a,x;g,b	14	2	1	17	–	1	–	1
f;b	1	1	1	3	–	–	–	–
Total	147	70	15	232	15	24	59	98
Km(1 +)	87	41	10	138	10	13	29	52
Km(1 –)	70	36	8	114	5	11	32	48
Total	157	77	18	252	15	24	61	100

[a] Excluded phenotypes. Caribs: Sandy Bay, Gm(a,x;b0,1,3,4,5,g5;2), Gm(f,a;g;1), Gm(a, x;b0,1,c3;A2m NT), Gm(f,a,x;b0,1,3,4,5,g,g5;1), Gm(a,x;b0,1,4,(b3,5?), g,g5;1,2), (Gm(a;b0,1,4,5,(c?), g,g5;1,2), Gm(a;b0,1,4, (b3,5?), c3,g,g5;1,2), Gm(a,x;b0,1,5 (b3-4-), c3,g,g5;1,2); Fancy, Gm(a;b0,1,3,4,5,c3,g,g5;1,2), Gm(a,x;b0,1(b3,4,5?),c3, g.g5;A2m NT); Owia, Gm(a;b0,1,3,4,5,c3,g,g5;2), Gm(f,a,x;b0,1,3,4,5,g5;1), Gm (f,a,x;b0,1,3,4,5,g5;1,2), Gm(a, (x);b0(b1,4,5?), g,g5;1), Gm(a;b3,4,5(b0,1?), c3,g, g5;1), Gm(a,x;b3,(b0,1,5?), c3,g,g5;A2m NT). Creoles: Fancy, Gm(a,x;b0,1,3,4,5,c3, g5;2), Gm(f,a;b0, (b1,3,4,5?), c3;1); Owia, Gm(a;b0,1(a;b0,1(b4?), c3;2), Gm(a;b3,4, 5, (b0,1?), g5; ND). NT, not tested; ND, not detected.
[b] b = b0,1,3,4,5.

G3m(g − g5 +) (Owia, Black Caribs, one; Sandy Bay, Black Caribs, two). This phenotype, G3m(g−g5 +) with either Gm(z,a) or Gm(z,a,x), has been reported by both van Loghem *et al.* (1977) and Rivat *et al.* (1978).

A total of 58 unselected Creoles from Belize City were tested for G2m(n).

Table 4. Immunoglobulin Haplotype Frequencies of Caribs and Creoles from Belize[a]

	Caribs			Creoles			
	Stann Creek	Punta Gorda	Total	Stann Creek	Punta Gorda	Belize City	Total
N	277	187	464	48	25	115	189
z,a;b0,1,3,4,5,u,v	0.601	0.520	0.568	0.542	0.360	0.504	0.495
z,a;b0,1,c3,5,u	0.124	0.126	0.125	0.156	0.100	0.165	0.153
z,a;b0,1,4,5,c3,u,v	0.052	0.044	0.049	0.010	0.020	0.052	0.037
z,a;b0,3,5,s,v	0.022	0.020	0.021	0.052	0.040	0.026	0.034
z,a,g,u,v	0.087	0.131	0.105	0.083	0.080	0.087	0.085
z,a,x;g,u,v	0.096	0.126	0.108	0.042	0.120	0.056	0.061
f;b0,1,3,4,5,u,v	0.018	0.032	0.024	0.115	0.280	0.109	0.132
x^2	24.61	10.96	15.79	4.15	NT	19.07	35.69
d.f.	12	15	17	3	–	12	14
P	0.017	NS	NS	NS	–	NS	0.002
Km^1	0.336	0.345	0.340	0.272	0.200	0.302	0.279

[a] NT, Not tested; NS, not significant.

Table 5. Immunoglobulin Haplotype Frequencies of Caribs and Creoles from St. Vincent[a]

	Caribs			Creoles	
	Sandy Bay	Owia	Total[b]	Fancy	Total[c]
N	147	70	232	59	98
z,a;b0,1,3,4,5,u,v	0.265	0.443	0.319	0.491	0.474
z,a;b0,1,c3,5,8	0.082	0.083	0.066	0.225	0.202
z,a;b0,1,4,5,c3,u,v	0.050	0.017	0.053	0.004	0.089
z,a;b0,3,5,s,v	0.014	0.036	0.019	0.025	0.025
z,a;g,u,v	0.245	0.143	0.209	0.119	0.082
z,a,x;g,u,v	0.235	0.214	0.228	0.008	0.025
f;b0,1,3,4,5,u,v	0.109	0.064	0.106	0.127	0.102
x^2	27.36	8.06	19.25	6.44	9.20
d.f.	14	8	16	4	8
P	0.016	NS	NS	NS	NS
Km^1	0.332	0.321	0.327	0.276	0.307

[a] Glm (z) presumed to be present from previous studies.
[b] Includes Fancy.
[c] Includes Sandy Bay and Owia.

In general G2m(n) was associated with the European haplotype $Gm^{f;b}$ [seven of 14 Gm(f;b)-positive sera], as previously reported (Schanfield and Fudenberg, 1975). However, four of 44 $Gm^{f;b}$-negative sera with African haplotypes were unexpectedly G2m(n)-positive. These included one each Gm(z,a;b;b0,1,3,4,5; 1,2). Gm(z,a;n;b0,1,3,4,5,g;1,2), Gm(z,a,x;n;b0,1,3,4,5,g;1,2), and Gm(z,a; n;b0,1,3,4,5,c3,g;1). Unfortunately, in the absence of family data it is not possible to define the haplotypes involved; however, G2m(n)-positive haplotypes are not usually found in Africans (Schanfield and Fudenberg, 1975).

A number of sera were excluded from the calculation of Gm haplotype frequencies. Some of them appear to represent rare haplotypes previously reported, as discussed later. Further, due to the large numbers of reagents used to define the St. Vincent phenotypes, many new phenotypes were defined due to variation in serological reactivity among antisera with the same specificity. To keep the results for both Belize and St. Vincent comparable, discrepancies due to antisera not used in both series were eliminated. Detailed analysis of the various G3m(b) reagents and different G3m(c) reagents will be the subject of a separate publication.

Examples of the phenotype Gm(a;b0,1,3,4,5,c3,g,g5) A2m(2 or 1,2) were found in Stann Creek (Black Carib, one; Creole, one), Belize City (Creole, one), Fancy (Black Carib, one), and Owia (Black Carib, one). These may represent examples of the uncommon African haplotype $Gm^{z,a;g,b}$ (Schanfield and Fudenberg, 1975; van Loghem et al., 1978). The phenotype Gm(a,x;b0,1,3,4, 5,g5;2) was found in Sandy Bay, and a Fancy Creole had the phenotype Gm(a, x;b0,1,3,4,5,c3,g5;2). These may all be examples of the uncommon African haplotype $Gm^{z,a,x;b}$ (van Loghem and Martensson, 1968; van Loghem et al., 1978). Other sera were excluded because their phenotypes could not be defined on the basis of known haplotypes; these are listed in Tables 2 and 3.

In general, no significant differences in Gm haplotypes or Km^1 frequencies were detected within the Black Carib and Creole populations of Belize or St. Vincent. However, the Black Carib groups differed from the coresident Creoles. The Black Caribs of Belize had marginally significantly higher frequencies of $Gm^{z,a;b}$ ($z = 1.61$, $P = 0.05$) and $Gm^{z,a,x;g}$ ($z = 1.80, P = 0.036$) and a significantly lower $Gm^{f;b}$ frequency ($z = 3.51$, $P = 0.0002$) than the Belize Creoles. The Black Caribs of Belize show greater similarity to the Black Caribs of Livingston, Guatemala, than to Creoles of Belize (see Table 6). The Black Caribs of St. Vincent had significantly higher frequencies of $Gm^{z,a;g}$ ($z = 2.73$, $P = 0.003$) and $Gm^{z,a,x;g}$ ($z = 4.72$, $P = 0.001$) and lower frequencies of $Gm^{z,a;b}$ ($z = 2.99$, $P = 0.002$) and $Gm^{z,a;b,c3,5}$ ($z = 2.62$, $P = 0.004$) than the St. Vincent Creoles. There were no significant differences in Km^1 frequency between Black Carib and Creole from Belize or St. Vincent.

Comparing the Black Caribs of Belize to the Black Caribs of St. Vincent yields several highly signficant differences. The Black Caribs of Belize have significantly more African haplotypes ($z = 7.65$, $P = 0.0001$ for all haplotypes

Table 6. Immunoglobulin Haplotype Frequencies in Selected Populations

IgG 1 IgG 3	z,a b	z,a b,c3,5	z,a b,c3	z,a[a] b,s	f b	z,a[b] g	z,a,x g	z,a b,s,t	Km[1]
Caribs									
Guatemala[c] (187)	0.495	0.118	0.067	0.029	0.011	0.134	0.131	—	0.401
Africans									
Senegal									
Bedik[d] (787)	0.727	0.208	e	0.118	0.003	0.025	—	f	0.389
Gambia									
Mendaur[g] (307)	0.820	0.115	0.023	0.042	—	—	—	—	0.375
Keneba[g] (822)	0.793	0.167	0.004	0.035	—	0.001	—	—	0.419
Upper Volta									
Kurumba[h] (150)	0.716	0.187	0.030	0.060	—	0.007	—	—	0.360
Nigeria									
Mixed[i] (214)	0.677	0.203	0.061	0.051	—	0.017	—	—	0.374
Cameroon									
Fali[h] (81)	0.698	0.154	0.093	0.056	—	—	—	—	0.379
French Antilles[j] (57)	0.517	0.193	0.035	0.009	0.158	0.053	0.026	—	NT[p]
Surinam[h] (521)	0.596	0.264	0.031	0.089	0.005	0.007	0.005	—	NT[p]
Caucasians									
U.S.[k] (146)	0.006	—	—	—	0.695	0.202	0.093	0.003	0.097
Spain[l] (186)	0.019	—	—	—	0.677	0.218	0.086	—	0.096

Amerindians										
Dominica										
Carib[m]	(99)	0.102	0.012		0.028	0.079	0.455	0.323	—	0.405
Mexico										
Maya[h]	(768)	0.036	0.022	—	0.002	0.122	0.649	0.123	0.044	NT[p]
Panama										
Guaymi[n]	(486)	0.008	—	—	—	0.008	0.670	0.314	—	0.544
Surinam										
Carib[o]	(257)	0.060	0.085	0.045	0.021	0.021	0.534	0.227	0.006	0.365
Arawak[o]	(194)	0.052	0.016	—	0.003	0.010	0.656	0.261	0.003	0.380

[a] In the absence of testing for G3m(s and t), Gm^a,b^3 is presumed to represent $Gm^{z,a;b,s}$.
[b] Includes $Gm^{z,a;g}$ plus $Gm^{z,a;g,b}$.
[c] Crawford et al. (1981). Sample size N is given in parentheses.
[d] Bouloux et al. (1972).
[e] Detected but no frequency estimate.
[f] Not reported but tested.
[g] Steinberg and Cook (1981), pp. 154–202.
[h] Van Loghem (1971).
[i] Van Loghem et al. (1978).
[j] Rivat et al. (1978).
[k] Stevenson and Schanfield (1981).
[l] Schanfield et al. (1981).
[m] Harvey et al. (1969).
[n] Gershowitz and Neel (1978).
[o] Geerdink et al. (1974).
[p] NT, Not tested.

Table 7. The GmA2m Phenotype and Haplotype Distributions in Caribs from St. Vincent[a]

	1−	1,2	−2	Total
a;b	0	11	19	30
a;b,c3	1	0	14	15
a;b,s	0	3	1	4
a;g,b	3	10	5	18
a,x;g,b	2	30	2	34
f,z,a;b	2	11	0	13
a;b0,1,c3	0	0	1	1
a;b0,1,4,5,c3	0	0	4	4
a;b,c,s	0	0	1	1
a;g,b0,1,c3	0	4	2	6
a,x;g,b0,1,c3	1	4	1	6
f,a;b,c3	1	5	0	6
a;g,b0,1,4,5,c3	2	3	0	5
a,x;g,b0,1,4,5,c3	0	4	1	5
a;g,b0,3,5,s	1	0	0	1
a,x;g,b0,3,5,s	0	0	0	1
f,a;b,s	1	0	0	1
a;g	6	3	1	10
axg	34	6	0	40
f,a;g,b	3	2	0	5
f,a,x;g,b	12	4	0	16
f;b	3	0	0	3
Total	72	101	52	225

Gm;	Am	
z,a;b0,1,3,4,5;	1	0.058
	2	0.268
z,a;b0,1,c3,5;	1	0.022
	2	0.045
z,a;b0,1,4,5,c3;	1	0.009
	2	0.044
z,a;b0,3,5,s;	1	0.009
	2	0.009
z,a;g;	1	0.157
	2	0.052
z,a,x;g	1	0.177
	2	0.051
f;b0,1,3,4,5;	1	0.106

[a] b = b0,1,3,4,5.

pooled), while the Black Caribs of St. Vincent have significantly higher frequencies of Amerindian and European haplotypes: $Gm^{z,a;g}$ ($z = 3.53$, $P = 0.0002$), $Gm^{z,a,x;g}$ ($z = 3.73$, $P = 0.0001$), and $Gm^{f;b}$ ($z = 3.93$, $P = 0.0001$). In contrast, the Creoles of Belize and St. Vincent are not significantly different from each other for Gm haplotypes. No significant differences in Km^1 frequencies were detected between Belize and St. Vincent Black Caribs and Creoles.

3.2. Admixture Estimates of Ethnic Composition

Elsewhere in this volume it is suggested that genetic data can be utilized to resolve or support questions of ethnohistorical reconstruction (Chapter 19). This chapter utilizes immunoglobulin allotypes (Gm) to explore specific ambiguities in the ethnohistorical reconstruction of the sequence of the genetic contributions to the Black Carib gene pool. Due to variation in sample sizes and unknown patterns of gene flow and genetic drift, it is difficult to attempt an explanation of all the variation in ethnic composition in the Black Carib and Creole communities of St. Vincent and Belize. However, the reported results can support or refute certain historical hypotheses, such as the origin of the European admixture in the Black Caribs. In Belize it is possible that the European component in the Black Caribs could be due to hybridization with either Creoles or Europeans. If one uses Creole $Gm^{f;b}$, $Gm^{z,a;g}$, and $Gm^{z,a,x;g}$ frequencies, the estimates of Amerindian admixture are lower but not significantly different in pattern from those obtained by assuming direct European gene flow. Therefore, either route of admixture is possible, and in this case the ethnohistorical ambiguity cannot be resolved. In the case of St. Vincent Island, European gene flow through the Creoles does not appear to be an adequate explanation of the observed distribution of Gm phenotypes. The St. Vincent Creoles and Black Caribs have similar amounts of European admixture yet very different proportions of African and Amerindian genes.

3.3. Population Structure

Figure 1 diagrammatically illustrates the genetic structure of the nine Carib and Creole populations in the Caribbean and Central America based upon nine immunoglobulin haplotypes. These populations are compared to the three "parental" composite groups that contributed genetic material to the Black Carib and Creole communities. The first two scaled eigenvectors account for

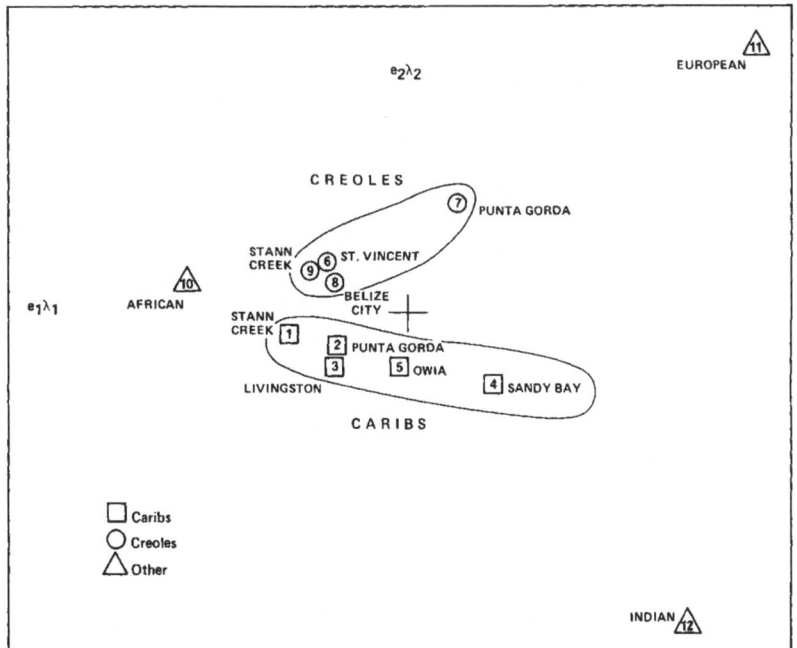

FIGURE 1. Two-dimensional least squares "genetic map" of nine Black Carib and Creole populations compared to European, Indian, and African composite groups.

Table 8. Estimation of Ethnic Composition of Caribs and Creoles[a]

| Population | African[b] | European[c] | Creole[d] | Amerindian | | |
				I[e]	II[f]	III[g]
Belize						
Caribs						
Stann Creek	0.799	0.027	0.165	0.174	0.179	0.163
Punta Gorda	0.710	0.049	0.294	0.241	0.248	0.220
Total	0.763	0.037	0.220	0.200	0.207	0.186
Creoles						
Stann Creek	0.755	0.171	NC	0.074	0.114	NC
Punta Gorda	0.520	0.428	NC	0.052	0.061	NC
Belize City	0.747	0.167	NC	0.086	0.091	NC
Total	0.719	0.202	NC	0.079	0.082	NC
St. Vincent						
Caribs						
Sandy Bay	0.411	0.167	1.069	0.422	0.437	0.378
Owia	0.579	0.098	0.627	0.323	0.325	0.291
Total	0.457	0.162	1.039	0.381	0.392	0.335
Creoles						
Total	0.790	0.156	NC	0.054	0.055	NC

[a] NC, Not calculated.

[b] $M_{African} = Gm^{z,a;b} + Gm^{z,a;b,c3,5} + Gm^{z,a;b,c3} + Gm^{z,a;b,s}/1.0$.

[c] $M_{European} = Gm^{f;b}(mixed)/Gm^{f;b}(European)$.

[d] $M_{Creole} = Gm^{f;b}(Carib)/Gm^{f;b}(Creole)$ (Belize or St. Vincent).

[e] $M_{Indian} = 1 - M_{African} - M_{European}$.

[f] $M_{Indian} = [Gm^{z,a;g} + Gm^{z,a,x;g}(mixed) - M_{European}]$
       $\times [Gm^{z,a;g} + Gm^{z,a,x;g}(European)]$
       $\times [Gm^{z,a;g} + Gm^{z,a,x;g}(Indian)]^{-1}$

[g] Same as preceding except European frequencies based on M_{Creole} and appropriate Creole haplotype frequencies.

93% of the observed variation (eigenvector 1–57%, eigenvector 2–36%). Sandy Bay (population 4) exhibits closest genetic affinity to the Amerindian groups (12), while Punta Gorda Creoles (7) appear to have experienced considerable European (11) gene flow. These conclusions are further supported by the admixture estimates based upon *Gm* in this chapter (see Table 8) and blood markers described in Chapter 16, which indicate that almost 44% of the Sandy Bay gene pool is of Amerindian origin, while the Punta Gorda Creoles exhibit almost 43% European admixture. Similarly, Stann Creek Caribs (1) are closer to the African (10) parental group, and, in fact, the ethnic composition of its gene pool contains almost 80% African ancestry.

Figure 2 provides a plot of the *Gm* haplotypes responsible for the dispersion of the populations plotted in Fig. 1. Notably, $Gm^{f,b}$ separates the European populations from all other groups, while $Gm^{z,a;b}$ contributes most to the

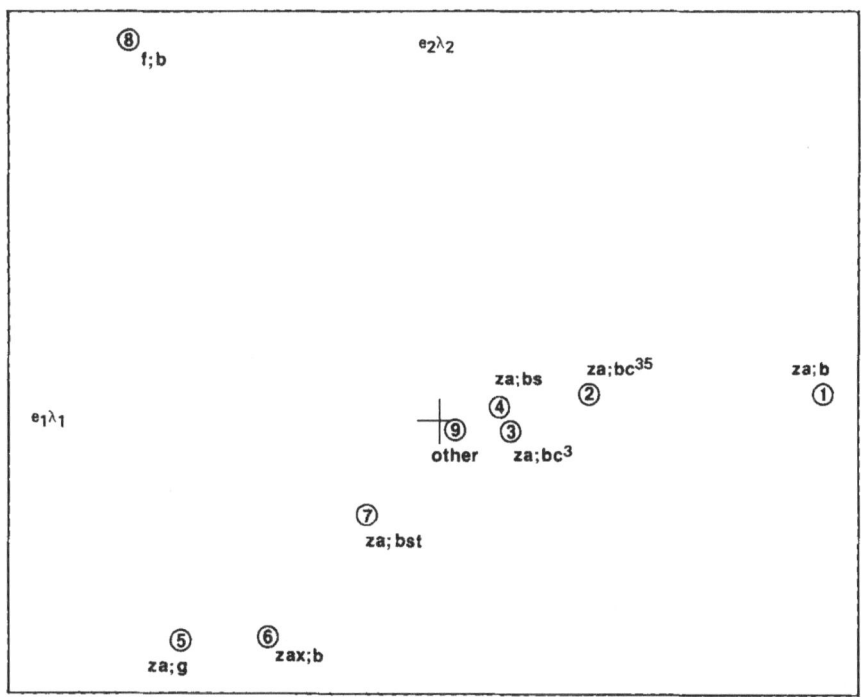

FIGURE 2. Least squares representation of nine immunoglobulin haplotypes corresponding to the "genetic map" shown in Fig. 1.

separation of the African groups. The Amerindian parental group is characterized by the haplotypes $Gm^{z,a;g}$ and $Gm^{z,a,x;b}$. These two haplotypes are responsible for separating the St. Vincent Island Caribs (Sandy Bay) from other groups.

Other African markers, $Gm^{z,a;b,s}$, $Gm^{z,a;b,c,3,5}$, $Gm^{z,a;b,c3}$, and $Gm^{z,a;b,s,t}$, add little to the separation of the groups.

In Fig. 3, the first scaled eigenvector accounts for 46.3% of the variation but clearly separates the Black Caribs from the Creoles. The second eigenvector ($e_2\lambda_2 = 37\%$) appears to cluster population subdivisions on the basis of geography, with the Sandy Bay and Owia Black Caribs diverging genetically from the Belizean communities. There is greater variation observed among the St. Vincent populations than in the more homogeneous Belizean and Guatemalan Black Caribs. In contrast, the Creole communities are tightly clustered, except for Punta Gorda (7), whose genetic uniqueness is influenced by a miniscule sample size. Among the Creoles, it is interesting to note that the St. Vincent sample has considerable affinity for Belize City and Stann Creek communities. Apparently, the European component remains fairly constant among the Creoles, while the Amerindian contribution varies from St. Vincent to Central American populations. This explanation of the genetic relationships observed in Fig. 3 is supported by the A-matrix plot in Fig. 4. The $Gm^{z,a;g}$ and $Gm^{z,a,x;g}$ distinguish

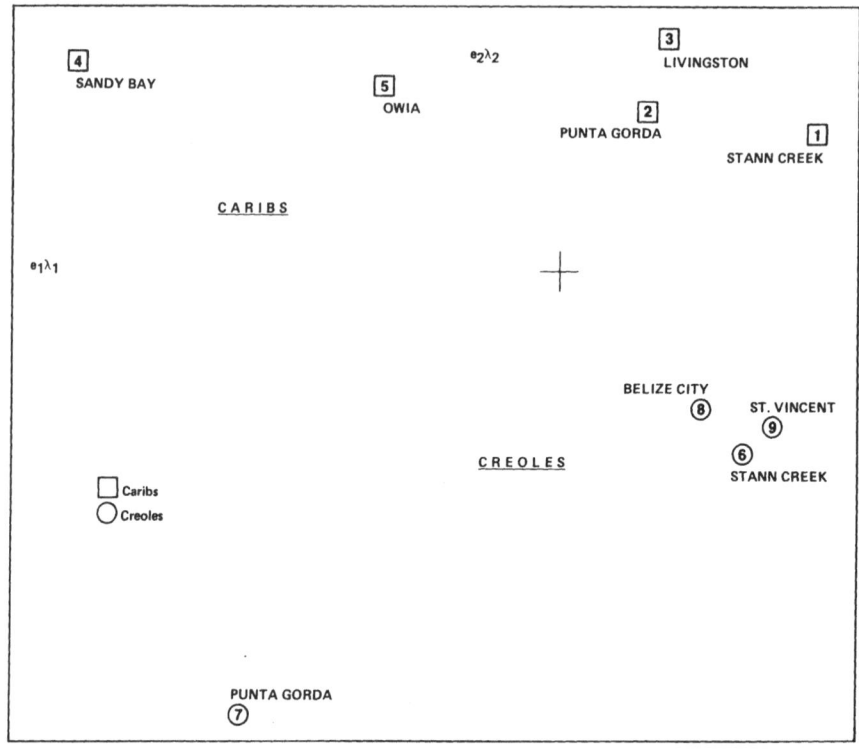

FIGURE 3. Least squares reduction "genetic map" of the nine Black Carib and Creole populations based upon eight immunoglobulin haplotype frequencies.

the Black Carib populations, while $Gm^{f;b}$ is instrumental in separating Punta Gorda from the remainder of the Creoles.

Wright's F_{ST} has been widely used as a measure of gene frequency differentiation between population subdivisions. It is computed by the formla

$$F_{ST} = \frac{\sigma_p^2}{\bar{p}\bar{q}}$$

where σ_p^2 is the variance of p across subdivisions and $\bar{p}$ is the weighted mean of p across subdivisions. Harpending and Jenkins (1974) have shown that the average value of the diagonal elements r_{ii} of the R matrix is an estimate of the mean genetic heterogeneity F_{ST}. An R_{ST} value of 0.095 for the Black Caribs and their parental groups is similar in magnitude to the values computed by Wright for the major races of the world. The R_{ST} value of 0.027 for the Black Caribs and Creoles is equivalent to those values observed for subdivided Papago groups (Workman and Niswander, 1970) and the Pygmies (Cavalli-Sforza, 1969). This apparent differentiation of gene frequency variances is exacerbated by varying degrees of admixture and hybridization.

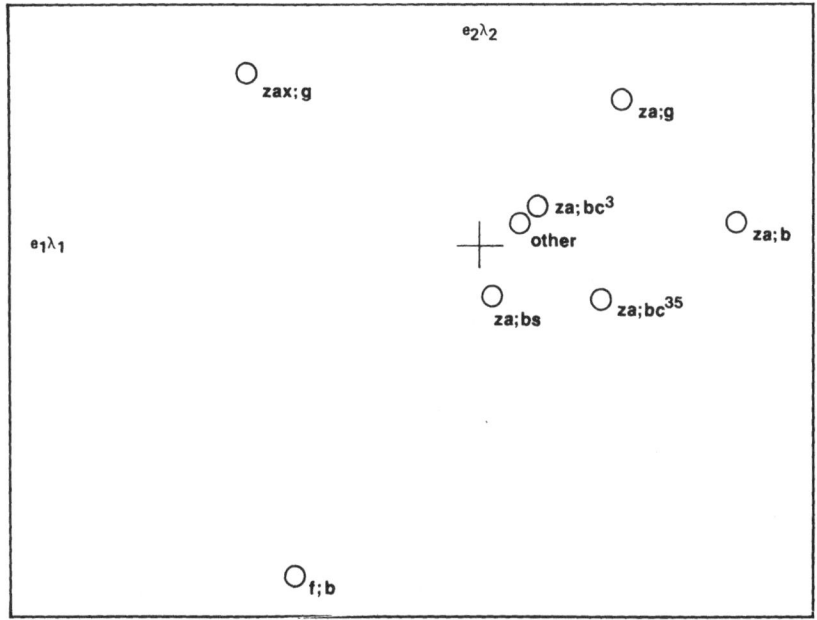

FIGURE 4. Dispersion of eight immunoglobulin haplotypes corresponding to the "genetic map" shown in Fig. 3.

4. Conclusions

1. As seen elsewhere in this volume (Chapter 16), based on other polymorphic systems, the St. Vincent populations are more heterogeneous genetically than are the Black Caribs on the mainland of Central America. This genetic heterogeneity is due primarily to variation in amounts of admixture (Amerindian and European) among subpopulations, followed by reproductive isolation.

2. The gene pool in the Black Carib population at Sandy Bay, St. Vincent Island, contains a greater proportion of Amerindian genes than any of the mainland Carib or Creole groups. This suggests that either the original Black Carib population contained more Amerindian genes than are presently observed in the mainland Black Caribs, or founder effect or drift has occurred, and the remaining St. Vincent population is not representative of the original Black Caribs.

3. The *Gm* haplotypes suggest that the majority of the component observed in the Black Carib gene pool was present in the founding populations prior to their deportation from St. Vincent.

4. If it is assumed that all of the European genes have been introduced into the mainland Black Carib gene pool through Creole–Black Carib interethnic mating, a total of 22% of the genes came by this route.

5. If the cumulative mainland gene flow is 22%, the rate per generation approaches 1% from Creole to Black Carib and Black Carib to Creole.

6. There is no proposed ethnohistorical explanation for the similar European haplotype frequencies observed among the Caribs and Creoles on St. Vincent Island. Apparently, the European component was added to the St. Vincent Carib populations subsequent to the deportation of the Black Caribs in 1797. The gene flow into the Black Caribs must have been of low magnitude and must have occurred when the remaining population was very small.

7. Immunoglobulins appear to be the most reliable markers for studying genetic structure of bi- or triracially hybridized populations. A comparison of eigenvectorial representations of the genetic structure of Black Carib and Creole populations, *Gm*'s versus blood group markers, reveals that *Gm*'s separate these groups more clearly than the traditional markers.

ACKNOWLEDGMENTS

The authors would like to thank R. Baylerian, G. Berman, C. Cousins, T. Kehoe, S. Schoeppner, and D. Valentine for technical assistance, and M. Blanc, D. Brazier, S. Litwin, L. Rivat, A. G. Steinberg, E. van Loghem, and R. Wistar for donations of rare reagents.

This work was supported in part by a grant from the Research and Education Trust of the Milwaukee Blood Center and Research Grant HL23654.

References

Bouloux, C., Gomila, J., and Langaney, A., 1972, Hemotypology of the Bedik, *Hum. Biol.* **44**:289–302.

Brazier, D. M., and Goldsmith, K. L. G., 1968, Frequency of certain Gm and Inv factors in the United Kingdom, *Nature* **219**:193.

Cavalli-Sforza, L. L., 1969, Human diversity, *Proc. XII Int. Congr. Genet.* **31**:405–416.

Crawford, M. H., Gonzalez, N. L., Schanfield, M. S., Dykes, D. D., Skradski, K., and Polesky, H. F., 1981, The Black Caribs (Garifuna) of Livingston, Guatamala: Genetic markers and admixture estimates, *Hum. Biol.* **53**:87–103.

Fleiss, J. S., 1973, *Statistical Methods for Rates and Proportions*, Wiley, New York.

Gallango, M., and Arends, T., 1965, Frecuencia de los Factores Gm(a) y Gm(x) en Espanoles Residentes en Venezuela, *Acta Client. Venez.* **16**:18–22.

Geerdink, R. A., Nijenhuis, L. E., van Loghem, E., and Sjoe, E. L. F., 1974, Blood groups in Trio and Wajana Indians from Surinam, *Am. J. Hum. Genet.* **26**:45–53.

Gershowitz, H., and Neel, J. V., 1978, the immunoglobulin allotypes (Gm and Km) of twelve indian tribes of Central and South America, *Am. J. Phys. Anthropol.* **49**:289–302.

Harpending, H. C., and Jenkins, 1973, Genetic distances among South African populations, in *Methods and Theories of Anthropological Genetics* (M. H. Crawford and P. L. Workman, eds.), pp. 177–199, University of New Mexico Press, Albuquerque.

Harpending, H. C., and Jenkins, T., 1974, !Kung population structure, in *Genetic Distance* (J. F. Crow and C. F. Denniston, eds.), pp. 137–161, Plenum, New York.

Harvey, R. G., Godber, M. J., Kopec, A. C., Mourant, A. E., and Tills, D., 1969, Frequency of genetic traits in the Caribs of Dominica, *Hum. Biol.* 41:342–364.

Lalouel, J. M. 1973, Topology of population structure, in *Genetic Structure of Populations* (N. E. Morton, Ed.), pp. 139–149, University of Hawaii Press, Honolulu.

Lawler, S., and Lele, K. P., 1961, Some comments on the Gm serum groups, in *Proceedings, 8th Congress, European Society Hematology, Vienna*, Paper 220.

Rivat, L., Rivat, C., Cook, C. E., and Steinberg, A. G., 1978, Gm(28), Un nouvel allotype du systeme Gm present sur les IgG3: Interet particulaire de son etude dans les populations negroides, *Ann. Immunol. (Inst. Pasteur)* 129:33–45.

Schanfield, M. S., 1971, Population studies on the Gm and Inv antigens in Asia and Oceania, Ph.D. thesis; University of Michigan, Ann Arbor, Michigan, available from University Microfilms, Ann Arbor.

Schanfield, M. S., and Fudenberg, H. H. 1975, The anthropological usefulness of the IgA allotypic markers, in *Biosocial Interrelations in Population Adaptation* (F. Johnston, ed.), pp. 105–114, Mouton, The Hague.

Schanfield, M. S., Baylerian, R., Maiguez, J., and Carbonell, F., 1981, Immunoglobulin allotypes in European populations. IV Gm, Am and Km allotypic markers in Valencia, Spain, *J. Immunogenet.* 8:529–532.

Steinberg, A. G., 1977, A Human antibody to Gm(26): An antigen usually present on the γ-3 chain of IgG when Gm (15) is absent, *Vox Sang.* 33:266–269.

Steinberg, A. G., and Cook, C. E., 1981, *The Distribution of the Human Immunoglobulin Allotypes*, Oxford University Press, Oxford.

Stevenson, J. C., and Schanfield, M. S., 1981, Immunoglobulin allotypes in European populations III. Gm, Am and Km allotypes in people of European Ancestry in the United States, *Hum. Biol.* 53:521–542.

Van Loghem, E. 1971, Stability of Gm polymorphism, in *Human Anti-Human Gamma-globulins* (R. Grubb and G. Samuelson, eds.) pp. 29–37, Pergamon, New York.

Van Loghem, E., and Grobbelaar, B. G., 1971, A new genetic marker of human IgG[3] immunoglobulins. Evolutionary dissociation of Gm allotypes, *Vox Sang.* 31:405–410.

Van Loghem, E., and Martensson, L., 1968, Gm(x) in Negroes, *Vox Sang.* 21:405–410.

Van Loghem, E., Blanc, M., and de Lange, G., 1977, Human IgG3 allotypes, with special reference to a new allotype related to G3m(g)(G3m21), *J. Immunogenet.* 4:371–383.

Van Loghem, E., Salimonu, L., Williams, A. I. A., Osunkoya, B. O., Body, A. M., de Lange, G., and Nijenhuis, L. F., 1978, Immunoglobulin allotypes in African Populations, I. Gm–Am Haplotypes in a Nigerian population, *J. Immunogenet.* 5:143–147.

WHO Committee on Human Immunoglobulin Allotypes (1976), Review of the notation for the allotypic and related markers of human immunoglobulins, *Eur. J. Immunol.* 6:599–601.

Workman, P. L., and Niswander, J., 1970, Population studies on Southwestern Indian Tribes. II. Local genetic differentiation in the Papago, *Am. J. Hum. Genet.* 22:24–49.

19

Genetic Population Structure of the Black Caribs and Creoles

ERIC J. DEVOR, MICHAEL H. CRAWFORD, and V. BACH-ENCISO

1. Introduction

In recent years, reduced-space least squares representations of the distribution of gene frequencies have come to be a standard method available to human population geneticists (Cannings and Cavalli-Sforza, 1973; Jorde, 1980). Such representations, derived from the spectral decomposition of matrices of normalized gene frequency covariances, are referred to as genetic structures (Harpending and Jenkins, 1974; Workman, *et al.*, 1973). However, these so-called "genetic maps" are of limited evolutionary significance unless accompanied by information independent of the allelic frequencies, such as patterns of demographic, environmental, or historical factors (Workman *et al.*, 1976; Harpending and Ward, 1982). For the most part, since the processes creating the observed gene frequency patterns have usually been in place for at most only a few generations, the requisite independent data consist of written or verbal histories. Rarely do archeological or paleontological sources have any direct bearing on interpretation, save for large-scale relationships over long time spans. Consequently the relevant interpretive framework for human population structure is composed almost exclusively of near-past historical, social, and economic processes.

ERIC J. DEVOR • Department of Psychiatry, Washington University School of Medicine, St. Louis, Missouri 63178. MICHAEL H. CRAWFORD and V. BACH-ENCISO • Laboratory of Biological Anthropology, University of Kansas, Lawrence, Kansas 66045.

The Black Caribs (Garifuna) of Central America are a case in point, in which independent social and historical data are essential for interpretation of the genetic structure. With reference to specific social and historical patterns, particularly to unique historical events, we will present the current genetic population structure of several Black Carib groups as derived from a number of red cell antigens as well as serum proteins and enzymes. We will show that the interplay of gene frequency distributions and historical data reveal a consistent and understandable population structure. Further, the present study indicates that the principal factors determining this structure are a series of unique migratory events resulting in the unequal incorporation of genes from several different indigenous groups across the array.

2. Biosocial History of the Black Caribs

The biosocial history of the Black Caribs can be characterized by a series of gene pool amalgamations and fissions. Initially, the Amerindian portion of the Black Carib gene pool arose from a mixture of Arawak-speaking Indians, who originally peopled the Lesser Antilles, and an invasion of Carib Indians expanding from South America. Shipwrecked and escaping West African slaves further added to this biracial melange on St. Vincent Island. Thus, the original Black Carib gene pool consisted of an admixed Indian ancestral group and a heterogeneous West African component.

The first fission of this population occurred in 1797, when the British deported the Black Carib survivors of a long war of attrition to Roatan. Those who avoided capture were the founders of our St. Vincent Island sample. The population underwent further fission and possibly some admixture on Roatan, when the majority of the Black Caribs migrated to the mainland of Central America in 1798.

The population history of the Black Caribs on the mainland of Central America consists of rapid expansion, possible admixture, and fission (see Davidson in Chapter 2 of this volume for a discussion of the Black Carib expansion). The Trujillo Bay migrants had formed five villages by 1810 according to Vallejo (1893; cited in Chapter 2). The gene pool underwent further fission with the movement of some Black Caribs eastward into Mosquitia. Another group of Black Caribs settled in British Honduras and founded Stann Creek in 1827 (Dunn, 1828; cited in Chapter 2). Through a series of migrations and fissions, this Black Carib gene pool from St. Vincent Island expanded to form at least 54 communities located from Stann Creek (Dangriga) to La Fe, Nicaragua, in 180 years (see Chapter 2). There is some evidence that the Black Caribs may have admixed with other West African groups who had settled the coast of Honduras and Roatan. In particular, French-speaking blacks from Haiti who were settled near Trujillo would have some cultural affinities to the Black

Caribs. In part, this would help explain the phenomenal rate of expansion and growth of the population from several thousand in 1797 to a currently estimated total of 80,000 persons.

3. Materials

Blood specimens were collected during a series of field trips to Guatemala (1975), Belize (1976), and St. Vincent Island (1979) by teams from the University of Kansas. The results of the blood analysis for Livingston, Stann Creek, Punta Gorda, Belize City, Fancy, Sandy Bay, and Owia are contained in Chapter 16 of this volume. Additional gene frequencies for Limon, Seine Bight, and Roatan were compiled by Weymes (Chapter 14) and Custodio *et al.* (Chapter 15).

4. Analytical Methods

4.1. Relationship Matrices

A number of different methods exist by which a genetic characterization of members of a subdivided population may be analyzed. If the concern of the analysis is to study the pattern of gene frequency variation, an array of allelic frequencies is converted to a normalized relationship matrix R of dimension $L \times L$, where L is the number of populations, villages, or samples. The observed, or sample, kinship coefficient between any two groups i and j is given by

$$r_{ij} = \frac{1}{k} \sum^{k} \frac{(P_i - \bar{P}_L)(P_j - \bar{P}_L)}{\bar{P}_L(1 - \bar{P}_L)} \qquad (1)$$

where k is the number of alleles in the array and $\bar{P}_L$ the average allelic frequency (Workman *et al.*, 1973). As noted by Harpending and Jenkins (1973), $\bar{P}_L$ may be taken as an estimate of an "underlying" mean gene frequency P.

The resulting relationship matrix R of kinship coefficients has several interesting properties. Where the value of r_{ij} is positive, the aggregate gene frequencies of populations i and j are more similar than the average similarity of all pairs of populations in the array. Conversely, where r_{ij} is negative, the aggregate frequencies are less similar (Workman *et al.*, 1973). In addition, the average value of the diagonal elements r_{ii} of the R matrix is an estimate of the mean genetic heterogeneity F_{ST}, or Wahlund's F (Harpending and Jenkins, 1974; Workman *et al.*, 1976). The R matrix can be used to compare the patterns of gene frequencies among groups with patterns predicted from other sources, such as migration, geography, and history.

Elements of the R matrix may also be used to compute a more direct measure of genetic distance. A squared quasi-Euclidean distance is derived from the R matrix by

$$d_{ij}^2 = r_{ii} + r_{jj} - 2r_{ij} \qquad (2)$$

for each pair of groups i and j. This distance is related to the G^2 measure of Sanghvi (1953). Other measures of genetic distance are available, such as those of Edwards (1971) and Nei (1974), but, as pointed out by Barrai (1974) and Workman *et al.* (1976), the correlation among these various methods is high.

4.2. Genetic Maps

Another use of the R matrix is in the construction of "genetic maps." This is a more satisfactory, visual method of comparing gene frequency patterns with predictions based on other sources. The maps are simply least squares representations of the relationship matrix (Harpending and Jenkins, 1973). By this method the variance in the R matrix is subsumed, in a cumulative manner, under L eigenvectors and L corresponding eigenvalues, where L is the number of groups in the original array. The "map" is then produced by plotting each group on a grid whose axes are the eigenvectors representing the greatest proportion of the variance in the R matrix. The eigenvector axes are scaled by the square root of the corresponding eigenvalues in order to equalize the scale of projection (Lalouel, 1973). The distance properties of this latent root and vector method were first discussed by Gower (1966).

As an aid to interpretation of the distribution of populations on the genetic maps, equal scale maps of the distribution of alleles in reduced space may also be produced. The relationship matrix required is derived from the transpose of the initial $K \times L$ matrix of allelic frequencies. The new R matrix is dimensioned $k \times k$, where k is the number of alleles (Harpending and Jenkins, 1973). By comparing the reduced space representation of alleles, scaled by the square root of the k eigenvalues, with that of the populations, the specific alleles responsible for population dispersion may be observed.

In using genetic maps, however, two cautions should be observed. First, loci without dominant alleles contain a greater amount of information than do loci with dominance. Also, common alleles tend to contain more information than do rarer alleles (Harpending and Jenkins, 1973). However, with regard to the second consideration, it has been demonstrated that rare alleles with high variance can exert considerable influence in the reduced space and may cause distortions in the relative position of groups (Devor, 1978).

4.3. Mean Per-Locus Heterozygosity

Another graphical method that utilizes the R matrix computed by eq. (1) has been developed by Harpending and Ward (1982). This method is based upon an intuitive, but not often stated, assumption regarding the relationship between genetic distance and heterozygosity. Equation (2) shows that the genetic distance between any two groups i and j is derived via a linear relationship among the elements of the normalized gene frequency covariances in the R matrix. Harpending and Ward have shown that the expected value of any diagonal element of the R matrix is

$$E(r_{ii}) = \frac{x_{ii} - \bar{X}}{\pi(1 - \pi) - \bar{X}} \tag{3}$$

where x_{ii} is the gene frequency variance in the ith population, $\bar{X}$ is the weighted mean of all entries, and π is the allelic frequency in an assumed parental population. Thus, the genetic distance between any two populations i and j computed from an R matrix via Eq. (2) is a distance *relative* to the distances from populations i and j to the ancestral population.

The relationship between the expression in Eq. (3) and heterozygosity is simply that if H_i is the average heterozygosity of the ith population and H_π is the average heterozygosity of the ancestral population, x_{ii} represents decremental values of heterozygosity relative to the ancestral group via

$$E(H_i) = H_\pi - x_{ii} \tag{4}$$

By combining eqs. (3) and (4), the linear relationship between "distance from centroid" and average heterozygosity becomes obvious:

$$E(r_{ii}) = \frac{H_\pi - \bar{X}}{H_\pi - \bar{X}} - \frac{E(H_i)}{H_\pi - \bar{X}} \tag{5}$$

Now, if $H_{\hat{p}}$ is the expected heterozygosity in a random mating population with gene frequencies $\hat{p}$, Harpending and Ward show that Eq. (5) becomes

$$r_{ii} = \frac{H_{\hat{p}} - H_i}{H_{\hat{p}}} \tag{6}$$

and, solving for H_i,

$$H_i = H_{\hat{p}} - H_{\hat{p}} r_{ii} \tag{7}$$

which is a linear relationship between the heterozygosity of the ith population and that of the ancestral group $H_{\hat{p}}$ with a coefficient $(1 - r_{ii})$, where r_{ii} is the distance of the ith population from the centroid of the array. Thus, it can be seen that the farther away a group is from the centroid, the higher its value of r_{ii}, and, consequently, the lower its heterozygosity should be relative to the average of the array.

This relationship is intuitive when one considers that, among the members of a subdivided population, those groups more centrally located tend to have higher within-group heterozygosity, while peripheral groups tend to have higher between-group heterozygosity. This is simply a paraphrase of the standard model developed by Wright (1931, 1943, 1951) with the exception that heterozygosity is here considered pairwise relative to overall mean heterozygosity. One further assumption, which is also not often stated, bearing on the development of this model is that systematic pressure is uniform in the array [see, for example, Morton (1973)]. Any nonrandom migration or differential admixture among subdivisions will constitute a violation of the assumption of uniform systematic pressure and distort the linearity of the relationship. As a result, local groups subject to more or less systematic pressure than the average of the array will not lie on the line predicted by Eq. (7). Herein, of course, lies the usefulness of this linearity.

Under the assumption of uniform systematic pressure, the relationship between the values of r_{ii} and the heterozygosity of the corresponding populations should be a uniform negative regression with slope $-H_{\bar{p}}$ and intercept $H_{\bar{p}}$. Thus, any deviations from the prediction may be assessed directly by use of a simple graph. The statistic used is mean per-locus heterozygosity $\bar{H}_i$ calculated from the observed allelic frequencies by

$$\bar{H}_i = 1 - \sum \frac{p_k^2}{K} \tag{8}$$

where k is the number of alleles and K the number of loci (Crawford and Devor, 1980). The values of $\bar{H}_i$ and r_{ii} can then be plotted as in Figs. 3 and 6. Groups that are more heterozygous than predicted by the regression line can be assumed to be less isolated from systematic pressure than their "genetic distance" suggests. Conversely, groups less heterozygous than predicted can be assumed to be more isolated. Such deviations from prediction are due almost exclusively to violations of the tenet of uniform systematic pressure in the array. Positive deviations are usually due to admixture, while negative deviations are due to isolations and drift.

5. Black Carib Population Structure

Differences and similarities in patterns of gene frequency distributions both within and between groups in a subdivided population must be assessed in the context of information independent of the gene frequencies themselves. Such independent sources are usually ethnohistorical and are composed of migration histories, information on political systems, economic factors, and social dynamics. Once the ethnohistorical context is established with reasonable certainty, various genetic similarities and dissimilarities among the groups may be ascribed to one or both of the standard microevolutionary processes, i.e., drift and gene flow. That is, the "static," present-day gene frequency patterns can be linked to dynamic causal processes through the specific histories of the groups in question.

This view of population structure does not, of course, deny the role of mutation and selection. However, these latter two processes rarely come into consideration in explanation to the extent of the former two. In the present case of the population structure of the Black Caribs, with a time depth of less than two centuries, drift in the guise of founder effect and gene flow in the form of admixture appear sufficient to relate ethnohistory to observed gene frequency distributions.

The population structure of the Black Caribs, represented by 10 populations over 13 alleles of three gene loci (ABO, Rhesus, MNSs), is presented in Fig. 1. The first two scaled eigenvectors are seen to account for 58.4% of the gene frequency variance in the array. Further, they are nearly equal in discriminating power, with e_1 accounting for 30.7% and e_2 for 27.7%. The position of the groups in the reduced space shows clearly that the first axis $(e_1\sqrt{\lambda_1})$ distinguishes those Carib groups residing on St. Vincent Island from those on Roatan Island and nearby coastal Belize. This separation conforms well with the known history of these subgroups. The St. Vincent population became isolated from the others in 1797. The coastal populations subsequently arose from a migration from Roatan Island in 1798 (see Chapter 2).

The distribution of groups along the second axis $(e_2\sqrt{\lambda_2})$ in Fig. 1 is less obvious. However, the reduced space representation of the alleles used to

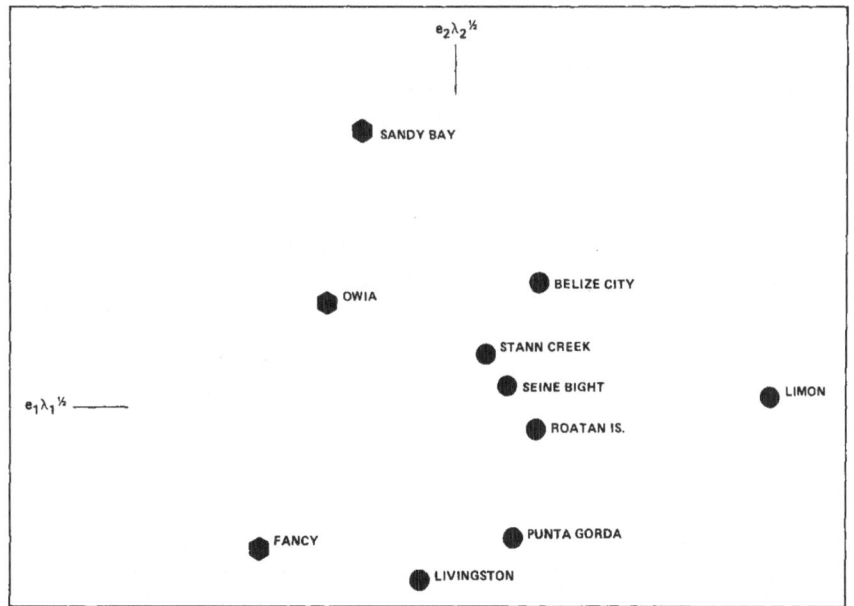

FIGURE 1. Least squares reduction "genetic map" of the 10 Black Carib populations based upon allelic frequencies for the ABO, Rhesus, and MNSs loci. St. Vincent Island populations are represented by the hexagons, all other populations by circles.

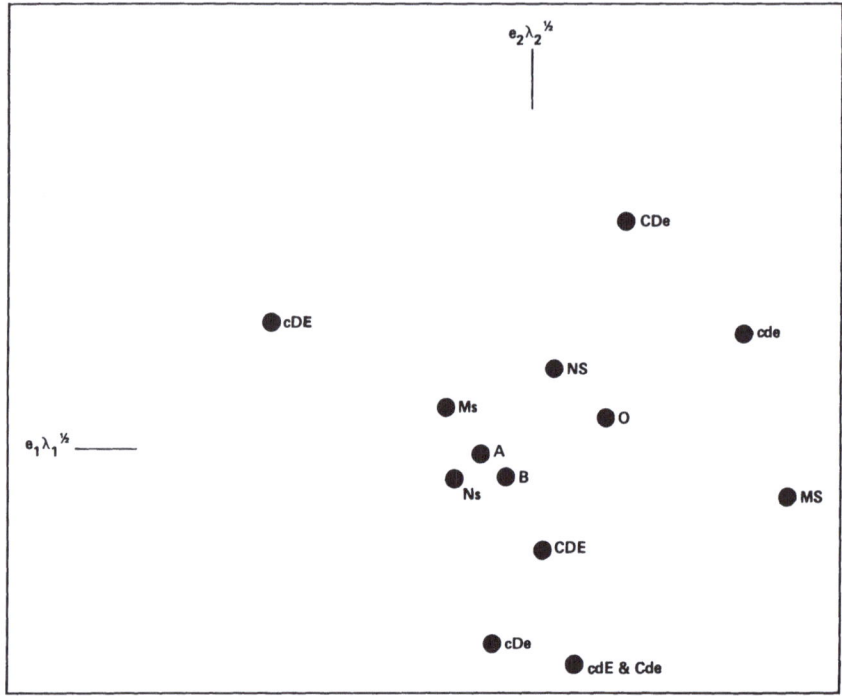

FIGURE 2. Least squares reduction "genetic map" of the 13 alleles of the ABO, Rhesus, and MNSs loci corresponding to the "map" in Fig. 1.

compute the "genetic map," which is presented in Fig. 2, shows that two of the Rhesus haplotypes, *CDe* and *cDe*, are major discriminators along the second axis. The *CDe* haplotype is rare among groups of African origin, while the *cDe* haplotype is much more common. The exact opposite situation obtains with reference to indigenous American Indian groups (Mourant *et al.*, 1976). Thus, it appears that a conclusion that the distribution of groups along the second scaled eigenvector is being conditioned by differential admixture with Amerindian and West African populations is warranted. Historically, those Black Caribs who migrated from Roatan to the Honduran coast could easily be distinguished from the local peoples they contacted (Bard, 1855). Over time, however, the Black Caribs continually interbred with these indigenous peoples so that, by the mid-20th century, all such coastal groups appeared as a homogeneous population with distinctly African characteristics (Crawford *et al.*, 1981; Gonzalez, 1969). These African characteristics were further enhanced by the assimilation of Haitians and black slaves as they made their way into the coastal communities. However, the results depicted in Fig. 1 show that this process of assimilation was not uniform, that certain Black Carib enclaves, notably Livingston, Guatemala, and Punta Gorda, Belize, are much more African than others. Another possible explanation of the observed variation in the degree of African admixture is that some of the founder groups contained a higher proportion of West African alleles.

Interestingly, it can be seen from Fig. 1 that the pattern of the samples from St. Vincent Island shows more pronounced differentiation than that of the other groups, even though the populations of Roatan and coastal Belize are separated by much greater geographical distances than are the St. Vincent groups. This would suggest that the populations of St. Vincent are more socially isolated than one would expect on the basis of geographic proximity.

The apparent social insularity of the St. Vincent groups is further suggested by the relationship between mean per-locus heterozygosity $\bar{H}_i$ and "distance from centroid" r_{ii}, shown in Fig. 3. Those groups suspected of receiving greater systematic pressure than average, that is, Sandy Bay and Owia on St. Vincent Island and Belize City, Stann Creek, and Limon on coastal Belize, all display

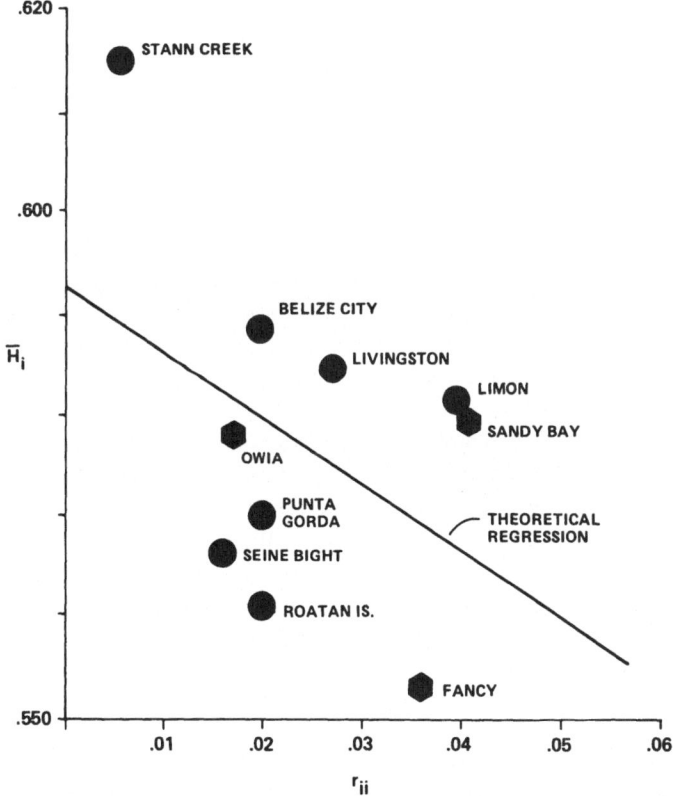

FIGURE 3. Plot of mean per-locus heterozygosity $\bar{H}_i$ against distance from the centroid r_{ii} of the relationship matrix for 10 Black Carib populations based upon allelic frequencies for the ABO, Rhesus, and MNSs loci. St. Vincent Island populations are represented by hexagons, all other populations by circles.

greater heterozygosity than predicted, with the exception of Owia, which shows slightly less. Also, the population of Livingston, Guatemala, a group that has a significant African component, is somewhat more heterozygous than expected. The insularity of the St. Vincent groups is best shown by the population of the village of Fancy. The inhabitants of this village, who characterize themselves as "Creole" as distinct from Carib, are the least heterozygous of any group in the array. In fact, the frequency of the Rhesus haplotype cDe ($p = 0.5658$), a clear African marker, is the highest among all groups sampled. One must conclude from these data that the self-representation of the inhabitants of Fancy as Creole is correct. These results further suggest why both Fancy and Owia are more isolated from one another, and from Sandy Bay, than their geographic relationships would indicate. First, the northern coast of St. Vincent Island is far more rugged than is the coast of Belize, and thus travel over short distances on St. Vincent is much more difficult than is travel over the larger distances elsewhere. Second, there is a distinct social differentiation between Carib and Creole on St. Vincent Island. Thus, Fancy, as the most African group on the island, is socially isolated as well as geographically remote. Owia retains a significant Creole population and is therefore subdivided, with the Creole component remaining socially isolated and the Carib component maintaining ties with Sandy Bay. It is Sandy Bay, however, that reflects most accurately the original population mix that produced the Black Carib (see Chapter 3 for details of the original population mixture).

A relatively great amount of genetic differentiation among the three St. Vincent Island populations in the face of their close geographical proximity would seem to conflict with a basic commonsense notion that pervades the study of human population structure: that groups residing proximally should be more alike genetically than two groups farther apart. This fundamental tenet lies at the heart of the theory of population structure first introduced by Wright (1931). However, this commonsense idea assumes that all other things are equal, such as migration, topography, and sociopolitical systems. In the case of St. Vincent Island, there are the mitigating factors of severe terrain, which restricts movement, and of social isolation, which together approximate the effect of greater distance between the groups. On the coast of Belize the situation is just the opposite. An earlier, unpublished study of ours on genetic differentiation among the villages of Livingston, Punta Gorda, and Stann Creek and the Belize City Creole population showed a correlation between pairwise genetic distances and pairwise geographical distances of $r = 0.89$. This extremely high correlation is due to the fact that all Black Carib villages lie on the coast, and roads are almost nonexistent (see Chapter 2). Therefore, the geography of migration between villages is one-dimensional, conforming exactly to the shape of the coast line. Here, there are no mitigating factors to distort the commonsense distance relationship.

Overall, geography plays a very small role in Black Carib population

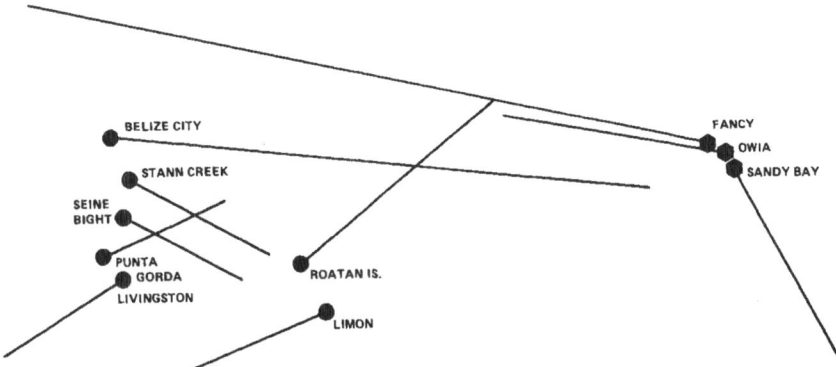

FIGURE 4. Maximum congruence rotation of "genetic distance" on geographical distance for 10 Black Carib populations based upon allelic frequencies for the ABO, Rhesus, and MNSs loci and straight-line map distance. Geographical locations are approximate and indicated by the hexagons for St. Vincent Island and by circles for the coastal groups. Maximum correlation between coordinates is $r_c = 0.36$.

structure. The primary reason for this is that the pairwise distances between any of the St. Vincent groups and any other group in the array are nearly 10 times greater than any other possible combination. Since these groups all share a common biological origin on St. Vincent Island, subsequent long-distance migrations should not have had any great affect upon genetic relationships over the short time spans involved. This is seen to be the case in Fig. 4, where the correlation between pairwise genetic distances and pairwise geographical distances is $r = 0.36$. However, there is still a large amount of genetic differentiation. This is due to the differential admixture cited earlier and not to any geographical influence, save for the fact that migrants are likely to encounter genetically different indigenous groups as a result of such movement.

As a result of the availability of additional gene frequency data for a few of the Black Carib groups, a second set of analyses were performed on these groups. This involved eight populations over 41 alleles from 14 genetic loci. In addition to the ABO, Rhesus, and MNSs loci, those of several serum proteins and enzymes, such as haptoglobin, group-specific component, transferrin, phosphoglucomutase, and adenylate kinase, were included. The resulting "genetic map" presented in Fig. 5 is interesting in that the refinement obtained from the use of more detailed genetic information is negligible. The first two scaled eigenvectors account for 59.6% of the total variation in the array, a modest 1.2% increase over the previous analysis using only three loci. The primary difference between the two is that, if anything, the differentiation between the St. Vincent Island groups and the other groups is somewhat clearer. This further suggests that the principal cause of the distinction is a result not of movement per se but of gene flow from the genetically different indigenous groups encountered in the two regions.

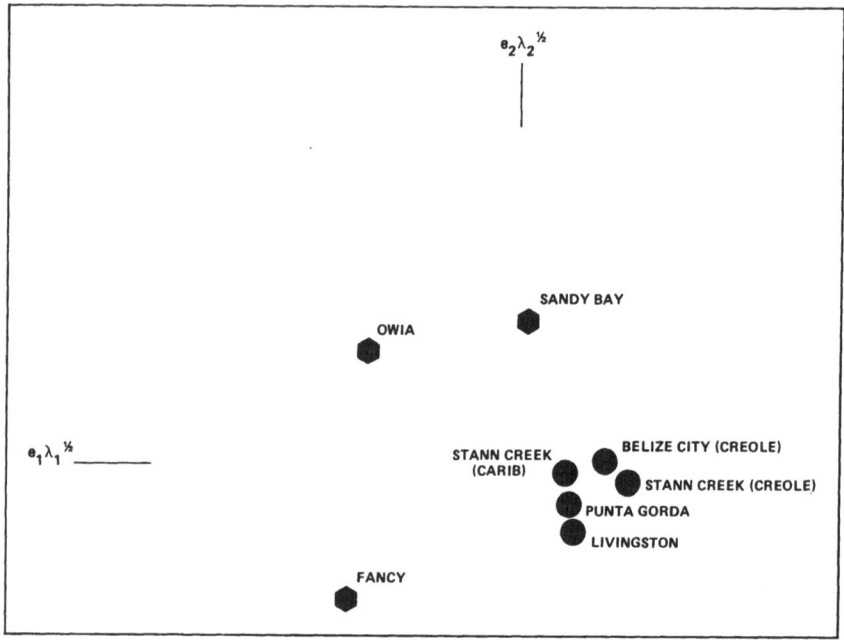

FIGURE 5. Least squares reduction "genetic map" of eight Black Carib populations based upon frequencies for 41 alleles from 14 loci. St. Vincent Island populations are represented by hexagons, the coastal populations by circles.

An interesting difference between the results from the two sets of data is seen in Fig. 6. There is, of course, a substantial decrease in mean per-locus heterozygosity in the second case, but this is to be expected from the addition of a large number of diallelic loci. However, independent of the magnitude of the mean heterozygosity in the array reflected by the $\bar{H}_i$ values, several groups (but not all) show a significant alteration in their relative heterozygosity to "distance from centroid" positions. These groups are Fancy and Owia from St. Vincent Island, which now show slightly higher heterozygosity than expected (see Fig. 3), and Sandy Bay from St. Vincent and Livingston, Guatemala, which now show slightly less. The reasons for these changes are not altogether clear, but it is likely that, unlike with the "gene maps," the addition of more detailed information and the group changes are creating a more "refined" picture of the relative relationships. On the basis of historical and geographical considerations, Fancy (St. Vincent) would likely be the most homogeneous group, as it is seen to be in Fig. 3. On the other hand, Belize City and Stann Creek, the least homogeneous by all considerations, remain so.

The changes in relative heterozygosities seen in Fig. 6 are most pronounced among those groups at the ends of the second scaled eigenvector in both Figs. 1 and 5, rather than those more centrally positioned. This indicates that the

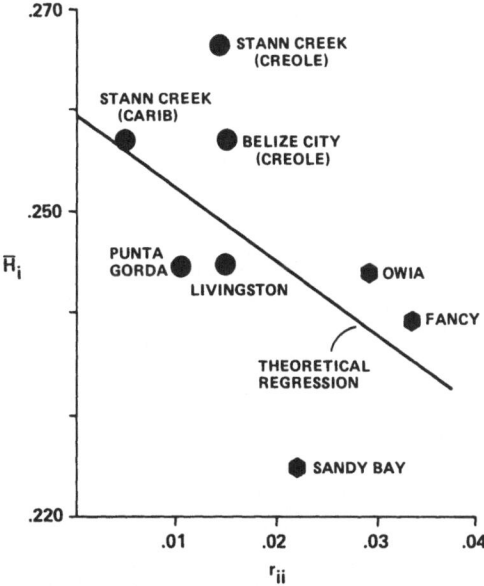

FIGURE 6. Plot of mean per-locus heterozygosity $\bar{H}_i$ against distance from the centroid r_{ii} of the relationship matrix from eight Black Carib populations based upon frequencies for 41 alleles from 14 loci. St. Vincent Island populations are represented by hexagons, the coastal populations by circles.

addition of more loci, particularly diallelic loci, has a greater effect upon samples that are most distinct from one another. In this case, the extreme differences are between the groups that are most African relative to the others, and those that are most Indian relative to the others. In particular, the greatest change is seen between the two most extreme populations, Fancy and Sandy Bay. Between these two the most significant difference is that Fancy is more heterozygous than Sandy Bay where the additional loci are concerned ($H_{\text{Fancy}} = 0.1614$; $\bar{H}_{\text{Sandy Bay}} = 0.1386$) and in particular at the hemolgobin locus, due to the presence of Hb^s in Fancy. These results suggest that this use of R matrix data is more sensitive to information contained in additional gene frequencies than is the method by which genetic maps are produced.

6. Discussion

The genetic population structure of the Black Carib groups presented here is seen to reflect the unique history of the Black Caribs as a whole. Genetic maps derived from red cell antigens and from the addition of serum proteins and enzymes indicate that the Black Caribs of St. Vincent Island, the historical source of all Black Caribs, are today a somewhat distinct subpopulation relative to the other groups studied. The most likely reason for this distinction is a microevolutionary phenomenon resulting from the extensive migrations that have characterized groups derived from the original St. Vincent population. As the Black Caribs moved from St. Vincent Island to Roatan Island and subsequently to the coast of Belize, Guatemala, and Honduras, the small migratory groups encountered genetically different and diverse indigenous and African populations. Gene flow from these local populations into the various Black Carib groups served to differentiate the Caribs in a few generations. The effect of this nonuniform systematic pressure has been to distinguish the migrant populations of Belize, Guatemala, and Honduras from the nonmigrants on St. Vincent Island.

Among the coastal populations, Creoles from Belize City and Stann Creek appear to be the most admixed. The most isolated (i.e., least admixed) groups are those from Punta Gorda, Belize, and Livingston, Guatemala. Of the St. Vincent Island populations presented here, the Sandy Bay gene pool contains the highest proportion of Indian genes and is genetically the most distinct of the Black Carib populations. However, the St. Vincent groups show a greater amount of differentiation than do the coastal populations and show some contradictory results. This is due to the fact that they have been considered in relation to the coastal populations with whom they share little in terms of either migratory or biological histories since 1797.

Although it is widely acknowledged that ethnohistory and historical demography are essential to the interpretation of the observed genetic patterns in human populations, genetic information is rarely employed to clarify ambiguities in ethnohistorical reconstruction. One such ambiguity concerns Squier's (1855) report of considerable phenotypic variation among the Black Caribs of Honduras. He described some individuals possessing predominantly Amerindian physical characteristics, such as straight black hair and "saffron colored skin," while others in the same community exhibited West African phenotypes with dark skin pigmentation. Yet, Gonzalez, during a survey of Black Carib communities of Guatemala and Honduras in the 1950s and 1960s (Crawford *et al.*, 1981), noted relative morphological homogeneity, with the absence of Amerindian features. This apparent contradiction may be explained through the genetic analyses of the Black Caribs of St. Vincent and the coastal mainland communities of Central America.

The genetic data suggest the following ethnohistorical reconstruction. At the time of deportation to Roatan in 1797, there was considerable pheontypic variation among the Black Caribs, since approximately 50% of the gene pool was of Amerindian origin. The migrants to Roatan and Honduras encountered West African communities, which in turn were incorporated into the Black Carib gene pool. In particular, the French-speaking Haitians that resided on the Bay of Trujillo, and shared a common French colonial experience with the Black Caribs, apparently hybridized with the new arrivals. One result of this admixture was the rapid increase of the African and diminution of the Amerindian component in the Black Carib gene pool. This reconstruction is supported by the genetic admixture estimates, which indicate that the Black Caribs of Sandy Bay are approximately 50% Amerindian, while communities such as Livingston in Guatemala contain less than 20% Indian admixture. An additional factor contributing to the genetic composition of the Black Carib communities is the founder effect. Most of the Black Carib villages were founded by miniscule numbers of persons.

Finally, the genetic data presented here support Kern's contention (Chapter 6) that the Black Caribs experienced considerable interethnic marriage. Specific support is found in the presence of the albumin Mexico variant (Al^{Me}) among the mainland Black Caribs together with its absence among the St. Vincentian groups, indicating gene flow from the coastal Amerindian populations.

References

Bard, S. A., 1855, *Adventures on the Mosquito Shore*, J. Blackwood, London.

Barrai, I., 1974, Indicators of genetic distance, in *Genetic Distance* (J. F. Crow and C. F. Denniston, eds.), pp. 1–4, Plenum, New York.

Cannings, C., and Cavalli-Sforza, L. L., 1973, Human population structure, in *Advances in Human Genetics*, Vol. 4 (H. Harris and K. Hirschhorn, eds.), pp. 105–171, Plenum, New York.

Crawford, M. H., and Devor, E. J., 1980, Population structure and admixture in transplanted Tlaxcaltecan populations, *Am. J. Phys. Anthropol.* **52**:485–490.

Crawford, M. H., Gonzalez, N. L., Schanfield, M. S., Dykes, D. D., Skradski, K., and Polesky, H. F., 1981, The Black Caribs (Garifuna) of Livingston, Guatemala: Genetic markers and admixture estimates, *Hum. Biol.* **53**:87–103.

Devor, E. J., 1978, Genetic variation in transferrin alleles of rhesus macaques, *Macaca mulatta*, *Am. J. Phys. Anthropol.* **48**:165–170.

Edwards, A. W. F., 1971, Distance between populations on the basis of gene frequencies, *Biometrics* **27**:873–881.

Gonzalez, N. L., 1969, *Black Carib Household Structure*, University of Washington Press, Seattle.

Gower, J. C., 1966, Some distance properties of latent root and vector methods used in multivariate analysis, *Biometrika* **53**:325–338.

Harpending, H. C., and Jenkins, T., 1973, Genetic distances among Southern African populations in *Methods and Theories of Antbropological Genetics* (M. H. Crawford and P. L. Workman, eds.), pp. 177–199, University of New Mexico Press, Albuquerque.

Harpending, H. C., and Jenkins, T., 1974, !Kung population structure, in *Genetic Distance* (J. F. Crow and C. F. Denniston, eds.), pp. 137–161, Plenum, New York.

Harpending, H. C., and Ward, R., 1982, Chemical systematics and human populations, in *Biochemical Aspects of Evolutionary Biology* (M. Nitecki, ed.), pp. 213–256, University of Chicago Press, Chicago.

Jorde, L. B., 1980, The genetic structure of subdivided human populations: A review, in *Current Developments in Anthropological Genetics*, Vol. 1 (J. H. Mielke and M. H. Crawford, eds.), pp. 135–208, Plenum, New York.

Lalouel, J. M., 1973, Topology of population structure, in *Genetic Structure of Populations* (N. E. Morton, ed.), pp. 139–149, University of Hawaii Press, Honolulu.

Morton, N. E. (ed.), 1973, *Genetic Structure of Populations*, University of Hawaii Press, Honolulu.

Mourant, A. E., Kopeć, A. C., and Domaniewska-Sobczak, D., 1976, *The Distribution of the Human Blood Groups and Other Polymorphisms*, Oxford University Press, London.

Nei, M., 1974, A new measure of genetic distance, in *Genetic Distance* (J. F. Crow and C. F. Denniston, eds.), pp. 63–76, Plenum, New York.

Sanghvi, L. D., 1953, Comparison of genetical and morphological methods for a study of biological differences, *Am. J. Phys. Anthropol.* **11**:385–404.

Squier, E. G., 1855, *Notes on Central America*, Harper, New York.

Workman, P. L., Harpending, H. C., Lalouel, J. M., Lynch, C., Niswander, J. D., and Singleton, R., 1973, Population studies on Southwestern Indian tribes. VI. Papago population structure: A comparison of genetic and migration analyses, in *Genetic Structure of Populations* (N. E. Morton, ed.), pp. 166–194, University of Hawaii Press, Honolulu.

Workan, P. L., Mielke, J. H., and Nevanlinna, H. R., 1976, The genetic structure of Finland, *Am. J. Phys. Anthropol.* **44**:341–368.

Wright, S., 1931, Evolution in Mendelian populations, *Genetics* **16**:97–159.

Wright, S., 1943, Isolation by distance, *Genetics* **28**:114–138.

Wright, S., 1951, The genetical structure of populations, *Am. Eugen.* **15**:323–354.

20

Anthropogenetics in a Hybrid Population

The Black Carib Studies

DEREK F. ROBERTS

1. Introduction

Volume 1 in this series examined aspects of the theory of anthropological genetics and Volume 2 applied that theory in a series of studies illustrating different points from different populations. There was lacking a single full case study, in which one population was examined intensively. To do this was the object of the present volume, and what an interesting population was chosen by Professor Crawford for this purpose! The Black Caribs are said historically to derive from intermixture between West Africans and Carib—Arawak Indians. At the end of the 18th century the population was split; a small group remained on the island of St. Vincent, a founder group of perhaps 100 individuals from whom the present population of 1000—2000 derive; the bulk of the original population, however, after forced deportation, made their way to the Central American mainland, establishing an initial settlement in Trujillo, Honduras, whence they spread along the coast and intermixed with Creoles to give the present population of some 80,000. As Professor Crawford mentions in the Preface, the choice of this population was partly fortuitous and partly deliberate; his previous studies had been carried out where groups had diverged some 400 and 4000 years ago, and a third group was required for comparison where known divergence had occurred more recently. The Black Caribs fulfilled such a requirement. The birth of the idea of this investigation and the development of the relevant

DEREK F. ROBERTS • Department of Human Genetics, University of Newcastle upon Tyne, Newcastle upon Tyne NE2 4AA, England.

fieldwork are sketched in the Preface, which also describes the incorporation of
contributions from an independent research group working on similar problems.

2. Sociocultural Background

The first section of this volume sketches those social, historical, cultural,
and demographic details so essential for the understanding of the biology of the
population. Chapter 2 by Davidson states the facts with commendable academic
detachment and leaves the reader to imagine the bewilderment and emotions of
the Caribs uprooted from St. Vincent, the consternation of the few Spanish
coastal settlers near and among whom they were resettled, and the types of
pressure that caused them to disperse. The linear distribution of small settlements along the coast, with all but three villages touching coastal waters and
with distances between villages averaging 5–15 miles, provides at first sight a
model geographical situation for the occurrence of unidimensional gene flow,
until the cultural habits of the population are remembered — their widespread
traveling, far-flung but welcoming kin, trading system, etc. The questions leap
to mind immediately. How will these interact? Will genetic divergence or homogeneity prevale?

The review by Gullick in Chapter 3 of the Caribs of St. Vincent shows how
difficult it is to obtain an accurate assessment of the size of this population, the
small numbers to which it and parts of it declined from time to time, and the
many difficult episodes (raids, wars, riots, deportations, forfeiture of land,
epidemics, storms) that make one appreciate the resilience of the population.
The implications are twofold. First, any quantitative genetic evolutionary
analysis relying on demographic information is unlikely to be accurate, and if
an approximation is attempted it will require support from other, indirect
genetic methods. Second, there was ample scope for random events to influence
the genetics of the population; will it be possible to quantify the extent of such
influence?

For Gonzalez (Chapter 4), migration is the key to understanding Garifuna
culture and society. Not only did the American contribution to the peopling of
the New World initiate new types of society, but the expectation of living in
more than one location during one's lifetime must have far-reaching social and
biological implications both for the society and for the individual. Her case
study in Livingston provides a clear illustration of the central role of the woman,
her children, and the other members of her family. Such "consanguineal households" provide stability in the absence of permanent males, which would be
virtually impossible in a system where the nuclear family household is the ideal.
She argues that the absence of pronounced African influence in the language of
the Garifuna of St. Vincent suggests that African ancestors joined the original
Indians sporadically in small numbers over a fairly long period of time, with the

Indians dominating numerically particularly in the earlier phases. Yet if the current social structure that she describes takes its origin from those early days, it would be expected that the predominant influences on the child would derive from its mother, including linguistic influence; this would provide at least a partial alternative interpretation and perhaps make for reconciliation of the linguistic evidence with the historical accounts that many Africans arrived from one or two shipwrecks. From the point of view of the genetic study, however, the effects of imbalance of the sex ratio and the mating pattern, by no means unusual in many advanced organisms, would offset each other: they would be expected respectively to increase, though negligibly, the rate of decay of genetic variability and to increase intrageneration variability. But what stands out so clearly from this chapter is that any attempt at evolutionary genetic analysis by pedigree in this population would be impossible.

In Chapter 5 Firschein shows very clearly some of the difficulties involved in applying data from an official census to biological problems. For example, the aberrant sex ratio that occurs in children as well as in adults is disquieting and though in this the census data are not contradicted by the registration records, both may share a common partial cause, underregistration and underenumeration, and one may ask how much reliance is to be placed on arguments based on such data. Nevertheless, interesting trends are suggested, for example, those to lower and delayed fertility, and it is good to see the changed pattern of survival, especially for the very young, though Firschein quite rightly draws attention to the implications of this for future population numbers. It is very satisfying that the distribution of high- and low-parity women in the population is closely approximated by that in the sample of women that he used in his hemoglobin studies, indicating its representativeness in this respect. Hence his hypothesis of the involvement of hemoglobin type in fertility, in sex ratio of offspring, and in their survival clearly requires further attention. The need for better and accurate recording of demographic data is paramount if the advantages and disadvantages of genotypes in this population in relation to survival and reproduction are to be unraveled.

If the extent of Garifuna genetic isolation is to be estimated, the importance of data on observed intermixture, rather than conjecture or statements based on "ideal" unions, is stressed by Kerns in Chapter 6. She notes that at the time of her fieldwork she considered intermixture a tangential issue, and hence the opportunity was missed to obtain samples on frequencies of unions in different localities. In her Table 4 for instance, if intraethnic means only Carib by Carib, and interethnic means Carib by other, then gene flow into rural village Carib is only 1.5%, representing quite an appreciable degree of isolation; the extent to which there was differential fertility between these two types of unions is a different matter. Comparisons with Table 6 and the literary sources that she cites, however, suggest possibly that this is a gross underestimation, or that there has been a reduction in the amount of intermixture since last mid-century, or that interethnic unions are more fertile, or that there are regional and local variations in intermixture amounts. Once again her study shows the difficulty of applying material collected in the course of census enumerations for purposes of genetic analysis. This same point is made by Cosminsky and Whipple in Chapter 7. They indicate a number of factors that make for differentiation or partial differentiation of the populations, but their section on attitudes toward intercultural relations provides the critical considerations. It is these that explain the idealized stereotype of endogamy and the pattern of the interethnic unions that occurs. Again from the genetic point of view the latter are of interest in that they suggest not only an appreciable amount of gene flow but also the possibility of differential gene flow of sex-linked genes.

3. Quantitative Biological Variables

Chapter 8, opening the section on morphology, provides a change of orientation. The data on growth show that there are real biological differences associated with the ethnic divisions that exist. To view the children's heights and weights against a background of standards from Europe and Africa may well be misleading, but comparison of the Garifuna with Creole children is valid. This shows consistent differences between the two: the Garifuna have lower mean weights and heights for age, a greater proportion of children fall in the less well-nourished categories, and more show poor growth. Possible explanations are found in the biocultural factors examined, especially the different frequencies of chronic diarrhea and of episodes of hospitalization with diarrhea, and into these differences elements of hygiene must enter. Similarly it is suggested that weaning is less efficient among Garifuna children, while the differences in child mortality and number of surviving children between the two populations, and between the households of children with good and poor growth, indicate that a fundamental variable is socioeconomic. Comparison with the life table data given by Firschein shows that the greatest mortality occurs in the first year of life, and is lower, though still high, during the weaning period (1–3 years), suggesting that in fact hygiene is the primary source of difficulty. This means genetically not only that selection by early differential mortality is likely within the populations, but also that there may be an element of interpopulation selection; the evolutionary consequences of these will be different. But certainly there is scope for search for genetic characteristics affecting and affected by such selection.

Chapter 9 on skin color provides further evidence of the differences between Garifuna and Creole populations; the Creoles are lighter and more variable at every wavelength, though this difference is not sufficient to account for the ability of local folk to assign an individual to one group or the other. The variability of both, however, is a clear indication of the genetic heterogeneity in each. The skin color data are the first to provide estimates of the amount of intermixture that has occurred, and the differences between the two populations, and between regional samples of the Garifuna, seem to be attributable to different admixture proportions — unless skin color is itself related to any differential selection or drift that may have occurred. Other factors, possibly environmental, developmental, and cultural, may of course be involved in the skin color results. But if they are, the extent of their influence appears slight, as is shown by the considerable similarity that occurs between the admixture estimates from skin color data and those from the *Gm* haplotypes and from blood groups. The implication is that a relatively simple genetic model based on several independent loci, with each locus having an equal and additive effect, seems reasonable for skin color. By contrast, the dental data (Chapter 10) show little differentiation between the two populations or localities. From an intensive multivariate analysis the similarity of the Honduras samples emerges as their outstanding feature, particularly by contrast to the variation that occurs in the Mexican material with which they are compared.

Lin's elegant comparison in Chapter 11 of anthropometric features of Garifuna in two localities, Livingston and St. Vincent, extracts the maximum from the data. Significant differences occur in almost every measurement between sexes, but these are less than those between populations of the same sex, and indeed the interaction of the two factors, sex-influenced variability and population-specific variability, produces a synergistic effect. Lin interprets these biological expressions as due to the history of isolation, interbreeding, and mating systems in general of the two populations. Of the 10 features best discriminating between the two sexes within populations, six occur in both communities. In these features are confounded the effects of intrinsic sex dimorphism and environmental variation due to occupational differences, and little can be attributed otherwise to genetic differences. Among the population discriminators, six out of the first 10 occur in both males and females. It is in these perhaps that some genetic element may be the more important, since, as later chapters show, the two populations have come to differ genetically, though again the possibility of phenotypic molding by local environment cannot be ruled out. It is interesting how few of the classical anthropometric dimensions devised for taxonomy appear among the 10 population discriminatory variables (Table 6).

In Chapter 12 on blood pressure, assessment of the extent of genetic influence is attempted by an interesting combination of methods, hybrid analysis and familial aggregation. The fact that the latter is restricted to parent—child and sib correlations inhibits precise analysis and indeed the differences that exist between the mother—child and father—child correlations, unfortunately on rather restricted sample size, and their generally low levels, suggest appreciable environmental influence. The table of gene frequencies indicates the intermediacy of the St. Vincent sample between West African and combined

Carib–Arawak, giving further support to the extent of intermixture mentioned in Chapter 9. The suggestion of an increase in blood pressure with age, similar to that in another hybrid group (American blacks) is interesting by comparison with the relative slightness of such trends in indigenous African communities, but there is no internal evidence that there is any association between hypertension and the proportion of the genotype derived from African sources. The variation in blood pressure with body dimensions is not surprising, though the suggestion that the relevance of fat varies between sexes is, and the limited success of discrimination by anthropometry between normotensive and hypertensive reminds one of the many variables that are also important in blood pressure not reflected in body dimensions. The suggestion that heritability may be higher for diastolic than systolic pressure clearly deserves further attention, while the suggestion in other studies that there may be some major gene effects associated with marker loci would be worth examining in this population.

In the dermatoglyphic data the first surprising feature is the limited intra-population variability in ridge count, considering the histories of the populations. In the population comparisons the trend is also toward homogeneity, and local variation is rather low key, except for the distinction of Punta Gorda in digital and total ridge counts, in frequency of pattern types, and in the comparison of dermatoglyphic with geographical distance, into which again possibly small sample size enters. The fact that similar patterns of dermatoglyphic relationships emerge irrespective of whether distances are calculated from the occurrence of pattern types or through sophisticated multivariate distance measures suggests the reality of the patterns found. However, the differences between sexes pose a problem as always and one wonders if the differences in population affinities suggested by the two sexes possibly reflect the internal migration patterns. As regards the genetic interpretation of the characters considered, the recurrence of the same underlying universals of dermatoglyphic variation as the authors have demonstrated in other populations suggests that some order is at last coming into the variability that is dermatoglyphics.

4. Genetic Variation

Chapter 14 by Weymes and Gershowitz opens the genetic section and provides from hemoglobin and enzyme studies an immediate objective answer to the amount of admixture, showing a contribution from Africans of 75.6%, from American Indians of 23.9%, and from Europeans of 0.5%, close to those from skin color and serology. Moreover, the amounts of admixture in the several population samples they examine seem to be similar. Indeed, the general similarity of the several samples is clear from the genetic distance analysis, though within this general homeogeneity there is the indication that the gene pools at settlements within each pair (Hopkins with Punta Gorda, and Seine Bight with

Stan Creek) are more similar to each other than are those between the pairs of settlements.

Chapter 15 points out some of the problems in attempting to use genetic data to establish amounts of intermixture, particularly founder effects, drift, and natural selection. It complements the preceding chapter by giving blood group gene frequencies. Much of the discussion of selection in humans has taken place with respect to the abnormal hemoglobins, and it is appropriate that a full chapter (Chapter 17) be devoted to the sickle cell carriers. There is a clear heterogeneity in their frequency among the seven communities tested, and partly this appears to be associated with the level of malarial infestation. The implication is that selection is intensely rapid, or migration cannot have been totally random with respect to abnormal hemoglobin, or that one's ability to withstand the effects of malaria affects the decision of whether or not to migrate and where to. The data presented on fertility are still not definitive, for, if it is the genotype of the fetus that is a factor in its survival, then the second parent also needs to be taken into consideration, and so does the duration of the union: West African studies doing so indicated the advantage of unions of normal homozygotes with heterozygotes.

The definitive study of the immunoglobulin phenotypes in the several samples from Belize and St. Vincent of Black Carib and Creole is most informative. There is no doubt about the predominance of the African haplotype, and European and Amerindian haplotypes are also shown to be present. This is the first definitive confirmation by the genetic data that the three continental populations did indeed contribute to Black Carib origins. There are significant gene frequency differences between the Black Caribs of Belize and St. Vincent, the former having more African haplotypes and the latter more Amerindian and European. The Creoles of the two localities do not differ from each other. Moreover, the Black Carib groups differ from the coresident Creoles in each locality. The specificity of the *Gm* groups allows exploration of detailed hypotheses of admixture, for example, whether the European component in the Black Caribs could be due to hybridization directly with Europeans or indirectly through Creoles. In Belize the indirect route of admixture is possible. In St. Vincent it is not. Overall, the St. Vincent populations are more heterogeneous genetically than are the mainland Black Caribs, and this heterogeneity is due primarily to variation in amounts of admixture among the local populations, followed by reproductive isolation.

Chapter 19 on genetic structure draws together the genetic and historical parts of the study. In view of the limited time depth, it is suggested that founder effect, drift, and gene flow by admixture are sufficient to explain the present genetic characteristics of the Black Carib and of the heterogeneity that exists among their several communities. The genetic distinction of St. Vincent from the other Black Caribs conforms to the known history, while the differences among the local groups suggest differing degrees of African admixture. There is a contrast between the greater heterogeneity of the St. Vincent populations and the lesser heterogeneity on the mainland. The St. Vincent populations appear to be more isolated than expected from their close geographical proximity, and this is related to the difficult terrain, which restricts movements between villages, and to their social isolation. On the coast of Belize there is by contrast a high correlation of genetic distance with geographic distance between communities. Apart from the St. Vincent and other Black Caribs, a second major source of heterogeneity comes from the variation in extent of African and Amerindian admixture – Black Caribs of Sandy Bay are 50% Amerindian, while those of Livingston are less than 20% Amerindian.

Not only does history help explain the population genetic structure, but the genetic structure may also be employed to clarify the historical reconstruction. Those Black Caribs in St. Vincent avoiding the deportation retained a sufficiency of genetic heterogeneity, with approximately 50% of their gene pool being of Amerindian origin. The migrants to the mainland encountered the essentially African communities with whom fusion occurred and their genes were incorporated into the Black Carib gene pool so that there was a rapid increase of the African and diminution of the Amerindian component.

5. Conclusion

From this remarkable and full study of the Black Caribs, a population with a complex history of which the major features are known, and their neighbors the Creoles, much of value has emerged: establishment of the extent of individual variation within each of the populations, the extent of the variation between communities within populations, the pattern of that variation and how it varies from one characteristic to another, and how it relates to the ethnohistory. The study shows so clearly what an improvement in depth of understanding comes with multidisciplinary investigation by comparison with that obtained from each individual enquiry. Each of the original objects has been achieved and more. These were:

1. To estimate the admixture in the population. There is remarkable concordance among the estimates of the amounts of admixture obtained from the different characters investigated. Moreover, this provides the key to the evolutionary divergence that has occurred.

2. To measure genetic microdifferentiation. The extent of microdifferentiation is already appreciable, but the way in which it varies from character to character is particularly interesting. If differential intermixture explains the monogenic variation, why do the dermatoglyphic traits, in which genetic influence heavily predominates, show, like the dental features, so much less heterogeneity?

3. To elucidate the ethnohistory. As Chapter 19 shows, history helps to

explain the population genetic structure and the latter in turn helps to clarify historical reconstructions.

4. To understand the inheritance of complex morphological features. Here there remain intriguing questions. Growth pattern differences can be related to differential environmental challenge. Is, then, the variation among populations in morphometric characters related to this or to their genetic differences?

Of the problems now posed, one is the further examination of the inheritance of complex traits. Work so far has established that this population would be extremely useful for this purpose. From the nature of the breeding pattern of the population there must be many half-sibs, both paternal and maternal. Intensive analysis of such family material, adding data to those already collected in population samples in the present study, would be most rewarding in identifying the extent of their genetic determination.

A second main area is provided by a topic discarded in the present interpretation. The mortality data suggest ample differentials and the growth and morphometric data suggest differences among the populations, while the nutritional work suggests factors affecting these, and there are in addition highly significant local differences in frequency of abnormal hemoglobins as shown by Custodio and Huntsman (Chapter 17), no matter whether these are associated with malarial infestation or differential fertility. There is also the emerging pattern of other local gene frequency differences. If admixture differences and random events were, as has been argued, totally responsible, would the pattern of genetic variation on the mainland be quite so regular? The conditions on the mainland, with exposure to representatives of other populations and existing sizable settlements, were certainly not identical with those on the island: the extent to which they differed in selective pressures will never be known. Would it be worth asking again whether selection is occurring in specific features, or whether on the mainland it is perhaps in the direction of the total genotype? While the wielding of Occam's razor indicates that on existing data preference be given to the authors' interpretation, the alternative of some selection remains as something that is not yet definitely excluded.

An enormous amount has been achieved from the work so far. Yet it should be regarded as the beginning rather than an end. It has pointed to the questions that should now be asked, has sketched what the potential is for answering specific problems, and has shown what a remarkable opportunity to do so the Black Carib population presents. To do this of course the experience and data obtained in the present study will be invaluable, but the study itself has also shown the tools essential for such further enquiry: improved documentation and registration, not only numerical but also familial, with full pedigrees and recording of diagnoses and episodes of ill health, causes of death, etc. For it is against these that the genetic, morphological, performance, developmental, epidemiological, and similar factors will be profitably compared. This population is indeed rich for such studies.

Index